Primary Care of the Solid Organ Transplant Recipient

Christopher J. Wong

Editor

Primary Care of the Solid Organ Transplant Recipient

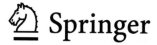 Springer

Editor
Christopher J. Wong
Department of Medicine
Division of General Internal Medicine
University of Washington
Seattle, WA
USA

ISBN 978-3-030-50631-5   ISBN 978-3-030-50629-2   (eBook)
https://doi.org/10.1007/978-3-030-50629-2

This Springer imprint is published by the registered company Springer Nature Switzerland AG
The registered company address is: Gewerbestrasse 11, 6330 Cham, Switzerland

Preface

Dear colleagues,

Being a primary care provider is one of the most rewarding practices in the field of medicine. We take care of the young and the old, the sick and the well, and everything in between. We build and grow long-term relationships with patients and their families. We work with patients to improve what they can, yet are still there for them when we cannot fix or cure their illness. And we learn—from our patients as they undergo their own personal and healthcare journeys, from our colleagues who teach us and push us to improve, and from our own successes and mistakes.

I suspect that most primary care providers—known for their breadth of knowledge and experience—do not begin their careers with a goal of caring for solid organ transplant recipients. In fact, it can be quite daunting to try to understand what these patients have gone through and partner with them to maintain and improve their well-being. It may seem like something best left solely to specialty care.

This book was created with the idea that primary care providers can and should have a role in the care of solid organ transplant recipients. At the University of Washington we have a robust solid organ transplantation program, and as a result our primary care practices have the pleasure to care for many solid organ transplant recipients. I have found that caring for solid organ transplant recipients is highly rewarding: it requires a high level of the practice of medicine—we need to understand anatomy, physiology, drug side effects and interactions, immunosuppression, and also psychosocial aspects of care. There are ample opportunities to make a positive impact, including managing the many complications suitable to primary care, assessing urgent care needs, and being an important source of continuity.

For this first edition I have sought the expertise of primary care providers and specialists who work with adult solid organ transplant recipients—the goal is to provide a source of information that a primary care provider may find useful. As such, we have tried to balance having enough information to be useful without including excessively detailed transplant care that would not be managed by a primary care provider. I recognize that the practice of medicine, especially transplantation medicine, will continue to evolve—therefore, ongoing collaboration with the transplant specialists should be a routine part of care for this patient population.

I thank and acknowledge my patients and their families; the students, residents, and fellows who train here; the transplant specialists who are always willing to teach us on top of their direct patient care duties; my incredible general internal medicine colleagues; and most of all my own family for their support.

Seattle, WA, USA   Christopher J. Wong, MD
April 2020

Acknowledgments

I would like to acknowledge Sumaiya Sathar, student assistant, for help with obtaining references; the solid organ transplant recipients whom I have been privileged to help care for; my fellow general internists for their inspirational teaching and wisdom; and the transplant specialists at the University of Washington for their clinical expertise and energy in teaching generalists about the care of this special population.

Contents

Contributors

Melissa A. Bender, MD Department of Family Medicine, University of Washington School of Medicine, Seattle, WA, USA

Gabrielle N. Berger, MD Department of Medicine, Division of General Internal Medicine, University of Washington, Seattle, WA, USA

Lauren A. Beste, MD, MSc, FACP Department of Medicine, Division of General Internal Medicine, University of Washington, Seattle, WA, USA

Richard K. Cheng, MD, MSc Department of Medicine, Division of Cardiology, University of Washington Medical Center, Seattle, WA, USA

Eleanor Curtis, MD, MPVM Department of Trauma, Burns and General Surgery, University of California, Davis, Sacramento, CA, USA

Iris C. De Castro, MD Department of Medicine, Division of Nephrology, University of Washington, Seattle, WA, USA

Tyra Fainstad, MD Department of Medicine, Division of General Internal Medicine, University of Colorado, Denver, CO, USA

Anna Golob, MD Department of Medicine, Division of General Internal Medicine, University of Washington, Seattle, WA, USA

VA Puget Sound Healthcare System, Seattle, WA, USA

Deborah Greenberg, MD Division of General Internal Medicine, Department of Medicine, University of Washington, Seattle, WA, USA

Katherine G. Hicks, MD Department of Medicine, Division of General Internal Medicine, University of Washington School of Medicine, Seattle, WA, USA

Christopher Knight, MD Department of Medicine, Division of General Internal Medicine, University of Washington, Seattle, WA, USA

Anne M. Larson, MD, FACP, FAASLD, AGAF Hepatology & Liver Transplantation, Division of Gastroenterology, University of Washington, Seattle, WA, USA

Erika D. Lease, MD, FCCP Department of Medicine, Division of Pulmonary, Critical Care, and Sleep Medicine, University of Washington, Seattle, WA, USA

Andy Y. Lee, MD Department of Medicine, Division of Cardiology, University of Washington Medical Center, Seattle, WA, USA

Leah M. Marcotte, MD Division of General Internal Medicine, Department of Medicine, University of Washington, Seattle, WA, USA

Vidang P. Nguyen, MD Cedars-Sinai Heart Institute, Cedars-Sinai Medical Center, Los Angeles, CA, USA

Kim O'Connor, MD Department of Medicine, Division of General Internal Medicine, University of Washington, Seattle, WA, USA

Genevieve L. Pagalilauan, MD Department of Medicine, Division of General Internal Medicine, University of Washington, Seattle, WA, USA

Cary H. Paine, MD Department of Medicine, Division of Nephrology, University of Washington, Seattle, WA, USA

Heidi Powell, MD Division of General Internal Medicine, Department of Medicine, University of Washington, Seattle, WA, USA

Lydia Sun, PharmD Department of Pharmacy, University of Washington Medical Center, Seattle, WA, USA

Christopher J. Wong, MD Division of General Internal Medicine, Department of Medicine, University of Washington, Seattle, WA, USA

Jennifer Wright, MD Department of Medicine, Division of General Internal Medicine, University of Washington, Seattle, WA, USA

Diana Zhong, MD Department of Medicine, Division of General Internal Medicine, University of Washington, Seattle, WA, USA

List of Abbreviations

AASLD	American Association for the Study of Liver Diseases
ACP	Advance care planning
ACR	Acute cellular rejection
AD	Advance directive
AIH	Autoimmune hepatitis
ARLD	Alcohol-related liver disease
AST	American Society of Transplantation (note can also refer to aspartate aminotransferase)
AUC	Area under the curve
AUDIT	Alcohol use disorders identification test
AZA	Azathioprine
BKVN	BK virus nephropathy
BMD	Bone mineral density
BMI	Body mass index
CAN	Chronic allograft nephropathy
CBT	Cognitive behavioral therapy
CDC	Centers for Disease Control
CMV	Cytomegalovirus
CNI	Calcineurin inhibitor
CPRA	Calculated panel reactive antibody
CsA	Cyclosporine
CT	Computed tomography
Cu-IUD	Copper-IUD
CVD	Cardiovascular disease
D/R	Donor/recipient (used to describe serologic status)
DAA	Direct-acting antiviral
DEXA	Dual-energy x-ray absorptiometry (also DXA)
DGF	Delayed graft function
DPOA-HC	Durable Power of Attorney for Healthcare
DSA	Donor-specific antibodies
DVT	Deep vein thrombosis

DXA	Dual-energy x-ray absorptiometry (also DEXA)
EBV	Epstein-Barr virus
ECG	Electrocardiogram
eGFR	Estimated glomerular filtration rate
EHR	Electronic health record
ERCP	Endoscopic retrograde cholangiopancreatography
ER	Emergency room
ESRD	End stage renal disease
EPTS	Estimated post transplant survival
F	Bioavailability
FSGS	Focal segmental glomerulosclerosis
GAD-7	General Anxiety Disorder -7
HAT	Hepatic artery thrombosis
HBV	Hepatitis B virus
HCC	Hepatocellular carcinoma
HCV	Hepatitis C virus
HIV	Human immunodeficiency virus
HLA	Human leukocyte antigen
IBW	Ideal body weight
ICU	Intensive care unit
IFTA	Interstitial fibrosis and tubular atrophy
IL	Interleukin
IPD	Invasive pneumococcal disease
IUD	Intrauterine device
KDIGO	Kidney Diseases Improving Global Outcomes
KDPI	Kidney donor profile index
LARC	Long-acting reversible contraception
LNG	Levonorgestrel
MBSR	Mindfulness-based stress reduction
MM	Malignant melanoma
MMF	Mycophenolate mofetil
MPA	Mycophenolic acid
MRCP	Magnetic resonance cholangiopancreatography
mTOR	Mammalian target of rapamycin
NAAT	Nucleic acid amplification test
NASH	Nonalcoholic steatohepatitis
NODAT	New onset diabetes after transplant (note also called post-transplant diabetes mellitus, PTDM)
NSAID	Non-steroidal anti-inflammatory drug
OPTN	Organ Procurement and Transplantation Network
OTC	Over the counter
PAK	Pancreas after kidney (transplant)
PBC	Primary biliary cholangitis
PCP	Primary care provider
PFT	Pulmonary function test

PHQ	Patient health questionnaire
POLST	Provider Orders for Life Sustaining Treatment (note similar abbreviations MOLST, POST, MOST, COLST, TPOPP)
PRA	Panel reactive antibody
PSC	Primary sclerosing cholangitis
PTA	Pancreas transplant alone
PTLD	Post-transplant lymphoproliferative disorder
PTSD	Post-traumatic stress disorder
rATG	Rabbit antithymocyte globulin
SCR	Subclinical rejection
SOT	Solid organ transplant
SOT recipient	Solid organ transplant recipient
SPK	Simultaneous pancreas-kidney (transplant)
SRTR	Scientific Registry of Transplant Recipients
$t_{1/2}$	Half-life
UPA	Ulipristal acetate
US MEC	United States Medical Eligibility Criteria

Chapter 1
Introduction

Christopher J. Wong

Why Primary Care?

Solid organ transplantation is a miracle of modern medicine. Transplant medicine has dramatically altered the natural history of end-organ failure—instead of death, there is life. While there are many potential complications, often solid organ transplant (SOT) recipients have excellent quality of life for their remaining years.

And yet, even after such a life-preserving intervention, there remains quite a bit of work to be done in order to maximize health and function of the transplanted organ and the well-being of the patient. While it may be convenient to believe that a solid organ transplant recipient's transplant center will provide all care that is needed, it is more likely that there will be at least some role for primary care. First, patients may live far from their transplant center and may need a local primary care provider for both urgent and chronic medical conditions. Second, patients often have a pre-existing relationship with their primary care provider prior to solid organ transplantation. Third, the number of surviving solid organ transplant recipients is increasing—transplant centers are not anticipated to have the resources to provide all care for this population.

Thus it is quite likely that primary care providers will play an important role in the care of solid organ transplant recipients. The balance of what aspects of care are performed by which provider should be a continued conversation between the transplant specialist and primary care provider. The transplant specialist typically will maintain immunosuppression and continue to assess function of the transplanted organ. Some transplant centers will follow patients closely even if the patients are doing well, while others may see patients yearly with the bulk of the patients' care returned to primary care and local specialists. For example, a liver

C. J. Wong (✉)
Department of Medicine, Division of General Internal Medicine,
University of Washington, Seattle, WA, USA
e-mail: cjwong@uw.edu

© Springer Nature Switzerland AG 2020
C. J. Wong (ed.), *Primary Care of the Solid Organ Transplant Recipient*,
https://doi.org/10.1007/978-3-030-50629-2_1

transplant recipient may return yearly to the liver transplant clinic, and be followed by a primary care provider and a local gastroenterologist in between those yearly visits, unless there are complications that would require a return evaluation sooner. Sometimes the transition back to primary care after the initial postoperative period is colloquially called "graduating."

Primary Care Roles in the Care of Solid Organ Transplant Recipients

While there will always be a vital role for the transplant specialist, primary care providers nevertheless are front-line in managing other illnesses that may arise in solid organ transplant recipients. Primary care providers who care for solid organ transplant recipients must be ever-vigilant in identifying and treating other complications and comorbidities.

- Is a solid organ transplant recipient's diarrhea from his or her mycophenolate, or is there a new cause of diarrhea, and if so, is it infectious or non-infectious?
- In a solid organ transplant recipient presenting with cough and shortness of breath, are these symptoms a sign of organ failure or an opportunistic infection, or just a viral upper respiratory infection?
- What medications should a solid organ transplant recipient be expected to be taking, and what side effects are likely?
- Will medication therapy for other conditions interfere with the patient's transplant drugs?
- When should the transplant specialist be consulted?

These questions can pose clinical challenges but are nevertheless important to the patient and rewarding to the provider. Caring for solid organ transplant recipients requires all the tools of a clinician to synthesize the presentation and determine the best evaluation and treatment.

In addition to new symptoms, primary care providers are front-line for delivering preventive health and care of chronic conditions to their patients. The primary care provider has an important role in making sure recommended screenings take place, modify screening as indicated, and be alert for metabolic complications and manage them appropriately. Questions might include:

- Should the recommended vaccination schedule be altered?
- How is cancer screening different in a solid organ transplant recipient?
- What metabolic problems, such as diabetes and osteoporosis, should be screened for?
- How should common conditions be managed differently in a solid organ transplant recipient?

How to Use This Book

This book is written with primary care providers in mind, as they try to sort out whether new symptoms and syndromes might represent a transplant-related complication, or, instead, fall into the category of routine primary care; as they navigate recommended preventive health and metabolic complications; and as they learn about complications specific to the transplanted organ. Many patients become experts in their own health, having taken quite a journey to make it through organ failure, transplant approval, and then successful organ transplantation. Primary care providers will take this journey with their patients and learn from the experience as well.

In this book, we hope to provide guidance for primary care providers in the rich and rewarding care of adult solid organ transplant recipients.

Chapter 2 covers a general overview of solid organ transplantation, including review of the pre-transplant course and taking a basic medical history of the patient after transplantation.

Chapter 3 addresses the basics of common anti-rejection medications used in solid organ transplantation and their common side effects. The authors discuss drug interactions for medications commonly used in the primary care setting.

Chapters 4, 5, 6, and 7 provide overviews of the care of kidney and kidney-pancreas, liver, heart, and lung transplant recipients. (Note that this book does not address combined heart-lung or small intestine transplantation.)

Chapter 8 is a review of infections in the solid organ transplant recipient. It includes discussion of select respiratory, gastrointestinal, urinary tract, central nervous system, and skin and soft tissue infections.

Chapter 9 provides a general approach to a set of common syndromes, including shortness of breath and cough, diarrhea, urinary tract symptoms, and skin lesions.

Chapter 10 addresses the important topic of cancer, a life-limiting complication in the immunosuppressed population.

Chapter 11 is an overview of metabolic complications including diabetes, hypertension, hyperlipidemia, gout, and osteoporosis, all of which are common in the solid organ transplant population.

Chapter 12 provides an overview of preventive health, highlighting similarities and differences between recommendations for solid organ transplant recipients compared to the general population.

Chapter 13 addresses palliative care, as solid organ transplant recipients may have important symptoms that impact quality of life, and discusses end-of-life issues.

This book does not need to be read cover-to-cover. The chapters specific to a transplanted organ will provide useful knowledge for primary care providers should they be involved in the care of patients with these transplanted organs. All providers may find useful the general overview chapter and the chapters on medications and complications. Those who see patients for urgent symptoms may find the chapters discussing common syndromes to be helpful, as well as the individual organ chapters as needed.

For this edition, we focus on heart, lung, liver, kidney, and pancreas transplants, and are not covering pediatric solid organ transplantation, small intestine, skin, and other organ transplants.

The goal of this book is to provide a framework and a starting point—as with any such clinical guidance, individualizing care based on the patient's unique circumstances is critical, and one must consult with the patient's specialty providers when the need arises. The care of solid organ transplant recipients is rewarding but requires background knowledge and clinical acumen—it is hoped that this book proves useful in furthering this care.

Chapter 2
Overview of Solid Organ Transplantation for Primary Care Providers

Diana Zhong and Christopher J. Wong

Introduction

Solid organ transplantation is increasing in prevalence. With each passing year, it becomes more likely that primary care providers will encounter patients who are recipients of a solid organ transplant.

In the United States, the number of solid organ transplantations has risen steadily over the past 20 years (Fig. 2.1), with 36,529 solid organ transplants performed in 2018 [1]. The greatest increases have been in liver and kidney transplants (Fig. 2.2). As the actuarial survival has also increased over this period of time, so too has the overall prevalence of living solid organ transplant recipients. It is estimated that as of 2017, there were approximately 220,000 kidney transplant recipients [2], 84,000 liver transplant recipients [3], 32,000 heart transplant recipients [4], and 14,000 lung transplant recipients [5] living in the United States. In total, the number of living solid organ transplant recipients could populate an entire mid-size US city.

Internationally, the World Health Organization estimated that a total of 135,860 solid organ transplants were performed in 2016—a number that has been increasing annually based on provisional data, including in the United States [6]. The majority of solid organ transplants worldwide occur in high-income countries, but transplantation is spreading to an increasing number of countries [7].

The demographics of organ transplantation continue to change. Age is no longer a contraindication to transplantation at many transplant centers; although practices vary by country and region, some countries are moving away from age-based criteria [8, 9]. Indeed, 21% of transplants in the United States in 2018 were received by recipients aged 65 and over [1]. Donor demographics are also changing: there is now expanded use of potentially higher risk, or "extended criteria" donors to help

D. Zhong · C. J. Wong (✉)
Department of Medicine, Division of General Internal Medicine, University of Washington, Seattle, WA, USA
e-mail: zhongd@uw.edu; cjwong@uw.edu

© Springer Nature Switzerland AG 2020
C. J. Wong (ed.), *Primary Care of the Solid Organ Transplant Recipient,*
https://doi.org/10.1007/978-3-030-50629-2_2

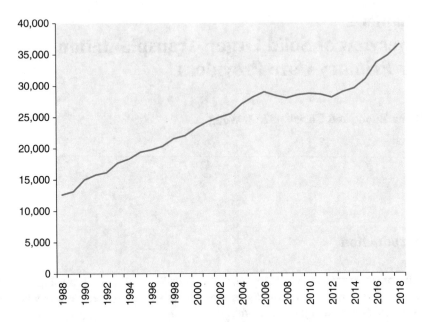

Fig. 2.1 Number of solid organ transplant recipients per year in the United States, 1988–2018. (Based on OPTN data from 2019, from https://optn.transplant.hrsa.gov/data/view-data-reports/national-data/. Accessed April 22, 2019)

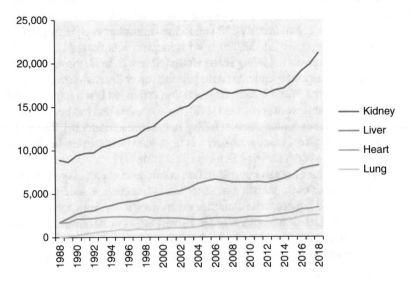

Fig. 2.2 Solid organ transplantation in the United States, by Organ, 1988–2018. *Kidney-pancreas, pancreas, heart-lung, and intestine transplantation data not shown. (Based on OPTN data from 2019, from https://optn.transplant.hrsa.gov/data/view-data-reports/national-data/. Accessed April 22, 2019)

reduce the number of patients on the transplant waiting lists. Extended criteria vary, but may include older age donors as well as the presence of potentially treatable viruses such as hepatitis C [10]. Terminology varies, and some transplant specialists recommend using the least stigmatizing terms to classify donor organs so that providers are not dissuaded from recommending suitable donations.

There are many implications for primary care. First, the volume of solid organ transplant recipients will likely lead to more primary, urgent, and emergent medical care taking place outside of a transplant center. For example, there are an estimated 244 kidney transplant centers in the United States [11]. These centers would have to deliver primary care to all 220,000 living kidney transplant recipients while also evaluating the pre-transplant population; it is preferable that patients could continue routine care with their own primary care providers. Second, patients often live far from their transplant center, making it more imperative to have effective local care. In the United Kingdom, the median distance to the transplant center for liver transplant recipients was 67 km [12]. A study of patients in the United States' Veterans Affairs healthcare system found that distance from the transplant center was inversely correlated with being waitlisted for transplantation—notably in that same study, the vast majority of pre-liver transplant candidates were over 100 miles from a transplant center [13]. In another study of patients in the United States listed for liver transplant, 28% lived over 100 miles from the transplant center [14]. While it is conceivable that some solid organ transplant recipients may move closer to a transplant center after transplantation, this percentage is likely to be small. Third, lessening age requirements and improved overall survival are resulting in an increasingly older population of solid organ transplant recipients. The general practitioner, experienced in the comorbidities of aging, is well-suited to provide care for these patients.

Pre-Transplant Evaluation

Overview

While this book focuses on the primary care of patients after receiving a solid organ transplant, knowledge of the pre-transplant process is useful in their ongoing treatment.

The pre-transplant process begins when a patient with end-stage organ failure is referred to a transplant specialist. This referral may arise from primary care, a specialist, or during an acute-care hospitalization. Pre-transplant testing can take place in a variety of settings, including outpatient clinics (not necessarily only in the transplant center) and inpatient hospital stays.

The transplant team typically includes a medical and surgical team (for example, a transplant hepatologist and a transplant surgeon, in the case of end-stage liver disease), as well as a social worker and other staff to assess social support and psychological health. Other specialists may be involved, such as an infectious disease specialist, psychiatrist, dietician, cardiologist, or pulmonologist, depending on the patient's needs and comorbidities. Testing generally includes laboratory studies, assessment of cardiac tolerance for surgery (other than for heart transplant), and cancer screening. Treatment often includes vaccinations and medication adjustments for medical optimization.

From there, a transplant committee evaluates a patient's candidacy for transplantation. The evaluation will include many factors, including the need for transplant, medical comorbidities, results of medical testing, suitability for major surgery, psychiatric evaluation, and other psychosocial considerations. If a patient is accepted as a candidate for transplantation, the patient is most commonly placed on a waiting list.

The transplant workup, evaluation, and candidate selection process vary depending on the transplant center, organ(s) affected, the patient's underlying disease, the urgency of transplantation, and many other individual patient factors. The information provided here is not intended to be comprehensive; rather, it will hopefully provide the primary care provider an overview of what the solid organ transplant recipient who presents to the outpatient clinic may have experienced prior to transplantation.

The pre-transplant evaluation is summarized in Table 2.1.

History and Exam

The initial pre-transplant medical evaluation will include a detailed history and physical exam. Active or chronic medical conditions are treated or optimized prior to transplantation. Severe medical conditions may be contraindications to transplantation, including untreatable significant dysfunction of another major organ system

Table 2.1 Pre-transplant evaluation

History and exam
Laboratory testing
Functional status
Nutrition and body mass index
Bone density
Cardiopulmonary assessment
Dental evaluation
Family planning (if applicable)
Infection screening
Immunizations
Cancer screening
Surgical evaluation
Psychosocial evaluation

(unless combined organ transplantation can be performed), uncorrected atherosclerotic disease with end-organ ischemia or coronary disease not amenable to revascularization, and other severe and uncorrectable diseases that may lead to a significantly shortened life expectancy [15, 16].

Laboratory Testing

Typical laboratory testing is shown in Table 2.2. In addition to routine testing, patients are evaluated for their risk of prior sensitization, including whether they have a history of blood or platelet transfusions, pregnancies, abortions, or previous transplants [15]. Patients are screened prior to transplant to help identify and treat active infections pre-transplant, to recognize infectious risks including latent infections, and to help prevent and manage post-transplant infections [17] (see "*Infections*" below).

Table 2.2 Typical pre-transplant laboratory tests

Routine tests [15, 18, 19]
Complete blood count
Kidney function and electrolytes
Liver function tests
Coagulation studies
Urinalysis and urine culture
Pregnancy test (if applicable)
Urine drug screen
Compatibility tests [15]
ABO-Rh blood type
Human leukocyte antigen (HLA) type
Panel reactive antibody assay (PRA)
Crossmatching
Infectious disease tests [17]
Human immunodeficiency virus (HIV): HIV antibody/antigen screening
Cytomegalovirus (CMV): CMV IgG
Hepatitis B virus (HBV): HBV surface antigen (HBsAg), HBV core antibody (HBcAb-IgM and IgG, or total core antibody), HBV surface antibody (HBsAb)
Hepatitis C virus (HCV): HCV antibody
HCV nucleic acid amplification testing (NAAT)
Epstein-Barr virus (EBV): EBV antibody (EBV viral capsid antigen IgG, IgM)
Toxoplasma gondii: *Toxoplasma* IgG antibody
Syphilis: available tests may vary by institution
Tuberculosis: Purified protein derivative (PPD) *or* Interferon gamma release assay (IGRA)
Additional testing if indicated by exposures and risk factors

Table 2.3 Pre-transplant cardiopulmonary screening tests

Most patients [21]:
Chest radiography (X-ray)
Electrocardiogram (ECG)
Depending on age and comorbidities, many patients will undergo further evaluation [21]:
Transthoracic echocardiogram (TTE)
Cardiac stress testing
Coronary angiography (if abnormal stress testing or echocardiogram)
Other testing considered may include [20]:
Cardiopulmonary exercise testing (CPET)
6-minute walk test (6MWT)
Noninvasive coronary CT angiography (CCTA)
Coronary artery calcium (CAC) score
Right heart catheterization
Some patients may have additional pulmonary evaluation with [18]:
Pulmonary function tests (PFTs)
Chest computed tomography (CT) scanning

Cardiopulmonary Screening

Screening is performed to evaluate for many cardiopulmonary conditions, including coronary artery disease, cardiomyopathy and heart failure, pulmonary hypertension, cardiac arrhythmias, valvular heart disease, and congenital heart disease [20]. Testing may vary by center, organ to be transplanted, and a patient's individual clinical features. Examples of cardiopulmonary testing are shown in Table 2.3.

Functional Status, Nutrition, and Bone Density

Poor functional status with limited rehabilitation potential may be a contraindication to transplantation. A patient's frailty can be assessed by whether they need assistance with activities of daily living (ADL), the sit-to-stand test, as well as whether they have unintentional weight loss and low physical activity [22]. Older age is increasingly not a contraindication by itself but is considered in the context of a patient's functional status and comorbidities [23].

Obesity can be a contraindication to transplantation. Patients are usually considered poor candidates for transplantation if they have a body mass index (BMI) ≥ 35 kg/m^2 for lung transplant candidacy and BMI ≥ 40 kg/m^2 for liver transplant candidacy. Conversely, malnourished patients are usually considered poor candidates as well [16, 18].

Most patients will have bone densitometry measured with dual-energy X-ray absorptiometry (DEXA). As patients will take chronic glucocorticoids post-transplantation, having baseline data is helpful for follow-up testing and management [18].

Dental Evaluation

A dental evaluation is performed to evaluate for dental abscesses, dental caries, buried roots, and gum disease. Dental problems can be a source of post-transplant infection. Dental procedures are performed prior to transplantation whenever possible [18].

Family Planning

Pregnancy in the first 12 months following transplantation is associated with both an increased risk of preterm delivery as well as graft dysfunction or rejection. It is therefore recommended to avoid pregnancy in the first year after transplantation [24]. A patient's family planning goals should be addressed prior to transplantation, including contraception. Intrauterine devices (IUD) are a preferred and effective method of contraception that will avoid interactions with medications—if placed prior to transplantation, identifying the type of IUD and date of implantation is needed for future management.

Organ-Specific Testing

Further organ-specific testing is performed in conjunction with specialist consultation. While all such testing is not necessary to review, especially if no longer relevant (e.g., the organ is removed), some tests may be helpful for future management. For example, a patient with end-stage liver disease will likely have had esophago-gastroduodenoscopy (EGD) performed to evaluate for esophageal varices—having the results of these evaluations may be useful for comparison if a repeat EGD is needed. Sometimes the workup for organ failure may uncover other syndromes that should be followed. For example, a monoclonal gammopathy may be identified during workup for chronic kidney disease; even if it was not the underlying etiology for the patient's kidney disease, it will still need to be followed post-transplantation. Finally, the explanted organ pathology may sometimes be useful. For example, a heart transplant recipient may have had negative biopsies, but on explant the finding of non-caseating granulomas may suggest sarcoidosis, a condition which could arise in other organs after transplantation.

Vaccines and Pre-transplant Prophylaxis

In most cases, the transplant team will attempt to make sure patients are as up to date as possible on vaccines *prior* to transplant [25]. Both inactivated and live-attenuated vaccines can be given to patients pre-transplant (unless otherwise contra-indicated), but live vaccines are contraindicated post-transplant due to risk of disseminated infection. Additionally, vaccines have variable immunogenicity after transplant due to immunosuppression and thus may be less effective. Therefore, the pre-transplant window is a crucial time for most vaccines to be administered, ideally earlier in a patient's disease course as immunogenicity can also decline due to the relative immunocompromise from organ failure. It is recommended that live vaccines be administered by ≥4 weeks prior to immunosuppression, and that inactivated vaccines be administered ≥2 weeks prior to immunosuppression [24, 26]. All vaccines that are appropriate for age, exposure history, and immune status should be administered prior to transplantation according to the Centers for Disease Control (CDC) guidelines. In addition to the usual vaccine schedule, there are further recommendations for patients awaiting solid organ transplantation, which include hepatitis A, herpes zoster, and pneumococcal vaccination, as shown in Table 2.4 [25]. If a patient is unable to receive vaccinations prior to transplantation, an infectious disease specialist will typically assist with post-transplant vaccination decisions. (For post-transplant guidelines, see Chap. 12).

Less common vaccines that may have been given prior to transplant include meningococcus, Bacille Galmette-Guerin (BCG), smallpox, anthrax, rabies, yellow

Table 2.4 Typical vaccination recommendations prior to solid organ transplantation[a]

Vaccine	Type	Evaluate for serologic response?	Notes
Influenza inactivated (IIV)	Inactivated	No	High-dose formulation often used
Influenza live-attenuated (LAIV)	Live-attenuated	No	Intranasal vaccine*
Hepatitis B	Inactivated	Yes	Various formulations (2-dose, 3-dose, or 4-dose series)
Hepatitis A	Inactivated	Sometimes	Sometimes given in combined formulation with Hepatitis B vaccine
Tetanus	Inactivated	No	
Pertussis (Tdap)	Inactivated	No	If no tetanus booster in the past 10 years, administer Tdap. At least one dose of acellular pertussis should be given in adulthood, especially women of child-bearing age and individuals in contact with infants.
Inactivated Polio	Inactivated	No	
H. influenzae type B	Inactivated	Yes	

Table 2.4   (continued)

Vaccine	Type	Evaluate for serologic response?	Notes
S. pneumoniae	Inactivated	No	There are two inactivated vaccines, PCV13 (Prevnar 13®) and PPSV23 (Pneumovax 23®). See CDC guidelines for details, as timing and dosing vary based on indication. Most solid organ transplant recipients should have received at last PPSV23 prior to transplant, as it is indicated for patients with chronic lung disease, chronic liver disease, and chronic heart disease. Some patients will have also received PCV13 as it is indicated for patients with chronic renal failure, or if they were immunosuppressed pre-transplant for other medical conditions [27]. PCV13 should be completed 8 weeks prior to PPSV23 [24]
Human papilloma virus (HPV)	Inactivated	No	Indicated for age 9–45 years
Measles, mumps, rubella (MMR)	Live-attenuated	Yes	
Varicella (VAR or Varivax®)	Live-attenuated	Yes	Given if not immune
Herpes zoster (recombinant zoster vaccine, RZV or Shringrix®)	Inactivated	No	Recommended for patients ≥50 years old. This is generally the preferred form of zoster vaccination due to its higher efficacy as compared with the live-attenuated vaccine, and because it is inactivated it will not delay transplantation
Herpes zoster (live zoster vaccine, LZV or Zostavax®)	Live-attenuated	No	Two doses should be administered ≥3 months apart, while considering that live vaccines should be given ≥4 weeks prior to transplant [24]

[a]Recommendations change and should be reassessed periodically. All live vaccines are only administered if the patient is not already severely immunocompromised
*The intranasal, live-attenuated influenza vaccine is not recommended for adults age 50 and over; guidelines for this vaccine have changed periodically

fever, Japanese encephalitis, typhoid, and cholera, depending on a patient's exposures and travel [25].

Infections

Transplant candidates are assessed for past infections and a detailed exposure history (travel, residence, occupation, lifestyle, animal, and environmental) [17]. In addition to the routine laboratory testing shown in Table 2.2, further testing may be performed for patients with certain exposures or from endemic areas, including assessment for *Strongyloides*, *Trypanosma cruzi*, and *Coccidioides* species [17, 28]. A rigorous separate screening process is used for potential organ donors.

HIV infection does not preclude receiving transplantation, though HIV should be well-controlled prior to pursuing transplantation [29]. Patients with hepatitis B and chronic hepatitis C can still be considered for transplantation but are evaluated for liver cirrhosis and considered for antiviral treatment prior to transplant [16, 23].

Viral serologies such as CMV and EBV testing can be used to guide donor selection and to stratify risk. Transplant recipients who are CMV seronegative are at higher risk for CMV infection if the donor is CMV seropositive; similarly, recipients who are EBV seronegative are at higher risk for EBV infection and post-transplant lymphoproliferative disorder (PTLD) if the donor is EBV seropositive. These cases require additional post-transplant monitoring and prevention strategies (see Chaps. 8 and 10) [17].

Colonization, Latent Infection, Chronic or Recurrent Infection, and Active Infection

Identification of infection risks can affect transplant candidacy and post-transplant treatment:

- *Colonization*: Microbial colonization can increase the risk of infection after transplantation. For example, a patient with cystic fibrosis awaiting lung transplantation may be colonized with multi-drug resistant strains of bacteria such as *Pseudomonas*, *Staphylococcus aureus*, *Stenotrophomonas*, and *Burkholderia*, as well as fungi such as *Aspergillus*. Patients are carefully evaluated to exclude active infection. Colonization with certain multi-drug resistant organisms or virulent organisms such as *Burkholderia* is associated with poor outcomes after transplantation and may be weighed as a consideration against transplantation [16]. Knowledge of this colonizing flora can aid in development of an individualized peri-transplant and post-transplant prophylactic antimicrobial regimen.
- *Latent infection*: Risk of recurrent infection is assessed and mitigated prior to transplantation. For example, a pre-transplantation history of active disease or seropositivity for coccidioidomycosis may warrant lifelong azole prophylaxis. In contrast, other endemic mycoses such as histoplasmosis are not routinely checked and do not directly alter management, but should be considered when evaluating a patient presenting with illness post-transplantation [17]. Patients with latent tuberculosis infection (LTBI) are ideally treated prior to transplantation [30].
- *Chronic or recurrent infections*: These infections generally require definitive treatment prior to transplantation. For example, patients with a history of severe and/or recurrent infection with *Clostridioides difficile* may receive secondary prevention with fecal microbiota transplant (FMT) or bezlotoxumab [31].
- *Active or uncontrolled infections*: These infections require treatment and often delay transplantation until the infection resolves or is controlled [17].

Cancer Screening

Pre-transplant evaluation requires age-appropriate cancer screening to be up to date. Patients with an active malignancy or recent history of malignancy will not be offered transplantation, as transplantation may not improve survival. Furthermore, immunosuppression increases the risk of malignancy post-transplant [32]. If a patient's cancer has been treated and the patient has been disease-free for a certain period of time, they may often be evaluated for transplantation [16, 19]. All patients should remain up to date on gender and age-appropriate cancer screening, which may include colonoscopy, mammogram, Papanicolaou (Pap) smear, skin examination, and additional screening if indicated for the patient's medical history (e.g., hepatocellular carcinoma screening for patients who have hepatitis B infection) [15].

Surgical Evaluation

A patient's surgical candidacy is a major component of the transplant evaluation, and factors in medical comorbidities as well as the patient's functional and nutritional status, as discussed above.

There are specific additional surgical considerations related to a patient's individual anatomy and history of prior surgeries and prior thromboses. Further workup such as CT scans or vascular studies may be warranted. Furthermore, depending on the organ site, there can be discussion of donor options (deceased, living, extended criteria donors). Specific comorbidities that confer especially high operative risk, such as portopulmonary hypertension in a patient with cirrhosis, will warrant evaluation with anesthesia and consultation with specialists [18]. A full discussion of the surgical evaluation is beyond the scope of this book.

Psychosocial Evaluation

The process of transplantation is fraught with difficult decisions and ethical dilemmas. Organs are a scarce resource. Although transplantation may be life-saving, patients are also encumbered by a lifelong need for medications, follow-up appointments, and management of care. Due to the immense post-transplant burden, the screening process for transplant candidacy encompasses many psychosocial factors, including having adequate social support, financial resources, and sufficient health literacy to be able to manage care. Unfortunately, these factors are often reflective of socioeconomic disparities [33].

Patients will be evaluated by a transplant social worker and often a transplant psychiatrist. There is not a universal evaluation metric, though several scoring scales exist [34, 35].

Patients will typically be evaluated for [34]:

- Treatment adherence and health behaviors
- Mental health history
- Substance use history
- Cognitive status and capacity to give informed consent
- Knowledge and understanding of their current illness
- Knowledge and understanding of current treatment options
- Coping abilities
- Social support
- Social history

Financial Evaluation

Depending on the country's health care system, the patient's insurance and the transplant center, financial approval may need to be secured at the beginning of the process to begin the transplant workup. In the United States, insurance coverage will be considered in terms of the costs of transplantation and post-transplantation care (including medication coverage), and the transplant center will typically have staff to assist with financial planning.

Psychiatric Evaluation

Patients with psychiatric disorders are required to have their diseases well-controlled prior to transplantation [16, 18]. Patients who are already taking psychotropic medications may need to have medications stopped or dose-reduced once transplant immunosuppression is introduced. For example, patients with bipolar disorder are often switched off of lithium to avoid postoperative metabolic shifts or renal insufficiency that could lead to medication toxicity. Such decisions should be made in conjunction with a transplant psychiatrist and a transplant pharmacist [36].

Depression and anxiety are common post-transplantation, either de novo or recurrent—knowing the patient's pre-transplant psychiatric history can be helpful with management after transplantation. Post-transplant patients have an increased risk of suicide and should be assessed regularly for mood disorders [37] (see Chap. 12).

Medication Adherence

Medication adherence is an important aspect of the psychosocial assessment. It is considered a contraindication to transplantation if a patient has current or a repeated history of medication non-adherence. Although a patient who has received a solid organ transplant will have passed adherence screening prior to transplant, data suggest that adherence may be an ongoing concern after transplantation. Rates of post-transplantation medication nonadherence have been reported to be up to 36% in kidney transplant recipients and 7–15% in other transplant types [38]. Younger patients may be at higher risk for medication nonadherence: Kidney transplant recipients who are older adolescents and young adults (aged 17–24 years) have the highest risk of graft failure irrespective of transplant age; this is felt in part to be related to higher rates of immunosuppressive therapy nonadherence [39].

Substance Use

Ongoing substance abuse or dependence is a contraindication to transplantation. Evaluation for transplant often includes screening tests for nicotine use, alcohol, and recreational drugs. Illness related to substance use may be the primary reason that a patient requires transplantation, such as alcoholic cirrhosis, or chronic obstructive pulmonary disease due to smoking. If a patient is able to be treated for substance use pre-transplant and has good prognostic factors, they may then be reassessed for transplant candidacy [16].

- Tobacco: Smoking is a contraindication to lung transplantation. For other organ transplantation, smoking cessation is strongly preferred as smoking is associated with worse outcomes post-transplantation including increased risk of graft loss, cardiovascular events, and malignancy [40].
- Alcohol: Patients with alcoholic cirrhosis who have ceased alcohol use (typically 6 months, but may vary by transplant center) may be assessed for liver transplantation. However, sobriety for a certain time period is often not sufficient, as a pattern of use and subsequent return to use may portend a high risk of returning to use after transplantation; rather, patients with serious alcohol use disorders are referred to formal alcohol treatment programs [18].
- Marijuana: Institutions have varying policies regarding marijuana, but in most cases usage is unfavorable [16, 41].
- Opioid use disorder: Patients who have a well-controlled opioid-use disorder treated with methadone may still be considered for solid organ transplantation, and it is not required for transplant listing that methadone doses be reduced or discontinued [18]. Treatment with buprenorphine-naloxone for opioid use disorder is not a contraindication, but a transplant pharmacist should be consulted for perioperative and postoperative management.

Transplantation

Patients who successfully complete the pre-transplant evaluation and are approved by the transplant committee are then placed on a waiting list, unless the case is considered emergent. The waiting process can be among the most difficult and stressful parts of the pre-transplant process. Despite yearly growth in the number of successful transplants performed, still more patients remain on the waiting list: in August 2019, over 124,000 individuals in the United States remained on the waiting list for an organ, over 3 times as many as were transplanted the year before [42]. Mortality while awaiting a transplant is significant; an estimated 20% of patients on the lung transplant waiting list will become too sick to transplant or die while on the waiting list [43, 44]. In addition to the numerical odds, the waiting process can be long and marked by worsening medical complications.

In some cases, patients are called for organ transplantation but do not receive an organ due to poor viability of the donated organ or other reasons—some patients have experienced several false alarms prior to transplantation.

Organ allocation and the initial transplant hospitalization are beyond the scope of primary care and are not covered in this book. Some patients have an uneventful course while others may have a difficult initial hospitalization. Early complications can include acute rejection, problems with the vascular or other anastomoses, thrombosis, and infection.

Returning to Primary Care

Patients who make it through the initial post-transplant hospitalization are usually discharged with prophylaxis against infections (see Chap. 8) and typically have a high dose of immunosuppression. In most cases, during the initial post-transplant period, patients will be cared for primarily by the transplant team.

After a period of time, the stable patient may "graduate" from the transplant program and be cared for by a community specialist along with a primary care provider. For example, a liver transplant recipient might return to primary care after 6 months and also be routinely followed by his or her local gastroenterologist; the patient may still return yearly to the transplant center (and more often if complications arise). The transition to primary care and local specialty care varies by transplant center, the patient's unique needs and preferences, and proximity to the transplant center.

Taking a Transplant History

When a solid organ transplant recipient enters (or re-enters) primary care, basic information should be obtained to optimize future care. The following data should be gathered (see Table 2.5) [45]:

Table 2.5 History-taking for the solid organ transplant recipient

History element	Example	Notes
Transplanted organ Indication Pre-transplant course	*Lung transplant, bilateral For cystic fibrosis, diagnosed at age 5 Prior to transplant, had repeat exacerbations Also has non-pulmonary complications of cystic fibrosis (sinusitis, history of intestinal obstruction)*	Pre-transplant course varies widely. For renal transplant recipients, helpful to know if prior history of dialysis and type of dialysis access
Time course	*Date of transplant (month/year)*	The time since transplantation may affect target drug levels and risk of infection and malignancy
Graft function	*Spirometry (date) FEV1, FVC. Last bronchoscopy, if performed (date) (results)*	Assessment will vary depending on the transplanted organ
Complications Surgery-related Infections Rejection episodes (acute or chronic)	*Bronchial stenosis, status post airway dilation × 2 Pneumonia in (month/year), bronchoscopy negative for rejection, fungal or viral infections; treated as community-acquired pneumonia No episodes of rejection*	If episodes of rejection, review treatment and doses (e.g., glucocorticoids, or increase in other immunosuppression)
Medications	*Tacrolimus 2 mg twice daily Mycophenolate mofetil 500 mg twice daily Prednisone 5 mg once daily*	See Chap. 3 If known, goal trough levels helpful to document
Serologic status Epstein-Barr Virus (EBV) Cytomegalovirus (CMV)	*EBV D+/R− CMV D+/R+*	D = Donor, R = Recipient The highest risk for EBV-related complications is in donor positive/ recipient negative patients CMV prophylaxis is often given in the initial post-transplant period, depending on serostatus of the donor and recipient, as well as the induction immunosuppression used. See Chap. 8
Metabolic complications	*Hypertension Hypomagnesemia Chronic kidney disease stage 3 Osteopenia: T-score −2.1, no history of facture*	See Chap. 11

Transplanted Organ

- Clearly listing the transplanted organ(s) and indication is helpful. Note that lung transplants can be single or bilateral. For kidney transplants, it is useful to document where the graft is located (usually in the lower pelvis—list which side). When applicable, the type of donor should be listed (kidney transplant recipients may have a living or cadaveric donor).
- Knowing the disease that led to organ transplantation is important, as it may recur in the graft. Examples include hepatitis C or autoimmune hepatitis that can develop again in the transplanted liver.
- A systemic condition or risk factor that led to organ transplantation may continue to affect other organ systems. Smoking may lead to chronic obstructive pulmonary disease and subsequent lung transplantation, but it may also be a risk factor for other cancers in the future. Cystic fibrosis may lead to lung transplantation, but its effects on the liver and gastrointestinal tract may continue. Alcohol use may recur in the liver transplant recipient, but even prior use may still be a risk factor for subsequent cancers.
- The pre-transplant course is often useful to review. Renal transplant recipients who have received hemodialysis may still have a fistula for access. Liver transplant recipients may have had recurrent gastrointestinal bleeding or encephalopathy, important considerations should graft failure occur.

Time Course

- As is discussed in Chap. 8, the time course after transplantation affects the general likelihood of opportunistic infections.
- Early infections (within the first month post-transplantation) are likely to be nosocomial or donor-derived, and are not typically encountered in primary care, as the patient will often primarily be in the care of the transplant team.
- In the 1–6 month time period, opportunistic infections can occur because of the higher levels of immunosuppression. Patients are usually still receiving the bulk of their care from the transplant team.
- After 6 months, community-acquired infections are common although some opportunistic infections still occur. For patients who experience a relatively uncomplicated post-transplantation course, many can transition the majority of their routine care to primary care around this time.
- If there is an episode of rejection that necessitates a higher level of immunosuppression, the time course is effectively "reset," with opportunistic infections becoming more likely.

Graft Function

- At primary care visits, providers should ask about symptoms of organ dysfunction.
- Surveillance studies of graft function should be reviewed. These tests are expected to be performed by the patient's specialist (typically either at the transplant center or by the local specialist). Function may be assessed by laboratory studies (creatinine in renal transplant recipients, hepatic function tests in liver transplant recipients), functional testing (spirometry in lung transplant recipients, echocardiograms in heart transplant recipients). Further testing varies by organ, transplant center, and individual patient, and may include imaging, biopsies, and immunosuppression levels.
- For more details, see organ-specific chapters (Chaps. 4, 5, 6, and 7).

Complications

- Surgery-related complications may include arterial or venous thrombosis, problems with vascular or other anastomoses, hernias, and surgical site infections. Organ-specific complications may occur. For example, hepatic artery thrombosis may occur early in liver transplantation; cardiac allograft vasculopathy is a unique form of coronary disease in the heart transplant recipient; lung transplantation can be complicated by airway stenoses requiring dilation.
- Opportunistic infections should be reviewed, including what organism, how the infection was confirmed, and what treatment was administered.
- Organ rejection should be asked about but also reviewed carefully in the medical record, as the presentation can vary widely. Sometimes organ rejection is asymptomatic and found on routine biopsy—therefore, patients may only be superficially aware of it.
- For more details, see organ-specific chapters (Chaps. 4, 5, 6, and 7).

Medications

- A thorough medication history should be taken, including supplements and non-transplant medications, as drug interactions are common. If patients see other providers who prescribe medications, those records should be obtained and reviewed.

- Adherence should be investigated. With good pre- and post-transplant education, patients are doubtless aware of the implications of having a transplanted organ and the importance of strict adherence to immunosuppressive medications. Nevertheless, many patients feel burdened not only by their transplantation and fear of graft rejection, but also by their medications, with concern for cancers and infections as a risk of their immunosuppression [46]. There is a significant post-transplant financial and emotional burden from medications, medical appointments, and hospitalizations [35, 46].
- Side effects should be addressed, both to help assess a patient's tolerance of their medications, but also as a factor potentially affecting adherence. Familiarity with common side effects of anti-rejection medications will facilitate history-taking about symptoms.
- Depending on the immunosuppression medication, the transplant specialist will be following medication levels. These are typically trough levels (i.e., immediately before the next dose). It is helpful to document the goal trough level if it is known.
- Anti-rejection medications are reviewed in Chap. 3.

Serologic Status

- Obtaining and documenting the EBV and CMV data for the recipient and the donor is useful, as it may affect viral prophylaxis (which will typically be managed by the transplant specialist) but also the risk of future infection or malignancy (See Chaps. 8 and 10).

Metabolic Complications

- Ask about and review the patient's chart for metabolic complications and comorbidities, including electrolyte imbalances, diabetes, hypertension, osteoporosis, and history of cancer (See Chap. 11).

Examination

- General physical examination should be performed as with non-transplant patients.
- Examine the surgical incision for signs of infection or hernia.
- Examine the transplanted organ system for signs of dysfunction.

  - The heart transplant recipient should have a thorough cardiopulmonary exam evaluating for signs of heart failure. The transplanted heart is denervated and

patients may not have classic angina if coronary artery disease occurs. Tachycardia may be a sign of rejection.
- The lung transplant recipient may have received a single or double lung transplant. Single lung transplant recipients may still have serious disease in the native lung. In the transplanted lung, rales or dyspnea may signal infection or rejection, but often rejection can be subtle without prominent exam findings.
- The liver transplant recipient should be examined for signs of cirrhosis; otherwise, dysfunction may not present on exam but instead be detected on laboratory findings. Splenomegaly may persist after transplantation.
- The kidney transplant recipient will typically have the transplanted kidney seated in the lower pelvis, often palpable on exam. The abdominal exam should be conducted with care—while one should look for signs of inflammation, one should not apply excessive pressure on the transplanted kidney itself.
- For more details, see Chaps. 4, 5, 6, and 7.

Establishing a Follow-Up Plan

- Patients who are doing very well—e.g., with a well-functioning graft, good adherence, and no history of graft rejection or opportunistic infections—might only need to see primary care and the transplant clinic yearly, with more frequent laboratory monitoring in between.
- Other patients who are at higher risk may continue quarterly visits, or even more frequently.
- Practice varies by transplant center and organ transplanted.
- Establish preventive health recommendations. Future metabolic testing should be assessed and coordinated with the transplant team. A plan for future immunizations should be made, and patients should be reminded that they can no longer receive live vaccines. For additional discussion, see Chap. 12.

Pearls

- *Inquire about the pre-transplant process.* Many patients will be forward-thinking and not wish to relive the pre-transplant process. However, if the primary care provider did not care for the patient pre-transplant, it can be useful to explore the pre-transplant course from the patient's perspective. For many patients, their life prior to transplantation is marked by years of chronic illness. The process of transplant evaluation can be a lengthy and harrowing one for many patients, and the subsequent wait for transplantation is yet another ordeal. Some patients have to travel great distances from their home. As organs are a scarce resource, the waiting process can be emotionally and psychologically difficult. Some patients have experienced healthcare-related trauma from intensive-care unit or other hospital stays.

Conversely, a smaller proportion of patients may have had a brief severe illness prior to transplantation. For example, a previously healthy patient presenting with acute fulminant liver failure may not have had the physical and psychological sequelae of chronic illness, or may have had limited primary care contact prior to transplantation.

- *Recordkeeping.* Gathering the pre-transplant and post-transplant information for a solid organ transplant recipient can be challenging, depending on the medical record system, whether the primary care provider and transplant specialists practice in the same healthcare system, and the culture of communication between providers. Ideally, the transplant team has summarized the pre-transplant evaluation in their documentation, with similarly detailed post-transplant surveillance in the medical record. However, obtaining additional records is sometimes required. These baseline tests can be very helpful as a basis of comparison if complications arise.
- *Communicate and consult early.* While one goal of this book is to improve the primary care provider's familiarity with the care of solid organ transplant recipients, even with the most meticulous care, the health of a solid organ transplant recipient can decline rapidly. If there is concern for graft dysfunction or an opportunistic infection, the primary care provider should consult with the transplant specialist. Many specialty centers have medical specialists who have additional expertise in transplant medicine (e.g., a transplant infectious disease specialist or a transplant pharmacist). It is recommended to review the expertise in one's local practice area, as well as the preferred consultants of the patient's transplant team. If there is uncertainty about an aspect of a patient's care, it is best to err on the side of communicating with the transplant team. Most transplant centers have a robust multidisciplinary team to help communicate and coordinate care.

Conclusion

Primary care providers have an increasingly vital role in the outpatient care of solid organ transplant recipients. While care of such patients can be complex, the ability to review a patient's prior transplant evaluations and assess the patient's current health status prepares the primary care provider to optimize future preventive care and address acute medical concerns.

References

1. Transplants in the U.S. by recipient age. U.S. transplants performed: January 1, 1988–March 31, 2019. Based on OPTN data as of April 21, 2019. https://optn.transplant.hrsa.gov/data/view-data-reports/national-data/. Accessed 22 Apr 2019.
2. Hart A, Smith JM, Skeans MA, Gustafson SK, Wilk AR, Castro S, Robinson A, Wainright JL, Snyder JJ, Kasiske BL, Israni AK. OPTN/SRTR 2017 annual data report: kidney. Am J Transplant. 2019;19(Suppl 2):19–123. https://doi.org/10.1111/ajt.15274.

3. Kim WR, Lake JR, Smith JM, Schladt DP, Skeans MA, Noreen SM, Robinson AM, Miller E, Snyder JJ, Israni AK, Kasiske BL. OPTN/SRTR 2017 annual data report: liver. Am J Transplant. 2019;19(Suppl 2):184–283. https://doi.org/10.1111/ajt.15276.
4. Colvin M, Smith JM, Hadley N, Skeans MA, Uccellini K, Lehman R, Robinson AM, Israni AK, Snyder JJ, Kasiske BL. OPTN/SRTR 2017 annual data report: heart. Am J Transplant. 2019;19(Suppl 2):323–403. https://doi.org/10.1111/ajt.15278.
5. Valapour M, Lehr CJ, Skeans MA, Smith JM, Uccellini K, Lehman R, Robinson A, Israni AK, Snyder JJ, Kasiske BL. OPTN/SRTR 2017 annual data report: lung. Am J Transplant. 2019;19(Suppl 2):404–84. https://doi.org/10.1111/ajt.15279.
6. Global Observatory on Donation and Transplantation, World Health Organization. Organ Donation and Transplantation Activities 2016. Data as of September 2018, requested disclaimer as follows: "The data and information presented here are published in order to promote transparency in transplantation activities. Whenever possible this information has been confirmed by official national sources. However, in some instances, there are still provisional estimates. It is therefore anticipated that some data presented may be modified without prior notice." Accessed 1 July 2019 at http://www.transplant-observatory.org/download/2016-activity-data-report/.
7. White SL, Hirth R, Mahíllo B, Domínguez-Gil B, Delmonico FL, Noel L, Chapman J, Matesanz R, Carmona M, Alvarez M, Núñez JR, Leichtmang A. The global diffusion of organ transplantation: trends, drivers and policy implications. Bull World Health Organ. 2014;92:826–35. https://doi.org/10.2471/BLT.14.137653.
8. UNOS Transplant Living. Frequently asked questions. Accessed 1 July 2019 at: https://transplantliving.org/before-the-transplant/frequently-asked-questions/.
9. Katvan E, Doron I, Ashkenazi T, Boas H, Carmiel-Haggai M, Elhalel MD, Shnoor B, Lavee J. Age limitation for organ transplantation: the Israeli example. Age Ageing. 2017;46(1):8–10. https://doi.org/10.1093/ageing/afw162.
10. Vodkin I, Kuo A. Extended criteria donors in liver transplantation. Clin Liver Dis. 2017;21(2):289–301. https://doi.org/10.1016/j.cld.2016.12.004.
11. http://www.nationalkidneycenter.org/treatment-options/transplant/find-a-transplant-center/.
12. Webb GJ, Hodson J, Chauhan A, O'Grady J, Neuberger JM, Hirschfield GM, Ferguson JW. Proximity to transplant center and outcome among liver transplant patients. Am J Transplant. 2019;19(1):208–20. https://doi.org/10.1111/ajt.15004.
13. Goldberg DS, French B, Forde KA, Groeneveld PW, Bittermann T, Backus L, Halpern SD, Kaplan DE. Association of distance from a transplant center with access to waitlist placement, receipt of liver transplantation, and survival among US veterans. JAMA. 2014;311(12):1234–43. https://doi.org/10.1001/jama.2014.2520.
14. Cicalese L, Shirafkan A, Jennings K, Zorzi D, Rastellini C. Increased risk of death for patients on the waitlist for liver transplant residing at greater distance from specialized liver transplant centers in the United States. Transplantation. 2016;100(10):2146–52. https://doi.org/10.1097/TP.0000000000001387.
15. Bunnapradist S, Danovitch GM. Evaluation of adult kidney transplant candidates. Am J Kidney Dis. 2007;50(5):890–8. https://doi.org/10.1053/j.ajkd.2007.08.010.
16. Weill D, Benden C, Corris PA, et al. A consensus document for the selection of lung transplant candidates: 2014--an update from the Pulmonary Transplantation Council of the International Society for Heart and Lung Transplantation. J Heart Lung Transplant. 2015;34(1):1–15. https://doi.org/10.1016/j.healun.2014.06.014.
17. Malinis M, Boucher HW, Practice ASTIDCo. Screening of donor and candidate prior to solid organ transplantation-guidelines from the American Society of Transplantation Infectious Diseases Community of Practice. Clin Transpl. 2019;33:e13548. https://doi.org/10.1111/ctr.13548.
18. Martin P, DiMartini A, Feng S, Brown R Jr, Fallon M. Evaluation for liver transplantation in adults: 2013 practice guideline by the American Association for the Study of Liver Diseases and the American Society of Transplantation. Hepatology. 2014;59(3):1144–65. https://doi.org/10.1002/hep.26972.

19. Pham PT, Pham PA, Pham PC, Parikh S, Danovitch G. Evaluation of adult kidney transplant candidates. Semin Dial. 2010;23(6):595–605. https://doi.org/10.1111/j.1525-139X.2010.00809.x.
20. VanWagner LB, Harinstein ME, Runo JR, et al. Multidisciplinary approach to cardiac and pulmonary vascular disease risk assessment in liver transplantation: an evaluation of the evidence and consensus recommendations. Am J Transplant. 2018;18(1):30–42. https://doi.org/10.1111/ajt.14531.
21. Sandal S, Chen T, Cantarovich M. The challenges with the cardiac evaluation of liver and kidney transplant candidates. Transplantation. 2019;104:251. https://doi.org/10.1097/TP.0000000000002951.
22. McAdams-DeMarco MA, Rasmussen S, Chu NM, et al. Perceptions and practices regarding frailty in kidney transplantation: results of a National Survey. Transplantation. 2019;104:349. https://doi.org/10.1097/TP.0000000000002779.
23. Adegunsoye A, Strek ME, Garrity E, Guzy R, Bag R. Comprehensive care of the lung transplant patient. Chest. 2017;152(1):150–64. https://doi.org/10.1016/j.chest.2016.10.001.
24. Cimino FM, Snyder KA. Primary care of the solid organ transplant recipient. Am Fam Physician. 2016;93(3):203–10.
25. Rubin LG, Levin MJ, Ljungman P, et al. IDSA clinical practice guideline for vaccination of the immunocompromised host. Clin Infect Dis. 2014;58(3):e44–100. https://doi.org/10.1093/cid/cit684.
26. Danziger-Isakov L, Kumar D. Vaccination of solid organ transplant candidates and recipients: guidelines from the American society of transplantation infectious diseases community of practice. Clin Transpl. 2019;33:e13563. https://doi.org/10.1111/ctr.13563.
27. CDC. Pneumococcal vaccination: summary of who and when to vaccinate. Secondary pneumococcal vaccination: summary of who and when to vaccinate 2017. https://www.cdc.gov/vaccines/vpd/pneumo/hcp/who-when-to-vaccinate.html.
28. Buchan CA, Kotton CN, ASTIDCo P. Travel medicine, transplant tourism, and the solid organ transplant recipient-guidelines from the American Society of Transplantation Infectious Diseases Community of Practice. Clin Transpl. 2019;33:e13529. https://doi.org/10.1111/ctr.13529.
29. Blumberg EA, Rogers CC, American Society of Transplantation Infectious Diseases Community of Practice. Solid organ transplantation in the HIV-infected patient: guidelines from the American Society of Transplantation Infectious Diseases Community of Practice. Clin Transpl. 2019;33:e13499. https://doi.org/10.1111/ctr.13499.
30. Epstein DJ, Subramanian AK. Prevention and management of tuberculosis in solid organ transplant recipients. Infect Dis Clin N Am. 2018;32(3):703–18. https://doi.org/10.1016/j.idc.2018.05.002.
31. Pouch SM, Friedman-Moraco RJ. Prevention and treatment of clostridium difficile-associated diarrhea in solid organ transplant recipients. Infect Dis Clin N Am. 2018;32(3):733–48. https://doi.org/10.1016/j.idc.2018.05.001.
32. Acuna SA, Huang JW, Scott AL, et al. Cancer screening recommendations for solid organ transplant recipients: a systematic review of clinical practice guidelines. Am J Transplant. 2017;17(1):103–14. https://doi.org/10.1111/ajt.13978.
33. Ladin K, Emerson J, Berry K, et al. Excluding patients from transplant due to social support: results from a national survey of transplant providers. Am J Transplant. 2019;19(1):193–203. https://doi.org/10.1111/ajt.14962.
34. Maldonado JR, Dubois HC, David EE, et al. The Stanford Integrated Psychosocial Assessment for Transplantation (SIPAT): a new tool for the psychosocial evaluation of pre-transplant candidates. Psychosomatics. 2012;53(2):123–32. https://doi.org/10.1016/j.psym.2011.12.012.
35. Dew MA, DiMartini AF, Dobbels F, et al. The 2018 ISHLT/APM/AST/ICCAC/STSW recommendations for the psychosocial evaluation of adult cardiothoracic transplant candidates and candidates for long-term mechanical circulatory support. J Heart Lung Transplant. 2018;37(7):803–23. https://doi.org/10.1016/j.healun.2018.03.005.
36. Surman OS, Cosimi AB, DiMartini A. Psychiatric care of patients undergoing organ transplantation. Transplantation. 2009;87(12):1753–61. https://doi.org/10.1097/TP.0b013e3181a754d4.
37. Heinrich TW, Marcangelo M. Psychiatric issues in solid organ transplantation. Harv Rev Psychiatry. 2009;17(6):398–406. https://doi.org/10.3109/10673220903463259.

38. Dew MA, DiMartini AF, De Vito Dabbs A, et al. Rates and risk factors for nonadherence to the medical regimen after adult solid organ transplantation. Transplantation. 2007;83(7):858–73. https://doi.org/10.1097/01.tp.0000258599.65257.a6.
39. Foster BJ, Dahhou M, Zhang X, Platt RW, Samuel SM, Hanley JA. Association between age and graft failure rates in young kidney transplant recipients. Transplantation. 2011;92(11):1237–43. https://doi.org/10.1097/TP.0b013e31823411d7.
40. Anis KH, Weinrauch LA, D'Elia JA. Effects of smoking on solid organ transplantation outcomes. Am J Med. 2019;132(4):413–9. https://doi.org/10.1016/j.amjmed.2018.11.005.
41. Levi ME, Montague BT, Thurstone C, et al. Marijuana use in transplantation: a call for clarity. Clin Transpl. 2019;33(2):e13456. https://doi.org/10.1111/ctr.13456.
42. Network OPaT. National data: Organ by state, current U.S. waiting list. Secondary national data: Organ by state, current U.S. waiting list 2019. https://optn.transplant.hrsa.gov/data/view-data-reports/national-data.
43. Valapour M, Lehr CJ, Skeans MA, et al. OPTN/SRTR 2016 annual data report: lung. Am J Transplant. 2018;18(Suppl 1):363–433. https://doi.org/10.1111/ajt.14562.
44. Ahya VN, Diamond JM. Lung transplantation. Med Clin North Am. 2019;103(3):425–33. https://doi.org/10.1016/j.mcna.2018.12.003.
45. Wong CJ, Pagalilauan G. Primary care of the solid organ transplant recipient. Med Clin North Am. 2015;99(5):1075–103. https://doi.org/10.1016/j.mcna.2015.05.002.
46. Ettenger R, Albrecht R, Alloway R, et al. Meeting report: FDA public meeting on patient-focused drug development and medication adherence in solid organ transplant patients. Am J Transplant. 2018;18(3):564–73. https://doi.org/10.1111/ajt.14635.

Chapter 3
Anti-rejection Medication Therapy in the Adult Solid Organ Transplant Recipient

Lydia Sun, Tyra Fainstad, and Christopher Knight

Introduction

Immunosuppressive medications reduce the risk of graft rejection, and without them, successful organ transplant would be impossible. Unfortunately, these medications also cause over half of transplant-related deaths, due to infections, cancer, and other risks related to long-term use [1]. Proper use and early recognition of adverse effects are crucial to a transplant recipient's health and survival. Once a patient is through the acute postoperative setting, primary care providers need to be comfortable recognizing adverse effects of immunosuppressive medications in order to provide well-informed, coordinated care with transplant specialists. They also have primary responsibility for managing interactions with new and existing medications [2].

Typical Immunosuppressant Course

The goals of immunosuppression are to prevent graft rejection, improve graft survival, while minimizing adverse effects including metabolic side effects, infection, and malignancy, in order to improve overall patient survival and quality of life (see

L. Sun (✉)
Department of Pharmacy, University of Washington Medical Center, Seattle, WA, USA
e-mail: lydsun@uw.edu

T. Fainstad
Department of Medicine, Division of General Internal Medicine, University of Colorado, Denver, CO, USA
e-mail: tyra.fainstad@cuanschutz.edu

C. Knight
Department of Medicine, Division of General Internal Medicine, University of Washington, Seattle, WA, USA
e-mail: cknight@uw.edu

© Springer Nature Switzerland AG 2020
C. J. Wong (ed.), *Primary Care of the Solid Organ Transplant Recipient*,
https://doi.org/10.1007/978-3-030-50629-2_3

Table 3.1 Goals of immunosuppression in transplant recipients

Prevent graft rejection
Improve graft survival
Improve patient survival
Minimize medication side effects
Improve patient quality of life

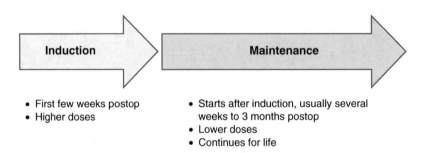

Induction

- First few weeks postop
- Higher doses

Maintenance

- Starts after induction, usually several weeks to 3 months postop
- Lower doses
- Continues for life

Fig. 3.1 Phases of anti-rejection medication use in transplant recipients

Table 3.1). Conventional maintenance regimens consist of a combination of immunosuppressive agents that differ by mechanism of action. A multidrug strategy maximizes overall effectiveness of the immunosuppressants, while also minimizing medication adverse effects [3].

Patients are typically treated with anti-rejection medications in two phases: induction and maintenance (see Fig. 3.1). In the induction phase, high doses of multiple immunosuppressants are given immediately postoperatively until a few weeks after transplantation. Immunosuppression is usually heavier in this period when the risk of rejection is higher due to a number of factors including preservation injury of the graft and sudden exposure of the recipient immune system to a load of foreign antigen. The maintenance phase starts several weeks to 3 months later and lasts through the life of the transplanted organ [4].

According to SRTR (Scientific Registry of Transplant Recipients) data from 2018, the triple regimen of tacrolimus, mycophenolate, and prednisone is the most common maintenance regimen at discharge, with use ranging from just over 60% in kidney transplant recipients, 63% in liver transplant recipients, to over 85% in lung and heart transplant recipients [5].

After 6–12 months, immunosuppression regimens are generally stably maintained, unless there is a specific reason, such as infection, malignancy, or drug toxicity, to reduce immunosuppression further. The optimal maintenance therapy in solid organ transplantation is not established, but immunosuppressant levels required to achieve a state of immune tolerance and graft survival differ between transplanted organs for unclear reasons [6]. As a general rule of thumb, lung, intestine and heart transplant recipients require a higher level of immunosuppression than kidney and liver recipients [6].

For the purposes of this chapter, we will focus on maintenance medications as these are primarily what the primary care provider will encounter.

Overview of Classes of Medications

The main classes of anti-rejection medications that are used for maintenance include calcineurin inhibitors, antiproliferative/antimetabolites, corticosteroids, and mammalian target of rapamycin (mTOR) inhibitors. High doses of corticosteroids are used early after transplantation, but are generally tapered as quickly as possible because of their long-term toxicity [7]. Mechanisms of action are shown in Table 3.2. Dosing, pharmacokinetics, and side effects are shown in Table 3.3.

Monitoring

Because most immunosuppressants have a narrow therapeutic index and blood concentrations vary significantly between individuals, therapeutic drug monitoring is essential to maintain efficacy while minimizing toxicity [7]. The calcineurin inhibitors (tacrolimus, cyclosporine) and mTOR inhibitors (sirolimus, everolimus) require routine therapeutic drug monitoring of trough concentrations as described in Table 3.3. A stable patient typically has laboratory studies drawn every 3 months after the first year, although this will be individualized based on center protocols and patient factors. Primary care providers should review the most recent laboratory testing—if there has been no testing in the past 3 months, then the patient and/or primary care provider should contact the transplant center, as the patient is likely overdue.

Table 3.2 Mechanism of action of common anti-rejection medications [1, 2, 7, 8]

Immunosuppressant	General mechanism of action	Specific mechanism of action
Calcineurin inhibitors Tacrolimus (Prograf®) Cyclosporine (Neoral®, Sandimmune®)	Inhibitors of T-cell activation (early)	Block IL-2 production
Antimetabolites Mycophenolate (Cellcept®, Myfortic®) Azathioprine (Imuran®)	Inhibitors of T-cell production	Block DNA (nucleotide) synthesis
Corticosteroids Prednisone Methylprednisolone	Non-specific inhibitors of immune function	Block IL-1 production
mTOR Inhibitors Sirolimus (Rapamune®) Everolimus (Afinitor®)	Inhibitors of T-cell activation (late)	Inhibit IL-2 activity and activation of cell cycle

IL interleukin, *mTOR* mammalian target of rapamycin

Table 3.3 Dosing, pharmacokinetics, and adverse effects of common immunosuppressant medications [1, 2, 7, 8]

	Immunosuppressant	Dosing monitoring	Pharmacokinetics: half-life ($t_{1/2}$) bioavailability (F)	Adverse effects	Comments
Calcineurin inhibitors	Tacrolimus (FK-506, Prograf®)	Dosing: 0.025–0.1 mg/kg PO Q12hrs Monitoring: target levels 5–15 ng/mL (trough)	$t_{1/2} \approx 8$ hours $F = 15$–30% (more predictable than cyclosporine)	Nephrotoxicity (related to dose and duration) • Acute nephrotoxicity is reversible • Chronic progressive renal disease is irreversible Electrolyte disturbance (related to reduction in renal blood flow) • Hyperkalemia • Hypomagnesemia Neurologic side effects • Headache • Tremor, paresthesias • Rare/serious: PRES (posterior reversible encephalopathy syndrome) Post-transplant diabetes Gastrointestinal toxicity • Diarrhea • Dyspepsia • Nausea, vomiting Metabolic/endocrine side effects: • Hypertension • Hypercholesterolemia	Neurologic side effects, gastrointestinal side effects, alopecia, and diabetes are more common with tacrolimus than cyclosporine Generic forms ARE bioequivalent The extended release formulation Envarsus® is not equivalent—dosing should be adjusted only by the transplant team

Cyclosporine (Gengraf®, Neoral®, Sandimmune®)	Dosing: 4–5 mg/kg PO Q12hrs (IBW) Monitoring: carriage return target levels 75–250 ng/mL (trough)	$t_{1/2} \approx$ 8–18 hours	Nephrotoxicity (related to dose and duration) • Acute nephrotoxicity is reversible • Chronic progressive renal disease is irreversible Electrolyte disturbance (related to reduction in renal blood flow) • Hyperkalemia • Hypomagnesemia Metabolic/endocrine side effects: • Hypertension • Hypercholesterolemia • Hirsutism	Hypertension, hypercholesterolemia, and hirsutism are more common with cyclosporine than tacrolimus Generic formulations of Gengraf® and Neoral® are also called "cyclosporine modified" Sandimmune® (cyclosporine non-modified): • Sandimmune® is NOT bioequivalent or interchangeable with Gengraf®/Neoral® • Most transplant recipients are started on Gengraf®/Neoral®. Only those patients transplanted prior to release of Gengraf®/Neoral® formulation are maintained on Sandimmune®

(continued)

Table 3.3 (continued)

	Immunosuppressant	Dosing monitoring	Pharmacokinetics: half-life ($t_{1/2}$) bioavailability (F)	Adverse effects	Comments
Antimetabolites	Mycophenolate (Cellcept, Myfortic®)	Dosing: Mycophenolate mofetil (MMF) or Cellcept® 250–1000 mg PO Q12hrs Mycophenolate sodium/ Mycophenolic acid (MPA) or Myfortic® 180–720 mg PO Q12hrs Monitoring: general routine use of mycophenolate therapeutic drug monitoring is not recommended on the basis of available evidence*	$t_{1/2} \approx 18$ hours	Gastrointestinal toxicity • Nausea, vomiting • Diarrhea (40%) • Abdominal pain Hematologic side effects • Leukopenia, anemia, thrombocytopenia	Contraindicated in pregnancy Use Cellcept® (MMF) for feeding tube administration because it is available in a liquid form. (Mycophenolate tablets should not be split, crushed, or chewed) Cellcept® (MMF) is a prodrug, and the first mycophenolate-based product developed Myfortic® (MPA) is active form Conversion: Cellcept® (MMF) 250 mg = Myfortic® (MPA) 180 mg While diarrhea is common, mycophenolate may rarely cause an illness similar to inflammatory bowel disease

Azathioprine (Imuran®)	Dosing: 1-2 mg/kg PO daily	Associated with more hematological toxicities than mycophenolate Gastrointestinal toxicity • Nausea, vomiting • Anorexia • Hepatotoxicity: increased transaminases, bilirubin, alkaline phosphatase Hematologic side effects • Leukopenia, anemia, thrombocytopenia	Older anti-proliferative agent used for maintenance therapy Rarely used due to increased rates of acute rejection vs. mycophenolate Disrupts DNA synthesis of de novo and salvage pathways May be used when: • Pregnancy is desired • Intolerable adverse effects with mycophenolate • Cost is an issue – approximately $40/month vs. $70–1000/month with mycophenolate • Patient has IBD (inflammatory bowel disease) or AIH (auto-immune hepatitis)

(continued)

Table 3.3 (continued)

	Immunosuppressant	Dosing monitoring	Pharmacokinetics: half-life ($t_{1/2}$) bioavailability (F)	Adverse effects	Comments
Corticosteroids	Prednisone, methylprednisolone	Dosing: Varies by organ transplanted and transplant center protocol Maintenance dosing is usually tapered to prednisone 5 mg daily or every other day		Short term (high dose) side effects: • Emotional lability, hallucinations • Insomnia • Heartburn, gastrointestinal bleeding • Hypertension • Hyperglycemia • Fluid retention • Facial swelling (moon facies) • Blurred vision Long term (low dose) side effects: • Muscle/joint weakness • Hyperglycemia • Weight gain (increased appetite) • Osteoporosis • Thinning of the skin • Rounded shoulders • Cataracts • Hypercholesterolemia • Acne	Tapering too quickly may lead to flare of underlying condition, or precipitate an episode of rejection Some centers will use steroid-free maintenance regimens in select patients, typically only in liver transplantation and less commonly kidney transplantation For select patients at high risk of adverse outcomes with any antibody induction, an induction using only corticosteroids may be used

| mTOR inhibitors | Sirolimus (Rapamune®) | Dosing: 1–5 mg PO daily

Monitoring: target levels 5–15 ng/mL (trough) | $t_{1/2}$ = 60 hours (113 hours in hepatic impairment) | Nephrotoxicity

Endocrine/metabolic
• Hypertriglyceridemia (45–57%)
• Hypercholesterolemia (20–46%)
• Posttransplant diabetes

Miscellaneous
• Delayed wound healing (inhibits smooth muscle proliferation)
• Mouth ulcers
• Rash
• Acne

Hematologic
• Leukopenia, anemia, thrombocytopenia
• HUS/thrombotic microangiopathy

Respiratory
• Pneumonitis
• Alveolar hemorrhage
• Pleural effusion

Cardiovascular
• Hypertension

Hepatotoxicity
• Increased transaminases, bilirubin

Gastrointestinal
• Diarrhea

Neuromuscular
• Arthralgia | Contraindicated in pregnancy |

(continued)

Table 3.3 (continued)

Immunosuppressant	Dosing monitoring	Pharmacokinetics: half-life ($t_{1/2}$) bioavailability (F)	Adverse effects	Comments
Everolimus (Afinitor, Zortress®)	Dosing: 0.75–5 mg PO Q12hrs Monitoring: target levels 3–8 ng/mL (trough)	$t_{1/2}$ = 30 hours	Adverse effects similar to sirolimus	Afinitor Disperz® (tablets for suspension) is NOT indicated in transplant recipients

*Drug levels only appropriate to assess adherence; there is no clear relationship between toxicity and exposure:
- Mycophenolic acid (MPA) trough 2–5mcg/mL
- Area under the curve (AUC) 30–60mcg/mL/hr

Monitoring is done via trough levels, which are drawn just prior to the next dose—for example, a patient who takes tacrolimus at 9 am and 9 pm may come to the lab to have blood drawn between 8–9 am (or between 8–9 pm if the laboratory is open). Trough levels correlate reasonably well with the area under the curve (AUC), with total AUC being an accurate measure of drug exposure [9]. Most solid organ transplant recipients are accustomed to knowing that they should be having trough levels drawn. However, if a patient has a non-trough blood level drawn, as might occur in an urgent-care or emergency department visit, then that level may need to be discussed with the transplant team, and likely would need to be redrawn as a trough level.

The frequency of drug level monitoring should be increased following dose adjustments, as well as in the following situations that a primary care provider may encounter (Table 3.4) [9]:

It is best to alert the transplant team when one of these situations occurs if they are not already engaged. While primary care providers may not be making routine dose adjustments, they are frequently involved with changes in interacting drugs, intercurrent illnesses, or changes in nutritional status.

The clinical utility of concentration monitoring for mycophenolate has been questioned as studies have uncovered conflicting results. There is no high level evidence of a strong association between troughs and outcome or between troughs and AUC; therefore, it is not very informative for adjusting doses or predicting toxicity [9]. Occasionally, providers will obtain mycophenolate levels to assess adherence due to unexpected acute rejection, validate dose reduction due to adverse gastrointestinal side effects, or in case of drug interaction [10].

Adherence can be a significant issue. As discussed previously (see Chap. 2), medication nonadherence has been reported in 7–36% of transplant recipients, with increased rates in younger kidney transplant recipients [11, 12]. Patients who are poorly adherent to immunosuppressive medications are more likely to experience graft failure or rejection, and if nonadherence is not discovered, they are at risk of further harm by changes in their immunosuppressive treatment that may not have been necessary if their doctor had known [3, 5]. Being aware of common side effects (see Table 3.3) can guide primary care providers in knowing what questions to ask.

Table 3.4 Indications to increase drug level monitoring in solid organ transplant recipients

Suspected adverse events or rejection
Deteriorating graft function
Route of administration or formulation changes
Discontinuation or addition of drugs known to interact with immunosuppressants
If the patient acquires a severe illness such as sepsis that may affect drug absorption/elimination
If nonadherence is suspected

Drug-related Complications

Immunosuppressive medications can cause complications from both direct side effects (renal insufficiency, diabetes, cardiovascular disease, and others as discussed in Chap. 11) as well as persistently low immune defenses (infections and malignancies) [13]. Specific drug-related complications and adverse effects are outlined in Table 3.3.

Infection is a common cause of morbidity and mortality among patients receiving immunosuppression. It is the second cause of death after cardiovascular disease. The risk of infection following transplantation depends on the recipient's degree of immunosuppression, epidemiologic exposures, and consequences of invasive procedures (see Chap. 8) [14].

The risk of malignancy is two- to fourfold higher in transplant recipients than age-, sex-, and race- matched individuals from similar geographic areas. Not only are cancers common, but they tend to be more aggressive and are associated with increased mortality among transplant recipients than in the general population [15]. (See Chap. 10).

The incidence of cancer is highest for malignancies related to viral infections, including non-Hodgkin lymphoma (Epstein-Barr virus), Kaposi sarcoma (human herpesvirus 8), liver (hepatitis B and hepatitis C viruses), and anogenital cancers (human papilloma virus). The increased risk of these cancers is related to impaired immune control of these oncogenic viruses [14]. Azathioprine and cyclosporine also directly enhance the carcinogenic effects of ultraviolet (UV) radiation via inhibiting DNA repair resulting in apoptosis of keratinocytes [15].

Drug Interactions [16, 17]

Interactions affecting drug metabolism are common in solid organ transplant recipients and typically involve specific elements of the cytochrome P-450 enzyme system (CYP) as well as P-glycoprotein (Pg-p). The combination of immunosuppressive drugs, which have a narrow therapeutic index, with medications for the treatment of common comorbidities such as dyslipidemia, infection, psychiatric conditions, and hypertension, can lead to life-threatening drug interactions. It is critical for primary care providers to understand these interactions, their impact on patient care, and management strategies [14]. A summary of common drug interactions is listed in Table 3.5.

Pregnancy and Breast-Feeding

Pregnancy is generally discouraged in the first year after transplantation, and afterward may be considered in select patients. Immunosuppression may need to be adjusted during pregnancy. The primary care provider should discuss the desire for

Table 3.5 Common drug interactions to consider in solid organ transplant recipients

Immunosuppressant	Interacting drug(s)	Mechanism	Consequences/management
Cyclosporine, tacrolimus, sirolimus, everolimus	*Antifungals:*		
	Ketoconazole	Inhibition of CYP3A4	↑ immunosuppressant levels, replacement of ketoconazole for other azole derivatives
	Fluconazole, voriconazole, itraconazole, clotrimazole	Inhibition of CYP3A4	Dose reduction of immunosuppressant is necessary; voriconazole – sirolimus combination is *contraindicated* (if must be used, 50–90% dose reduction of sirolimus and close monitoring)
	Antibiotics:		
	Clarithromycin, erythromycin, azithromycin	Inhibition of CYP3A4 QT prolongation	↑ immunosuppressant levels, additive risk for QT prolongation (assess baseline ECG, monitor routinely if antibiotic course is prolonged)
			Note: CYP3A4 inhibition is a more significant risk with clarithromycin and erythromycin and these are generally avoided
			QT prolongation is a more significant risk with azithromycin and may be used with caution if necessary
	Trimethoprim/sulfamethoxazole	Hyperkalemia	Additive risk for hyperkalemia (monitor closely)
	Rifampin	Induction of CYP3A4	↓ immunosuppressant levels

(continued)

Table 3.5 (continued)

Immunosuppressant	Interacting drug(s)	Mechanism	Consequences/management
	Fluoroquinolones	QT prolongation	Additive risk for QT prolongation (assess baseline EKG, monitor routinely if antibiotic course is prolonged)
	Antiviral agents:		
	Ritonavir	Inhibition of CYP3A4	↑ immunosuppressant levels
	Lipid lowering agents:		
	simvastatin, lovastatin	Increased statin exposure by calcineurin inhibitors, especially cyclosporine (inhibits CYP3A4)	↑ risk of myopathy and rhabdomyolysis Pravastatin or rosuvastatin are preferred, although other statins have been used successfully. If other statins considered, reduce dose to 50% *prior* to starting immunosuppressive medication and monitor for myopathy if uptitration required; discuss with transplant team (Note: all heart transplant recipients receive statin therapy) (see Chap. 11)
	Antihypertensive agents:		
	ACE-I/ARB	Nephrotoxicity	Additive risk for nephrotoxicity in combination with immunosuppression (Practices vary: dihydropyridine calcium channel blockers such as amlodipine, and sometimes beta blockers, are often used initially after transplant. In a stable patient, >3–6 months after transplantation, ACE-I and ARB may be used with careful monitoring of potassium and renal function)
	Diltiazem, verapamil	Inhibition of CYP3A4, formation of metabolic intermediate complex	↑ immunosuppressant levels; verapamil-sirolimus combination is associated with increased blood levels of verapamil
	Nifedipine	Inhibition of CYP3A4	↑ immunosuppressant levels

Drug	Mechanism	Notes
Carvedilol		↑ absorption of oral cyclosporine
Psychiatric medications:		
Carbamazepine, valproic acid	Induction of CYP3A4	↓ immunosuppressant levels
Selective serotonin reuptake inhibitors (SSRIs)	Inhibition of CYP3A4	↑ tacrolimus/cyclosporine levels
		Sertraline and escitalopram generally preferred due to fewer drug interactions
		Fluvoxamine *contraindicated* with tacrolimus/cyclosporine
		Citalopram may cause QT prolongation, should be used with caution; consider QTc monitoring
		Fluoxetine should be avoided; if necessary should consult with transplant team
		Note: SNRIs, mirtazapine, and bupropion generally acceptable with regard to drug interactions
Anti-gout medications:		
Colchicine	Unclear mechanism, possible inhibition of colchicine transport by Pg-p and/or inhibition of colchicine metabolism by CYP3A4	May increase colchicine levels; avoid use if possible
		After the immediate posttransplant period, short courses of colchicine can sometimes be used in patients for the treatment of acute gout if no other options
Herbal and natural products:		
St. John's wort	Induction of CYP3A4	↓ immunosuppressant levels
Grapefruit, pomelo, pomegranate, star fruit	Inhibition of CYP3A4	↑ immunosuppressant levels

(continued)

Table 3.5 (continued)

Immunosuppressant	Interacting drug(s)	Mechanism	Consequences/management
	Proton-pump inhibitors:		
	Omeprazole, lansoprazole, rabeprazole		Inhibition of CYP2C19. However, magnitude and clinical severity of interaction appear to be dependent on an individual patient's CYP2C19 and/or CYP3A5 genotypes	May increase immunosuppressant levels, but often tolerated in practice Patients with loss-of-function CYP2C19 and CYP3A5 genotypes at higher risk for more severe PPI-tacrolimus interaction
	NSAIDS:		
	Ibuprofen, naproxen, full dose aspirin		Nephrotoxicity	Additive risk for nephrotoxicity in combination with immunosuppression (avoid if possible, use acetaminophen)
Azathioprine	Allopurinol		Inhibition of xanthine oxidase	Life-threatening myelotoxicity (bone marrow suppression)
Mycophenolate	Cholestyramine		Inhibition of enterohepatic circulation	↓ mycophenolate levels
	Antiviral agents:		
	ganciclovir valganciclovir		Mycophenolate-glucuronide inhibits renal tubular secretion of ganciclovir	↑ ganciclovir/valganciclovir levels, ↑ risk of toxicity (nephrotoxicity, neutropenia, leukopenia)
Prednisone methylprednisolone	*Antifungals:*		
	ketoconazole, fluconazole, voriconazole, itraconazole		Inhibition of CYP3A4	↑ corticosteroid levels
	Antibiotics:		
	rifampin		Induction of CYP3A4	↓ corticosteroid levels
	Antiviral agents:		
	ritonavir		Inhibition of CYP3A4	↑ corticosteroid levels

pregnancy with solid organ transplant recipients who have a uterus and are of child-bearing age, especially if they are taking mycophenolate or mTOR inhibitors, both of which are contraindicated during pregnancy. In almost all cases, the patient should be referred back to their transplant specialist as well as an obstetric specialist (e.g., maternal-fetal-medicine or high-risk obstetrics specialist) who has experience with the transplant population. Often immunosuppressive drug levels are checked more frequently during pregnancy.

Breast-feeding cautions are similar to those during pregnancy, with mycophenolate and mTOR inhibitors generally avoided. Patients should work closely with their transplant team, as well as obstetrics and pediatrics. (Contraception is discussed in Chap. 12.)

Pearls for the Primary Care Provider

For the primary care provider who takes care of solid organ transplant recipients, the most important medications to be familiar with are tacrolimus, mycophenolate, and prednisone, as these comprise the most common immunosuppression regimen. At each clinic visit, adherence should be assessed in a nonjudgmental fashion, with recognition that pill burden and side effects may be factors in how consistently patients take their medications. Laboratory studies may be done at a different location, and the primary care provider may need to start exchanging information with the transplant specialist. It is useful to review the transplant specialist's documentation for what trough levels of medications are targeted, as patients do not always know. As primary care providers work more with this patient population, they will build relationships with the transplant team—these bridges are essential for when they need to communicate. New medications should be checked for drug interactions with the anti-rejection medications using available databases. If there is uncertainty, then it is advisable to contact the patient's transplant specialist. In larger centers, a transplant pharmacist may be available to field questions. Table 3.6 shows recommendations for medication assessment at outpatient visits.

Table 3.6 Checklist for assessing medication use outpatient clinic visits for solid organ transplant recipients

Ask about:
☐ Adherence ("how often do you miss a dose of ___?")
☐ Side effects (know and ask about common side effects)
☐ Supplements and prescriptions from other providers
Review:
☐ Transplant team's lab monitoring schedule, goal trough levels
☐ Potential drug interactions before starting any new medications

Conclusion

Success of a transplanted organ depends on many factors and can be enhanced under the care of an attentive primary care provider as well as with an adherent patient. Primary care clinicians can play a pivotal role in supporting the immuno-suppressive medication regimen by simplifying nontransplant medications, creating a psychologically safe atmosphere, and providing appropriate follow-up based on the patient's medical literacy [18, 19, 20]. Communication around medical prescribing between the primary care physician and transplant team is key to better patient outcomes and quality of life [20].

References

1. Halloran P. Immunosuppressive drugs for kidney transplantation. N Engl J Med. 2004;351:1215–29.
2. Enderby C. An overview of immunosuppression in solid organ transplantation. Am J Manag Care. 2015;21:S12–23.
3. Wiesner RH, Fung JJ. Present state of immunosuppressive therapy in liver transplant recipients. Liver Transpl. 2011;17(suppl 3):S1–9.
4. Mahmud N, Klipa D, Ahsan N. Antibody immunosuppressive therapy in solid-organ transplant: Part I. MAbs. 2010;2(2):148–56.
5. OPTN/SRTR 2018 Annual Data Report. Accessed online January 29, 2020 at: https://srtr.transplant.hrsa.gov/annual_reports/2018_ADR_Preview.aspx4.
6. Madariaga M, Kreisel D, Madsen J. Organ-specific differences in achieving tolerance. Curr Opin Organ Transplant. 2015;20(4):392–9. https://doi.org/10.1097/MOT.0000000000000206.
7. Moini M, Schilsky ML, Tichy EM. Review on immunosuppression in liver transplantation. World J Hepatol. 2015;7(10):1355–68. https://doi.org/10.4254/wjh.v7.i10.1355.
8. Mika A, Stepnowski P. Current methods of the analysis of immunosuppressive agents in clinical materials: a review. J Pharm Biomed Anal. 2016;127:207–31.
9. Christians U, Pokaiyavanichkul T, Tacrolimus CL. In: Burton ME, Shaw LM, Schentag JJ, Evans WE, editors. Applied pharmacokinetics and pharmacodynamics: principles of therapeutic drug monitoring. 4th ed. Philadelphia: Lippincott Williams & Wilkins; 2006. p. 563–94.
10. Nawrocki A, Korecka M, Solari S, Kang J, Shaw LM. Mycophenolic acid. In: Burton ME, Shaw LM, Schentag JJ, Evans WE, editors. Applied pharmacokinetics and pharmacodynamics: principles of therapeutic drug monitoring. 4th ed. Philadelphia: Lippincott Williams & Wilkins; 2006. p. 563–94.
11. Foster BJ, Dahhou M, Zhang X, Platt RW, Samuel SM, Hanley JA. Association between age and graft failure rates in young kidney transplant recipients. Transplantation. 2011;92(11):1237–43. https://doi.org/10.1097/TP.0b013e31823411d7.
12. Dew MA, DiMartini AF, De Vito Dabbs A, et al. Rates and risk factors for nonadherence to the medical regimen after adult solid organ transplantation. Transplantation. 2007;83(7):858–73. https://doi.org/10.1097/01.tp.0000258599.65257.a6.
13. Girlanda R. Complications of post-transplant immunosuppression. In: Andrades JA, editors. Regenerative medicine and tissue engineering. Chapter 33. InTech Open. 2013. dx.doi.org/10.5772/55614
14. Veroux M. Infective complications in renal allograft recipients: epidemiology and outcome. Transplant Proc. 2008;40:1873–6.

15. Doshi M. Cancer in solid organ transplantation, Chapter 16. Onco-nephrology curriculum. American Society of Nephrology. 2016
16. Manitpisitkul W. Drug interactions in transplant patients: what everyone should know. Curr Opin Nephrol Hypertens. 2009;18:404–11.
17. Monostory K. Metabolic drug interactions with immunosuppressants. In: Rsoulfas G, editor. Organ donation and transplantation: current status and future challenges. Chapter 20. London: IntechOpen; 2018. https://doi.org/10.5772/intechopen.74524.
18. Martin LR, Williams SL, Haskard KB, DiMatteo MR. The challenge of patient adherence. Ther Clin Risk Manag. 2005;1:189–99.
19. McCashland TM. Posttransplantation care: role of the primary care physician versus transplant center. Liver Transpl. 2001;7(Suppl 1):S2–12.
20. Hughes L. The transplant patient and transplant medicine in family practice. J Family Med Prim Care. 2014;3(4):345–54. https://doi.org/10.4103/2249-4863.148106.

Chapter 4
Primary Care of the Adult Kidney Transplant and Kidney-Pancreas Transplant Recipient

Cary H. Paine and Iris C. De Castro

Kidney Transplant Recipients

Introduction

The existence of dialysis as a widely available treatment for end-stage renal disease (ESRD) makes kidney failure unique when compared to other types of solid organ failure. Although significant advancements have been made in recent years with respect to mechanical support devices for heart failure, and to a lesser extent liver failure, these treatments pale in comparison to dialysis as a form of treatment for end-stage organ failure.

Still, dialysis is clearly not enough. While mortality trends for patients on dialysis have improved over time, with data varying by country, mode and intensity of dialysis, and patient age and comorbidities, still the overall mortality remains high. In the United States in 2010, overall 5-year survival for patients on hemodialysis was 42% [1]. In sharp contrast, the 5-year mortality with kidney transplantation is considerably better, and as such, transplantation is considered the treatment of choice for all suitable candidates with ESRD [2–4]. Furthermore, transplantation is endorsed by the Kidney Diseases Improving Global Outcomes (KDIGO) working group, and, in the United States, the Centers for Medicare and Medicaid Services is considering referral for transplantation as a quality metric [5, 6].

The first successful transplantation of a kidney from one human to another was performed in 1954 by Joseph E. Murray at the Peter Bent Brigham Hospital in Boston, MA. The left kidney was surgically removed from 23-year-old Ronald Herrick and implanted in his identical twin brother, Richard Herrick, who was suffering from kidney failure. Upon completion of the surgical anastomosis, the

C. H. Paine (✉) · I. C. De Castro
Department of Medicine, Division of Nephrology, University of Washington, Seattle, WA, USA
e-mail: chpaine@uw.edu; icastro@uw.edu

© Springer Nature Switzerland AG 2020
C. J. Wong (ed.), *Primary Care of the Solid Organ Transplant Recipient*,
https://doi.org/10.1007/978-3-030-50629-2_4

surgical team "removed the clamps on the vessels and Richard's blood began to flow into his new organ…urine began flowing briskly" [7]. Richard's condition improved dramatically within the first week after surgery and he went on to live for another 9 years with his brother's kidney before dying of a heart attack in 1963.

Since then, more than 450,000 kidney transplants have been performed in the United States. Kidney transplants account for nearly 60% of all solid organ transplantations performed in the last 30 years, and in 2019 alone 23,401 kidney transplants were performed in the United States (based on OPTN data as of January 1, 2020). In a typical year, more than two-thirds of the transplanted kidneys come from deceased donors, with the remainder coming from living donors, either related or unrelated to the recipient. Despite steady annual growth in the number of kidney transplants performed, as of January, 2020, there were 94,663 potential kidney transplant candidates actively listed and awaiting kidney transplant.

The increasing number of kidney transplantations performed, combined with improvements in post-transplant allograft and patient survival, have stretched the available infrastructure at kidney transplant centers, such that the long-term care of kidney transplant recipients has largely shifted to a multidisciplinary team. Accordingly, it is common practice for patients to be followed exclusively by the transplant center for the first 3–6 months after surgery, after which the majority of care is transitioned to the general nephrologist and primary care provider, both of whom will play a critical role in maintaining the function of the kidney allograft and the well-being of the patient in the years that follow. It is therefore essential that primary care providers be familiar with the unique issues and specialized care needs of kidney transplant recipients.

Pre-transplant Course

While this book focuses on the care of solid organ transplant recipients after transplantation, the pre-transplant clinical history is important to review.

- Indication: The optimal timing for kidney transplantation is uncertain. A person must have progressive, irreversible reduction in kidney function to be eligible for kidney transplantation. In the United States, candidates are eligible for kidney transplantation when the eGFR is ≤20 mL/min or when they are receiving chronic dialysis therapy. Often, nephrologists refer patients for pre-transplant evaluation when the eGFR is <30 mL/min especially when there is a clear decline in kidney function. This allows ample time for evaluation and to address relative contraindications. Also, an earlier referral gives the patient the opportunity to receive a transplant prior to needing dialysis.

  The most common causes of ESRD in the United States are diabetes and hypertension, followed by glomerulonephritis, obstructive nephropathy, cystic kidney disease, and other less common etiologies [8]. While it is always preferable to make a specific diagnosis, in some cases, the underlying cause of disease is unknown, as a patient may present to medical care with late stage disease, a diagnostic workup fails to elucidate a cause, or a kidney biopsy cannot be obtained. Unlike most other solid organ transplants, the native kidneys are typically not explanted to yield a pathologic diagnosis. Nevertheless, the original etiology of kidney failure is usually known prior to transplantation and has prognostic significance for the kidney transplant recipient. The underlying diagnosis may cause other organ system involvement (for example, cystic disease can involve the liver), and it may recur in the kidney allograft (for example, C3 Glomerulonephritis, FSGS, IgA Nephropathy, etc.) [9, 10].

- Pre-transplant treatment: Most patients who undergo kidney transplant are receiving treatment with dialysis at the time of transplant, although a small percentage may receive preemptive transplantation prior to dialysis initiation. The following information is helpful to obtain:
  - Pre-transplant dialysis: Both the number of years spent on dialysis prior to transplant and the dialysis modality—hemodialysis or peritoneal dialysis—have prognostic implications as it relates to post-transplant cardiovascular risk and overall mortality [11]. Increased time on dialysis before transplantation is associated with decreased patient and graft survival.
  - Dialysis access: Patients who were previously on hemodialysis may still have vascular access, such as an arteriovenous graft or fistula, which can develop complications over time even when not being used routinely for hemodialysis.
- *Waiting list*: After placement on the waiting list, the average wait time for a deceased donor kidney transplant in the United States is 3.6 years; however, there is considerable variability between different regions of the country [12]. Factors other than geography can also influence wait time, including recipient blood type and immune system sensitization [13]. Wait time for living donor kidney transplantation is typically much less, as it relies solely on the availability of a suitable donor.
  - *Allocation*: For other solid organ transplants, there exists no mechanical support system equivalent to dialysis. Therefore, organ allocation is prioritized based on need (severity of disease). For kidney transplants, however, deceased donors are allocated based primarily on time, such that the more time a potential recipient accrues on the waiting list, the more likely those potential recipients are to be transplanted [14]. This system is designed to favor the principle of equity, recognizing that treatment with dialysis can allow a patient to survive for many years after the onset of organ failure while waiting for a transplant organ.
  - Reducing inequality: In the United States, changes were made to the national kidney allocation system in 2014, in an attempt to address several systemic inequalities in the prior system [15]. Priority is now given to patients with sensitized immune systems for whom it can be difficult to find a suitable donor match. This has led to substantial improvements in rates of transplantations for highly sensitized individuals [16]. As late referral to a nephrologist is associated with reduced access to kidney transplantation [17], the new system now retroactively gives waitlist credit for time spent on dialysis prior to transplant referral, which has helped to improve transplant rates for ethnic

minorities that have traditionally had decreased access to care and decreased rates of timely transplant referral [18].

- Longevity matching: Not every donated kidney has the same projected longevity. In order to allocate kidneys deemed to be of higher quality to recipients with the longest post-transplant life expectancy, every donor is assigned a Kidney Donor Profile Index (KDPI) score which attempts to quantify how long an organ from that donor is expected to function, and, similarly, each recipient is assigned an Estimated Post-Transplant Survival (EPTS) score.

Anatomy

- Location: Kidney transplantation is a heterotopic procedure in which the native kidneys are left in place and the kidney allograft is placed in the extraperitoneal iliac fossa (see Fig. 4.1)
- Anastomoses: In the conventional approach, a curvilinear incision is made in the right or left lower quadrant of the recipient and the iliac vessels are exposed. The right

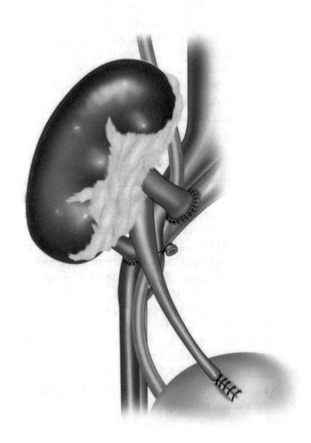

Fig. 4.1 Kidney transplant anastomoses. Shown is the end-to-side anastomosis of the donor renal vein to the recipient iliac vein or its branch (blue), the donor renal artery to the recipient iliac artery or its branch (red). (The external iliac vein and artery is commonly used; anastomoses may vary depending on a patient's anatomy.) The donor ureter is implanted into the bladder (brown). (From Forsyth, reprinted with permission [19])

side is often preferred because the right iliac vessels are more superficial and thus more easily accessed. End-to-side anastomoses are performed between the donor renal vein and the recipient's external iliac vein, followed by the donor renal artery and the recipient's external iliac artery. Less commonly, the surgeon may perform an end-to-side anastomosis between the donor renal artery and the recipient's common iliac artery, or an end-to-end anastomosis with to the recipient's internal iliac artery. The ureter is then implanted to the bladder. Although practice varies, many centers place a double-J ureteral stent to reduce pressure on the ureteral anastomosis in the early post-operative period, and then retrieve it 2–4 weeks after surgery.

- Occasionally, as in instances in which the allograft is too large to be easily placed in the pelvis, the kidney may be implanted intraperitoneally.

  Recipient nephrectomy is rarely performed but can be considered in cases of severe uncontrolled hypertension, large symptomatic polycystic kidneys, or recurrent kidney infections.
- A transplant from a deceased donor may include an aortic patch along with the renal artery—this longer length of donor vasculature can facilitate an easier anastomosis.

Immunosuppression Regimen

Advances in immunosuppression have been associated with improved graft survival and reduced rejection. Figure 4.2 shows 1-year graft survival, rejection within the first year, and introduction of immunosuppression medications over a 45-year period.

Immunosuppression typically occurs in two phases: induction and maintenance.

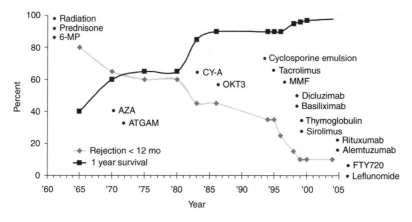

Fig. 4.2 One-year first cadaveric renal allograft survival and rejection episodes over time. "The time that various immunosuppression medications were introduced is indicated by their position on the graph." 6-MP 6 mercaptopurine, ATGAM horse anti thymocyte globulin, AZA azathioprine, CY-A cyclosporine, FTY720 fingolimod, MMF mycophenolate mofetil, OKT3 muromonab-CD. (From Zand et al. [20]. Reprinted with permission)

Induction Immunosuppression

Nearly all kidney transplant recipients require induction immunosuppression to mitigate the risk of acute rejection in the first few months after transplant. The choice of induction regimen considers the recipient's risk for rejection, infection, malignancy, predilection to adverse effects from the induction medication, and the transplant center's preferences. A recipient receiving a two-haplotype match from a living related donor, which confers substantially less risk of rejection, may require less initial immunosuppression.

In general, patients at higher risk for acute rejection tend to be younger, African American, or have an immunologic profile that confers higher than average rejection risk such as higher calculated panel reactive antibody (CPRA) or the presence of pre-formed donor specific antibodies at the time of transplantation (Table 4.1) [21]. The CPRA is based upon unacceptable HLA antigens to which the recipient has been sensitized and which, if present in a donor, would represent an unacceptable risk for the candidate or the transplant program. The CPRA is computed from HLA antigen frequencies among donors in the United States and thus represents the percentage of actual organ donors that express one or more of those unacceptable HLA antigens [22].

For patients at risk for acute rejection, a common practice is to administer lymphocyte-depleting antibody therapy. The most common agent used for induction in the United States is rabbit antithymocyte globulin (rATG). (Of note, rATG has been approved by the Food and Drug Administration only for the treatment of rejection, so although it is widely used for induction immunosuppression, this use is technically off-label.) rATG is created by immunizing rabbits with human thymocytes and then purifying the resultant polyclonal immunoglobulins which, when administered to a human recipient, will target T-cells and cause complement-mediated apoptosis. Protocols differ between centers with respect to dosing; the most conventional approach is to administer three doses: intraoperatively in conjunction with intravenous corticosteroids, followed by subsequent doses on post-operative days. Doses may be reduced or held if there is significant leukopenia, thrombocytopenia, or adverse effect, such as hemodynamic instability, temporarily related to drug administration.

Table 4.1 Possible risk factors for acute rejection [20]

The number of human leukocyte antigen (HLA) mismatches
Younger recipient age
Older donor age
African-American ethnicity (in the United States)
Panel-reactive antibody (PRA) >30%
Presence of a donor-specific antibody
Blood group incompatibility
Delayed onset of graft function
Cold ischemia time > 24 hours

Recipients at lower risk for rejection, or those who cannot receive lymphocyte-depleting therapy due to clinical contraindications such as prohibitive leukopenia, thrombocytopenia, or hypotension, are typically administered induction therapy with non-depleting antibodies. The most common non-lymphocyte depleting drug is basiliximab (Simulect®), an antibody directed against the IL-2 receptor (CD25). Basiliximab is dosed intraoperatively and on post-operative day four.

There is a large and growing body of literature comparing the efficacy of various induction immunosuppression regimens; a full appraisal of these studies is beyond the scope of this chapter. It has been clearly demonstrated that induction with rATG reduces the rate of acute rejection when compared with no induction, but is also associated with higher rates of leukopenia, thrombocytopenia, and CMV infection [23, 24]. IL-2 receptor antagonists have also been shown to be superior to placebo with respect to reducing the risk of acute rejection and allograft failure, but have been associated with a higher incidence of biopsy-proven, subclinical acute rejection when compared to other induction agents [25]. rATG appears to be superior to other forms of induction therapy, including horse-derived antithymocyte globulin (Atgam®), the anti-CD52 humanized, monoclonal antibody alemtuzumab (Campath®), and basiliximab with respect to the risk of acute rejection, particularly in high risk individuals [26–28]. Results are less clear with respect to risk for delayed graft function, long-term allograft survival, and mortality.

Familiarity with what type and dosage of induction immunosuppression is pertinent to primary care practice. While under the primary provider's care, the patient may be treated again with rATG if they develop moderate to severe cellular rejection. Also, it is important to note that the cumulative dose of rATG has been associated with higher incidence of post-transplant lymphoproliferative disorder (PTLD).

Maintenance Immunosuppression

Calcineurin inhibitors have formed the backbone of nearly all maintenance immunosuppression regimens for kidney transplant recipients since the 1980s.

- Most kidney transplant recipients will be treated with a three-drug regimen consisting of a calcineurin inhibitor, an antiproliferative agent such as mycophenolate mofetil, and a corticosteroid. In 2017, the most recent year for which data is available, more than 60% of patients were maintained on the combination of tacrolimus, mycophenolate, and a corticosteroid (Fig. 4.3).
- There has been an increased interest in using calcineurin-free and steroid-free protocols, with significant differences emerging between different transplant centers. The 2009 KDIGO practice guidelines support the use of a three-drug immunosuppressive regimen for most patients, but for patients of low immunological risk who receive induction immunosuppression, it is considered reasonable to consider discontinuation of glucocorticoids after the first week [21]. Programs vary widely in their adoption of such a strategy: in 2017, 30% of patients were maintained on steroid-free protocols with just tacrolimus and mycophenolate (Fig. 4.3).

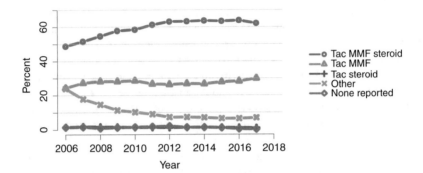

Fig. 4.3 Maintenance immunosuppressive regimens in kidney transplant recipients. Tac = tacrolimus, MMF = mycophenolate mofetil. (From Hart et al. [13]. Reprinted with permission)

- Tacrolimus versus cyclosporine: In the last two decades, tacrolimus has almost completely replaced cyclosporine as the calcineurin inhibitor of choice after kidney transplantation, with 92% of kidney recipients receiving tacrolimus and only 2% cyclosporine [13]. Compared to cyclosporine, the use of tacrolimus confers a significantly lower risk of acute rejection and a modest improvement in the rate of allograft failure at 6 months and all later time points [29–31]. Although tacrolimus is associated with slightly higher rates of side effects, including neurotoxicity, infections, and new onset diabetes after transplant (NODAT), these risks are generally thought to be offset by the superiority of tacrolimus with respect to preservation of allograft function [24]. Occasionally, a patient who experiences intolerable side effects from tacrolimus, such as severe neurotoxicity, may be switched to cyclosporine, although there is relatively little data to support this practice.
- Calcineurin inhibitor dosing: Dosing of tacrolimus or cyclosporine can vary significantly between patients due to genetic differences and the presence of other medications, both of which may affect drug metabolism. In general, tacrolimus is dosed twice daily with serial monitoring of 12-hour trough levels. There is an extended release, once a day preparation available as an alternative. Specific trough targets may vary depending on factors such as the type of induction immunosuppression, the risk of rejection related to the patient's immunophenotype, and the transplant center protocol. A common approach is to target a trough level of 8–10 ng/mL for the first 3 months and then a level of 5–7 ng/mL after 1 year post-transplant.
- Nephrotoxicity: The most common side effect of calcineurin inhibitors that can limit their long-term use is the development of nephrotoxicity in the kidney allograft. Alternate immunosuppression strategies have been proposed to help reduce or completely eliminate exposure to calcineurin inhibitors in select patients. The two most common calcineurin-free approaches involve the use of either mammalian target of rapamycin (mTOR) inhibitors such as sirolimus or everolimus, or belatacept, a selective blocker of T-cell co-stimulation. Although some centers use these agents as first-line components in their maintenance

immunosuppression regimens, the use of mTOR inhibitors as initial agents is generally discouraged, as it has been associated with increased rates of delayed graft function and poor wound healing [32]. Similarly, early use of belatacept has been associated with an increased rate of acute rejection within the first year, but a substantially higher eGFR thereafter [33, 34]. As such, the most common strategy is to start with a calcineurin inhibitor-based regimen and switch to an alternate agent if nephrotoxicity develops.

Table 4.2 summarizes common immunosuppression regimens in kidney transplant recipients. Protocols vary by transplant center and patient factors. For a general overview of anti-rejection medications, see Chap. 3.

Graft Function Surveillance

The typical approach to monitoring the function of the kidney allograft varies depending on the amount of time since transplant and the stability of allograft function.

- Immediate post-transplant period: While primary care providers are not likely to be involved in the patient's care, it is helpful to review the transplant records. In the first week following transplantation, kidney transplant recipients are monitored in the hospital, with daily measurement of the serum creatinine and quantification of the urine output, taking into consideration any residual pre-transplant urine production. *Immediate graft function* is defined as not requiring dialysis post-transplant, while *delayed graft function (DGF)* is defined as the need for dialysis within 1 week following transplant, excluding those patients that require a single dialysis procedure for acute hyperkalemia. Risk factors for DGF include increasing donor age and KDPI, male sex, increasing cold ischemia time, and

Table 4.2 Examples of immunosuppression regimens in kidney transplant recipients

Induction immunosuppression	Maintenance immunosuppression
Standard or high rejection risk:	Standard:
Rabbit antithymocyte globulin (rATG) + intravenous corticosteroids	Calcineurin inhibitor (tacrolimus or cyclosporine)
	Anti-metabolite (mycophenolate or azathioprine)
	Corticosteroid (prednisone)
OR	Others:
Alemtuzumab (Campath) + intravenous corticosteroids	Steroid-free[a]
	Calcineurin inhibitor (tacrolimus or cyclosporine)
	Anti-metabolite (mycophenolate or azathioprine)
Low rejection risk or unable to receive rATG:	Calcineurin-free[a]
Basiliximab (Simulect®) + intravenous corticosteroids	Mammalian target of rapamycin inhibitors (MTORi) (sirolimus or everolimus)
	Antimetabolite (mycophenolate or azathioprine OR
	Belatacept + mycophenolate + prednisone

[a]May have increased risk of rejection compared to other regimens

receipt of a deceased donor transplant as compared to an allograft from a living donor [13, 35, 36].

- First weeks to months post-transplant: After hospital discharge, in the first weeks to months post-transplant, the serum creatinine is monitored serially, usually once or twice per week, and is expected to decrease in the setting of a properly functioning allograft until it reaches steady state, at which time the post-transplant baseline creatinine is established. Some patients will never reach a "normal" post-transplant serum creatinine—the nadir will depend on such variables as the overall quality of the donor organ as well as donor-recipient size mismatch (a kidney from a smaller donor will yield a higher baseline creatinine when implanted in a larger recipient). During this time the recipient's urine is monitored for the presence of blood, which is expected initially but should resolve in the weeks following removal of the double-J ureteral stent, and proteinuria. The early onset of proteinuria, particularly when it is progressive in patients with a history of an underlying glomerular disease such as FSGS, can indicate recurrence of primary disease or de novo glomerular disease and should prompt further workup.

- Six months post-transplant and beyond: As time from transplant increases beyond 6 months, the need for regular surveillance of allograft function persists; however, the frequency of laboratory testing will decrease. It is in this period that the care of kidney transplant recipients is transitioned to the general nephrologist and the primary care physician. Although protocols vary by center and depending on specific patient variables, a typical kidney transplant recipient will require monthly testing of serum creatinine, electrolytes, complete blood counts, urinalysis, urine protein quantification, and immunosuppressive drug levels for at least the first 2 years and then not less than every 3 months thereafter. Primary care providers should be comfortable interpreting the results of these tests and should partner with transplant specialists when an abnormality triggers the need for further testing.

- Clinical evaluation: In addition to routine laboratory testing, patients should be seen and examined regularly, as many risk factors for allograft dysfunction and other post-transplant complications have easily identifiable manifestations on physical examination. As is the case with laboratory monitoring, if a patient is doing well the frequency of in-person follow-up visits may decrease as time from surgery increases, with most long-term follow-up patients requiring in-person visits approximately once every 3 months (Table 4.3). Close attention should be paid to assessment of peripheral volume status, including weight, as both volume excess and depletion may cause allograft dysfunction. Patients should be monitored for physical signs of medication toxicity, such as the development of tremor with calcineurin inhibitors, as there is often an association between the development of neurotoxicity and the incidence of nephrotoxicity [37]. Blood pressure should be monitored at every visit and patients should also be encouraged to measure blood pressure at home. Daily home blood pressure monitoring is standard practice in most programs for at least the first 3 months after transplant [38]. Patients may additionally be encouraged to continue monitoring home blood

Table 4.3 Suggested frequency of monitoring for stable kidney transplant recipients[a]	Time after transplant	Lab and immunosuppression monitoring frequency	Clinic visit frequency
	0–4 weeks	1–2 per week	1–2 per week
	4–12 weeks	Every 1 week	Every 1–2 weeks
	3–6 months	Every 2–4 weeks	Every 1–2 months
	6–12 months	Every 2–4 weeks	Every 2–4 months
	>1 year	Every 1–3 months	Every 3–6 months

[a]Protocols may vary by transplant center

pressure indefinitely at a frequency determined by the patient and the transplant center.

- Immune surveillance: Some transplant programs incorporate routine post-transplant immune surveillance in addition to general monitoring of allograft function. Historically, it was common to perform protocol-driven kidney biopsies. While some programs continue this practice, it is becoming less common as less invasive methods of surveillance are developed, shifting the risk/benefit ratio.
  - Donor-specific antibodies (DSA): The serial measurement of donor-specific antibodies has become increasingly popular as support for protocol biopsies has waned [39]. This is a semi-quantitative test that monitors the recipient's serum for presence and level of antibodies against donor HLA. Flow cytometry using microparticles ("beads") coated with recombinant or soluble HLA antigens representative of the donor HLA are used. Measurement of donor-specific antibodies for patients with apparently normal allograft function may allow for earlier detection of otherwise silent immunological phenomena and, when positive, may provide pre-clinical evidence of an allograft that is at risk for developing overt, clinical antibody-mediated rejection. By definition this type of protocol-driven testing is performed for all patients, even those with normal allograft function and is fundamentally different from testing that is done "for cause," as in the setting of worsening allograft function, at which time further specialized testing is strongly indicated regardless of surveillance protocol. Although primary care providers are not typically the ones ordering these more specialized tests, generalists should become familiar with the specific transplant center surveillance protocols.
  - Biopsies: Common indications for renal allograft biopsy are increasing creatinine and increasing proteinuria. Risk of performing kidney allograft biopsies has diminished over recent years, with the routine use of smaller gauge biopsy needles and ultrasound guidance for the biopsy procedure. The allograft kidney is located closer to the body surface than the native kidney, making localization of the organ for biopsy more straightforward than for native kidney [40]. Protocol biopsies, as opposed to "for cause" biopsies, are used by several centers for research purposes, in highly sensitized patients, and in patients on steroid- or CNI-free maintenance regimens. The purpose of protocol biopsies is to identify patients with subclinical rejection (SCR) and chronic allograft nephropathy (CAN) for whom treatment or immunosuppression adjustment may result

in improved allograft survival. Subclinical rejection is when there are histologic signs of rejection without overt clinical signs of allograft dysfunction such as increased creatinine or proteinuria. With newer and almost uniform use of induction immunosuppression, the incidence of subclinical rejection has declined. Protocol biopsies have not been shown to improve long-term graft function and the benefits of treating SCR detected by protocol biopsy in particular are not clear-cut [41]. Moreover, the optimal timing of protocol biopsies and reliable methods to quantify the histologic changes observed in biopsy specimens have yet to be determined. The cost, risk, and patient inconvenience of surveillance biopsies must be weighed against potential gains from early interventions guided by the findings [42].

Allograft Dysfunction

The differential diagnosis for kidney allograft dysfunction, which is typically evidenced by an increase in the serum creatinine or increase in proteinuria, is quite broad and influenced by the time since transplant. Just as with native kidneys, kidney allograft dysfunction can be characterized as acute or chronic and can range from mild to severe. It is important to remember that kidney transplant recipients remain at risk for all of the common medical conditions to which native kidneys are susceptible, including ischemic acute tubular necrosis and prerenal azotemia from intravascular volume depletion, as well as more specific causes of kidney allograft dysfunction such as surgical complications and rejection. Indeed, as patient and allograft survival continue to improve, transplant recipients are at increased risk of developing chronic allograft dysfunction due to common causes such as diabetic kidney disease and hypertension-related kidney disease [43].

Surgical Complications

Most surgical complications are diagnosed early in the post-transplant course and thus may not come to the attention of primary providers. Still, it is important to have some knowledge of specific complications that a patient has experienced, as there may be implications for the likelihood of developing downstream complications later on.

- Lymphoceles: At the time of transplantation, the recipient undergoes extensive dissection of the lymphatic network surrounding the iliac vessels. This can lead to the leakage of lymph and the formation of lymphoceles in approximately 5–15% of patients [44]. Lymphoceles often resolve without intervention, although sometimes will persist and may require drainage if there is compression of local structures including the ureter or the renal vein. Uncommonly, patients may develop chronic lymphedema after kidney transplant, thought to be related to impaired lymphangiogenesis. Several case reports have suggested that this may be more common in patients treated with mTOR inhibitors [45].

- Urine leak: Early urine leak is not uncommon, occurring in approximately 1–3% of kidney transplants [46]. Urine leak is usually diagnosed when serum creatinine fails to improve, and there is high post-operative output from the surgical drains adjacent to the kidney. Diagnosis can be made by measuring the creatinine level in the drain fluid; if the drain fluid contains urine, then the creatinine level will be considerably higher than the creatinine level measured in the serum. Urine leaks are commonly addressed with either ureteral stenting or surgical revision, and patients requiring more complicated revision may be at risk for future complications such as stenosis at the site of the ureteral anastomosis.
- Vascular: Vascular complications such as anastomotic stricture are one of the few anatomical complications that can develop many years after transplantation. As with native kidney renal artery stenosis, stenosis in the transplant renal artery can be associated with worsening hypertension and fluid retention with an exaggerated sensitivity to medications that interfere with the renin-angiotensin-aldosterone system, such as ACE inhibitors and angiotensin receptor blockers [47]. A bruit is sometimes present; however, the absence of a bruit does not rule out stenosis and the presence of worsening hypertension in a kidney transplant recipient should prompt further investigation including duplex ultrasonography of the transplanted kidney vasculature and consultation with the nephrologist involved with the patient's care.

Acute Rejection

As with many issues related to kidney transplantation, the type of rejection to which a kidney allograft is most susceptible depends on the time since transplantation.

- *Hyperacute rejection* is caused by preformed donor-specific antibodies, as in the case of an ABO incompatible donor. It presents immediately within the first hours after transplantation. This complication is relatively rare in the modern era of transplantation, as preformed antibodies will be routinely detected by the complement-dependent cytotoxicity (CDC) crossmatch, and a positive crossmatch is considered a contraindication to transplant.
- *Acute rejection* tends to present in the first weeks to months after transplantation, but it can also occur years after transplant especially when patients are not compliant with their immunosuppression regimen or new medications have resulted in sub therapeutic levels of immunosuppression. Acute rejection may be cellular—caused by the activation and proliferation of T-cells, antibody mediated—caused by the development of antibodies against donor HLA antigens, or both. Acute rejection may present with decreased urine output, allograft tenderness, or fever. However, in the era of modern immunosuppression, most episodes of acute rejection are asymptomatic and are identified only after an increase in the serum creatinine is observed. Creatinine elevation is generally thought to be a late marker for injury, at which time there is likely already considerable histological

injury—hence the move towards earlier detection strategies such as DSA monitoring protocols discussed above.

When there is suspicion for acute rejection—for example, an acute rise in the creatinine is found—the transplant team should be contacted urgently to discuss arranging a kidney biopsy. Standardized histological definitions for acute cellular and antibody-mediated rejection have been established by the Banff consortium [48, 49]. In general, acute cellular rejection is associated with the presence of inflammation in the renal tubules (tubulitis) and in the renal arteries (arteritis). Antibody-mediated rejection is suggested by the deposition of C4d, a split product in the complement cascade, in the peritubular capillaries, typically in association with donor-specific antibodies.

Treatment of acute rejection depends on the specific type of rejection (cellular vs. antibody-mediated) and the histological severity. Treatment for cellular rejection often mirrors induction immunosuppression, with mild cases receiving pulse doses of corticosteroids and more severe cases necessitating the use of lymphocyte-depleting antibody preparations such as rATG [50–52]. Treatment for antibody-mediated rejection also depends on severity, as determined both by histology and by antibody titers, and tends to target both the existing antibodies and the B-cells responsible for antibody production. Protocols vary between centers but will typically employ a combination of intravenous immunoglobulin (IVIG), anti-CD20 antibodies such as rituximab, and plasmapheresis [53].

Rejection episodes have important clinical and prognostic significance. The development of one episode of acute rejection increases the risk for subsequent rejection episodes. Furthermore, the cumulative effect of additional immunosuppressive agents used to treat rejection can significantly increase the risk of developing short-term infectious complications, as well as long-term complications such as malignancy (see Chaps. 8 and 10).

Chronic Allograft Nephropathy

The most common cause of kidney allograft failure after the first year is a poorly defined and incompletely understood entity that has historically been termed chronic allograft nephropathy, transplant glomerulopathy, or chronic rejection, and more recently has been referred to as chronic allograft injury [54, 55]. As there are no consensus clinical or histopathological criteria for this diagnosis, the exact incidence and pathophysiology remain uncertain. In general, a diagnosis of chronic allograft injury is made when there is allograft dysfunction after the first 3 months post-transplant and no evidence of acute rejection or acute drug-related injury. The histological criteria for diagnosis are complex, and under frequent revision; however, the hallmark of chronic allograft nephropathy is the development of interstitial fibrosis and tubular atrophy (IFTA) which may be graded as mild, moderate, or severe [46].

The mechanisms underlying the development of chronic allograft nephropathy are not fully understood; however, one unifying factor seems to be the presence of chronic inflammation in the allograft leading to progressive IFTA as described above [56]. Some of this inflammation is likely to be immune-mediated, as it has been observed that less well-matched allografts are more likely to develop chronic allograft nephropathy [57]. Moreover, removal of immunosuppression, as in cases of medication nonadherence, has been associated with the accelerated development of chronic allograft nephropathy, underscoring the importance of life-long immunosuppression [58].

Other Complications and Pearls

BK Nephropathy

BK virus, a ubiquitous human polyomavirus, is a unique cause of complications in kidney transplant recipients. Although most humans have been exposed to polyomaviruses, these viruses tend only to cause disease in immunocompromised individuals. In kidney transplant recipients, the following complications may occur:

- BK virus nephropathy (BKVN): BK virus nephropathy is a form of tubulointerstitial nephritis which occurs in the kidney allograft of approximately 5% of kidney transplant recipients [59].
  - Risk factors and pathophysiology: Primary BK virus exposure typically occurs at a young age via respiratory secretions. The virus persists in the renal epithelium and thus post-transplant complications associated with BK virus are thought most likely to be derived from the donor. Although retrospective studies have attempted to find an association with specific immunosuppressive regimens, the most significant risk factor for the development of BKVN appears to be a high degree of immunosuppression, regardless of the particular type or number of agents used [60, 61].
  - Clinical presentation and diagnosis: BKVN typically presents as a slow, progressive increase in the serum creatinine. Definitive diagnosis is made on kidney biopsy which will demonstrate the presence of characteristic histopathologic changes and a positive immunohistochemical stain for the SV40 antigen. A positive SV40 stain is highly specific for polyoma virus nephropathy but is less sensitive, owing to the patchy nature of BKVN and the potential for absent virus on a small sample of kidney tissue [62]. The diagnosis is supported by the presence of BK virus DNA in the urine and in the blood, as detected by quantitative PCR.
  - Screening: The presence of BK viruria and viremia should significantly predate the development of clinically evident BKVN. For this reason, it is common practice at most transplant centers to screen routinely for BK virus in the urine every 3–6 months during the first 2 years after transplant. When BK

viruria is detected in the setting of normal allograft function, it may prompt further testing for BK viremia, and/or preemptive reduction in immunosuppression.

- Treatment: When BKVN nephropathy is diagnosed, the mainstay of treatment is reduction in immunosuppression. Antiviral therapies such as leflunomide or cidofovir are sometimes used for persistent cases, although data is lacking and largely anecdotal [63].
- There are infrequent case reports of immunocompromised individuals developing BKVN in the native kidney—this evaluation may be challenging and is best left to the managing nephrologist [64].
- Ureteral stenosis is a relatively rare complication associated with BK virus. It can present with hematuria and hydronephrosis with or without increase in serum creatinine.

Cardiovascular Disease

When compared to the treatment of patients with ESRD with dialysis, kidney transplantation is associated with a significant decrease in the incidence of cardiovascular events. However, cardiovascular disease remains the leading cause of morbidity and mortality in kidney transplant recipients [65]. This risk is due in part to the prevalence of cardiovascular disease and comorbidities such as diabetes within the ESRD population, as well as exacerbation of risk factors such as hypertension and dyslipidemia by immunosuppressive medications. Furthermore, several studies have demonstrated significant variability in the rates of cardioprotective medication use among kidney transplant recipients, including angiotensin-converting enzyme (ACE) inhibitors/angiotensin receptor blockers (ARBs), statins, and aspirin [66].

Most kidney transplant recipients should be treated with a statin, regardless of post-transplant lipid levels, although it should be noted that the data to support this recommendation is limited. The only randomized, controlled trial to assess cardiovascular events in post-kidney transplant patients with dyslipidemia is the ALERT trial which randomized patients to receive either fluvastatin or placebo and showed a significant reduction in LDL in the treatment group, and a trend towards reduction of cardiovascular events that failed to reach statistical significance [67]. Several subsequent meta-analyses have shown a reduction in cardiovascular mortality with statin use in kidney transplant recipients, but results have been mixed with respect to all-cause mortality [68]. Still, despite the weak supporting evidence, it is the recommendation of the KDIGO work group that all post-kidney transplant patients be treated with statin therapy [69]. The optimal statin choice and dosing strategy is not known, but regardless of agent, it is generally recommended to start with a lower dose than that recommended for the general population in order to reduce the likelihood of adverse events. If the patient is treated with a calcineurin inhibitor (tacrolimus or cyclosporine) and statin therapy is indicated, then pravastatin or rosuvastatin are preferred as they have a lower risk of drug interaction, although other statins have also been used successfully (see Chap. 3).

Hypertension is common after kidney transplant and should be treated aggressively. Risk factors for hypertension include anatomical causes such as renal artery stenosis and the use of calcineurin inhibitors. In the absence of an anatomical lesion, pharmacological treatment should be used to target a blood pressure of less than 130/80 [68]. While the optimal antihypertensive agent is not known, in general the treatment of hypertension in transplant recipients should mirror that in non-transplant recipients, with the first-line agent typically being a dihydropyridine calcium channel blocker such as amlodipine, particularly in the first 6 months. The use of beta blockers for hypertension has fallen out of favor in the most recent American College of Cardiology (ACC)/American Heart Association (AHA) guidelines [70], although their use is still relatively common in kidney transplant recipients, as heightened concerns about side effects from diuretics, ACE inhibitors, or ARBs can limit use of these medications early after transplantation. ACE inhibitors and ARBs should be used cautiously in the early post-transplant period, as they carry some risk of decreased GFR due to renal arteriolar vasoconstriction, as well as hyperkalemia, both of which are exacerbated by calcineurin inhibitor use. However, ACE inhibitors and ARBs are generally well tolerated after 3–6 months post-transplantation and should be strongly considered in patients with proteinuria.

Diabetes

Diabetes is the number one cause of ESRD in the United States. Accordingly, diabetes is highly prevalent in kidney transplant patients. Even those patients without antecedent diabetes are at risk for developing diabetes post-transplant, with estimated rates of New Onset Diabetes After Transplant (NODAT) ranging from 5% to 50% at 1 year post-transplantation, although the incidence appears to be decreasing [13, 71]. NODAT is a distinct entity from the phenomenon of transient, glucocorticoid-associated hyperglycemia in the immediate post-transplant period. The development of NODAT is multifactorial and is associated with traditional risk factors for type 2 diabetes, including obesity and a positive family history of diabetes, as well as unique, transplant-specific risk factors including the use of certain immunosuppressive medications. Beyond glucocorticoids, calcineurin inhibitors have the strongest association with the development of NODAT, with several studies suggesting increased rates of diabetes with tacrolimus as compared with cyclosporine [72]. NODAT is managed similarly to diabetes in the non-transplant population, with a stepwise progression first focused on lifestyle modification followed by oral therapy and then insulin if needed to target a hemoglobin A1C of less than 7%.

Newer medications may be considered with caution as there is relatively less data in the post kidney transplant population.

The Kidney Transplant Recipient Presenting with an Increase in Creatinine

An elevated serum creatinine found on routine surveillance blood tests will likely be managed by the ordering nephrologist. However, there may be other times when an elevated creatinine is obtained on testing at other times, such as urgent care or emergency department visits. When a kidney transplant patient is found to have a creatinine that is elevated over baseline, if the time course is uncertain, then evaluation for typical causes of acute kidney injury is indicated, including assessment for pre-renal, intrinsic renal, and post-renal causes based on history, examination, and laboratory studies, as well as evaluating for infection. Additionally, one should strongly consider early consultation with the transplant nephrologist to determine whether evaluation for rejection is needed.

For a more general discussion of metabolic complications in solid organ transplant recipients, see Chap. 11. For further details pertaining to infectious complications, see Chap. 8.

Clinical pearls for the outpatient evaluation of kidney transplant recipients are shown in Table 4.4.

Table 4.4 *Clinical pearls for the primary care provider—evaluating kidney transplant recipients at outpatient clinic visits* (see text for details; also see Chap. 2 for discussion of general history-taking)

Initial visit:

  Review pre-transplant and initial post-transplant course: Indication for transplant, pre-transplant dialysis, dialysis access (if still present), type of donor, anatomic location of transplant, type of induction immunosuppression

  Creatinine nadir

  Early complications (delayed graft function, surgical complications, infection, rejection)

  Symptoms, exam, medications, laboratory studies similar to follow-up visits

Follow-up visits:

  Symptoms: Urine output, hematuria, pain, symptoms of volume depletion or excess, side effects of medications, symptoms of infection

  Exam: Blood pressure, heart, lung, abdomen exam, volume status

  Medications: Current regimen, adherence, side effects, goal trough levels

  Laboratory and other studies: Adherence to surveillance schedule set forth by the transplant team; surveillance for rejection (biopsy vs. donor-specific antibodies); creatinine, proteinuria, BK virus (if checked)

  Home blood pressure: Review readings (if being followed)

  Metabolic complications: Assess and treat

    If sudden worsening of hypertension, consider renal artery duplex

---

Pancreas Transplant Recipients

Introduction

Although there have been remarkable advancements in the medical treatment of diabetes mellitus in recent years, pancreas transplantation remains the only definitive treatment that allows for restoration of euglycemia without the potential risk of life-threatening hypoglycemia. As such, pancreas transplantation is the treatment of choice for patients with type 1 diabetes mellitus and select patients with insulin-dependent type 2 diabetes mellitus.

The first successful pancreas transplantation was performed in 1966 at the University of Minnesota by Drs. William Kelly and Richard Lillehei as part of a multi-visceral procedure that included the transplantation of a pancreas, duodenum, and kidney from a deceased donor to a patient with type 1 diabetes and diabetic nephropathy [73]. Blood glucose levels in the recipient were noted to decrease almost immediately upon completion of the surgery and the patient went on to live for 3 months before dying of an apparent pulmonary embolism. In the following years, as immunosuppressive strategies have improved, so too has the success of pancreas transplantation, such that in the last three decades there have been more than 32,000 pancreas transplantations performed in the United States based on OPTN data as of January 1, 2020. Interestingly, the number of annual pancreas transplantations in the United States peaked in 2014, with 1483 transplants performed, and then decreased steadily over the ensuing decade. In 2018, the most recent year for which data is available, there were 1015 pancreas transplants performed, with recent data suggesting 85–90% of allografts survive the first year [74].

Pancreas transplant recipients can be categorized as belonging to one of three distinct groups. The first, and largest category, are those patients with insulin-dependent diabetes mellitus and ESRD who receive a simultaneous pancreas-kidney (SPK) transplant from a single deceased donor. SPK transplants accounted for more than 80% of all pancreas transplantations last year. The second group includes those patients with ESRD who have already received a kidney transplant—typically a living donor kidney transplant—who undergo pancreas after kidney (PAK) transplantation. Both SPK and PAK recipients will require life-long immunosuppression for maintenance of the kidney allograft; therefore, the risk associated with the addition of pancreas transplantation is limited primarily to the increased surgical risk. The third group includes patients with relatively preserved kidney function who receive a pancreas transplant alone (PTA). These patients would not otherwise be receiving immunosuppressive therapy and thus there should be serious consideration in weighing the potential benefits of PTA, which include improved quality of life and decreased end-organ complications from diabetes, against the attendant risks inherent in committing an individual to life-long immunosuppression, including increased rates of infection and malignancy [75]. A fourth group of patients should be noted briefly, as isolated pancreatic islet cell transplantation has become a viable treatment option for some patients. However, this procedure remains experimental and must be performed as part of an FDA-approved clinical trial, the details of which are beyond the scope of this chapter.

Benefits of Pancreas Transplantation

There is some debate as to the long-term benefit of pancreas transplantation for treatment of insulin-dependent diabetes mellitus. It is generally agreed upon that SPK transplantation improves quality of life compared with kidney transplantation alone; however, the data regarding mortality is less clear and is limited by ethical considerations preventing randomized controlled trials of SPK versus kidney transplant alone [76, 77]. Still, it appears to be true that 4-year patient survival after pancreas transplant is better for all three groups—SPK, PAK, and PTA—when compared to individuals remaining on the waitlist [78]. Additionally, there is some evidence that pancreas transplantation can reduce the severity of end-organ complications associated with diabetes, including nephropathy, neuropathy, and atherosclerotic cardiovascular disease, particularly in instances in which the allograft is functioning properly and able to maintain euglycemia for more than 5 years [79–81]. This risk-benefit discussion will no doubt continue as medical treatments for diabetes are continually advancing.

Anatomy

Surgical technique for pancreas transplantation is the same, regardless of whether or not the patient is receiving a dual organ transplantation. The pancreas is removed from the donor complete with a small segment of duodenum (surgically closed at each luminal end) and placed in the pelvis of the recipient. In the United States, it is common to use systemic venous drainage with anastomosis to a branch of the iliac vein, as opposed to portal venous drainage. In theory, portal venous drainage is more physiologic and avoids the risks associated with systemic hyperinsulinemia; however, it has been associated with a higher risk of thrombosis and thus more than 90% of pancreas transplants in the United States use systemic venous drainage [82]. Drainage of pancreatic exocrine secretions is accomplished either by attaching the small duodenal segment to the bladder or to the small bowel in a side to side fashion. Historically, bladder drainage was preferred as it has the advantage of allowing for early detection of rejection via monitoring of urinary amylase levels; however, this technique has been associated with increased rates of multiple complications including the development of a hyperchloremic metabolic alkalosis, recurrent urinary tract infections, pancreatic leaks, and allograft pancreatitis [83]. Allograft survival rates appear to be similar regardless of drainage type. However, given the

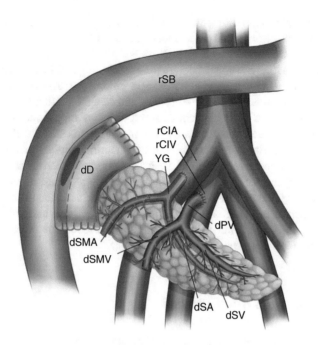

Fig. 4.4 Pancreas transplant anatomy. Surgical techniques vary. In this illustration, the arterial anastomosis is created by using a "Y graft" (YG), using the donor's common, internal, and external iliac artery, to connect the donor superior mesenteric artery (dSMA) and the donor splenic artery (dSA) into a single vessel that connects end-to-side to the recipient common iliac artery (rCIA). The donor superior mesenteric vein (dSMV) and the donor splenic vein (dSV) join the donor portal vein (dPV) intact, and the donor portal vein is anastomosed end-to-side to the recipient common iliac vein (rCIV) (venous anastomoses vary). The portion of the donor duodenum (dD) attached to the donor pancreas is anastomosed directly to the recipient small bowel (rSB). Other variations, such as bladder drainage of the exocrine pancreas, are not shown. (From Dillman and Elsayes [85], reprinted with permission)

reduction in associated complications, more than 80% of pancreas transplantations performed in the United States are enteric drained [84] (Fig. 4.4).

Immunosuppression

Immunosuppression strategies for pancreas transplantation closely mirror those for kidney transplantation. Nearly all transplant centers advocate induction immunosuppression for every pancreas transplantation, with the vast majority of pancreas recipients (more than 85%) receiving T-cell depleting antibodies such as rATG [86]. The remainder will typically receive IL-2 receptor antibodies such as basiliximab, although basiliximab has been associated with an increased rate of acute rejection within the first year when compared to rATG, so its use is generally reserved for those patients with strong contraindications to rATG [87].

Most patients undergoing SPK or PAK transplant will be maintained on a three-drug maintenance immunosuppression regimen including a calcineurin inhibitor, an antimetabolite (typically mycophenolate), and prednisone. As with kidney transplantation, there is significant variability between centers, particularly with respect to the long-term use of glucocorticoids. Approximately three fourths of pancreas transplant recipients will remain on triple immunosuppression for the life of the allograft [86]. Tacrolimus is the first-line calcineurin inhibitor of choice due to decreased rates of acute rejection and increased allograft survival at 1 year when compared with cyclosporine [88]. The popularity of alternate agents such as mTOR inhibitors has declined considerably in recent years, likely related to concerns about side effects such as proteinuria, poor wound healing, and dyslipidemia in patients with diabetes, such that fewer than 10% of pancreas recipients receive an mTOR inhibitor within the first year [84].

Allograft Function and Rejection

Freedom from insulin dependence is the hallmark criterion for pancreas allograft survival; however, it is generally agreed upon that the development of hyperglycemia is a late manifestation of allograft dysfunction. Because of the clinically silent nature of pancreatic dysfunction, routine laboratory monitoring is essential for surveillance of allograft function, with patients typically followed once or twice weekly for the first several months and then every 2–4 weeks thereafter for the first year. Most programs will perform serial monitoring of lipase, amylase, and fasting serum glucose. Some transplant centers will also perform routine monitoring of DSAs, as has become common for kidney transplant recipients. When recipients with a history of type 1 diabetes present with hyperglycemia or other evidence of allograft dysfunction, it is common to perform tests for anti-insulin, anti-islet cell, and anti-glutamic acid decarboxylase antibodies to assess for recurrent disease.

Most instances of allograft dysfunction, including those caused by acute rejection, are asymptomatic, although occasionally a patient will experience tenderness at the site of the allograft. Other nonspecific symptoms such as fever, malaise, or nausea can indicate allograft dysfunction. The most common laboratory abnormality is new elevation in pancreatic enzyme levels with or without new onset hyperglycemia. The differential diagnosis for elevated pancreatic enzymes should include acute pancreas allograft rejection, pancreas allograft vascular thrombosis, or stenosis as well as other causes of intraabdominal pathology including ileus, enzyme leak, small bowel obstruction, fluid collection, native pancreatitis, chemical-, alcohol- or hyperlipidemia-induced native or allograft pancreatitis, and infection including CMV pancreatitis and abscess.

When acute rejection is suspected based on laboratory findings or history, additional workup is warranted. This should include abdominal imaging, typically with ultrasound of the pancreas allograft with Doppler and a contrast enhanced CT scan of the abdomen and pelvis, followed by a biopsy when imaging is inconclusive. CT scan of the abdomen and pelvis can also detect if any inflammation is occurring in the native pancreas. In SPK recipients, it is common to first perform a kidney biopsy, as this procedure is less technically complicated than a pancreas biopsy and is associated with fewer complications. However, rates of discordance of up to 30% have been reported between kidney and pancreas biopsies, such that a pancreas biopsy should still be performed if results of the kidney biopsy fail to reveal a suitable explanation for pancreatic dysfunction [89].

When compared to kidney transplantation, acute rejection is much more common in pancreas transplant recipients, with an estimated 15–20% of patients experiencing an episode of acute rejection by 1 year [90, 91]. Randomized trials comparing treatment strategies for acute rejection in pancreas transplantation are lacking, so treatment protocols are typically based on the treatment of acute rejection in kidney transplant recipients. In general, acute cellular rejection is treated with corticosteroids and ATG, whereas acute antibody-mediated rejection is treated with the combination of plasmapheresis, IVIG, and rituximab. Response to treatment correlates with the extent of injury on biopsy, and outcomes tend to be better when pancreatic dysfunction is detected early.

Conclusion

Care of the kidney and kidney-pancreas transplant recipient requires a thorough review of the patient's transplant history, knowledge of typical transplant protocols and medications and their adverse effects, and meticulous evaluations of the patient combined with timely communication with the transplant team. Primary care providers can partner with nephrologists to take care of a range of issues for these patients, including metabolic and cardiovascular complications, as well as onset of new medical concerns. Indeed, the wide range of prescribing practices of cardiovascular medications suggests the need for more rigorous studies of the post-kidney transplant population. Collaboration between transplant specialists and primary care providers should be an ongoing process of research and clinical care to improve longevity and quality of life in kidney transplant recipients.

References

1. United States Renal Data System. Chapter 5: Mortality. In: 2017 USRDS annual data report: volume 2—ESRD in the United States. Accessed online 4 Oct 2019, at https://www.usrds.org/2017/download/v2_c05_Mortality_17.pdf.
2. Rabbat CG, Thorpe KE, Russell JD, Churchill DN. Comparison of mortality risk for dialysis patients and cadaveric first renal transplant recipients in Ontario, Canada. J Am Soc Nephrol. 2000;11:917–22.

3. Wolfe RA, Ashby VB, Milford EL, Ojo AO, Ettenger RE, Agodoa LY, Held PJ, Port FK. Comparison of mortality in all patients on dialysis, patients on dialysis awaiting transplantation, and recipients of a first cadaveric transplant. N Engl J Med. 1999;341: 1725–30.
4. Tonelli M, Wiebe N, Knoll G, Bello A, Browne S, Jadhav D, Klarenbach S, Gill J. Systematic review: kidney transplantation compared with dialysis in clinically relevant outcomes. Am J Transplant. 2011;11:2093–109.
5. Kidney Disease: Improving Global Outcomes (KDIGO) CKD Work Group. KDIGO 2012 clinical practice guideline for the evaluation and management of chronic kidney disease. Kidney Int Suppl. 2013;3:1–150.
6. Fowler KJ. Accountability of dialysis facilities in transplant referral: CMS needs to collect national data on dialysis facility kidney transplant referrals. Clin J Am Soc Nephrol. 2018;13(2):193–4. https://doi.org/10.2215/CJN.13741217.
7. Murray JE. The fight for life: Harvard Medicine. Accessed online 28 Jan 2020 at: https://hms.harvard.edu/magazine/science-emotion/fight-life.
8. United States Renal Data System. 2018 USRDS annual data report: Epidemiology of kidney disease in the United States. Bethesda: National Institutes of Health, National Institute of Diabetes and Digestive and Kidney Diseases; 2018. Accessed online 1 Jan 2020.
9. Wu C, Evans I, Joseph R, Shapiro R, Tan H, Basu A, Smetanka C, Khan A, McCauley J, Unruh M. Comorbid conditions in kidney transplantation: association with graft and patient survival. J Am Soc Nephrol. 2005;l16:3437–44.
10. Ramos EL, Tisher CC. Recurrent diseases in the kidney transplant. Am J Kidney Dis. 1994;24:142–54.
11. Meier-Kriesche H-U, Kaplan B. Waiting time on dialysis as the strongest modifiable risk factor for renal transplant outcomes: a paired donor kidney analysis. Transplantation. 2002;74:1377–81.
12. Hart A, Smith JM, Skeans MA, Gustafson SK, Wilk AR, Castro S, Robinson A, Wainright JL, Snyder JJ, Kasiske BL, Israni AK. OPTN/SRTR 2017 annual data report: kidney. Am J Transplant. 2019;19(Suppl 2):19–123. https://doi.org/10.1111/ajt.15274.
13. Sanfilippo FP, Vaughn WK, Peters TG, Shield CF, Adams PL, Lorber MI, Williams GM. Factors affecting the waiting time of cadaveric kidney transplant candidates in the United States. JAMA. 1992;267:247–52.
14. Organ Procurement and Transplantation Network Policies. Policy 8: allocation of kidneys. Effective date: 1/9/2020. Available online at: https://optn.transplant.hrsa.gov/media/1200/optn_policies.pdf.
15. Friedewald JJ, Samana CJ, Kasiske BL, Israni AK, Stewart D, Cherikh W, Formica RN. The kidney allocation system. Surg Clin North Am. 2013;93:1395–406.
16. Stewart DE, Kucheryavaya AY, Klassen DK, Turgeon NA, Formica RN, Aeder MI. Changes in deceased donor kidney transplantation one year after KAS implementation. Am J Transplant. 2016;16:1834–47.
17. Cass A, Cunningham J, Snelling P, Ayanian JZ. Late referral to a nephrologist reduces access to renal transplantation. Am J Kidney Dis. 2003;42:1043–9.
18. Stewart DE, Klassen DK. Early experience with the new kidney allocation system: a perspective from UNOS. Clin J Am Soc Nephrol. 2017;12(12):2063–5. https://doi.org/10.2215/CJN.06380617.
19. Forsythe JLR. Deceased-donor kidney transplantation. In: Oniscu G, Forsythe J, Pomfret E, editors. Transplantation surgery: Springer Surgery Atlas Series. Berlin: Springer; 2019.
20. Zand MS. Immunosuppression and immune monitoring after renal transplantation. Semin Dial. 2005;18:511–9.
21. Kidney Disease: Improving Global Outcomes (KDIGO) Transplant Work Group. KDIGO clinical practice guideline for the care of kidney transplant recipients. Am J Transplant. 2009;9(Suppl 3):S1–155.

22. Cecka JM. Calculated PRA (CPRA): the new measure of sensitization for transplant candidates. Am J Transplant. 2010;10(1):26–9. https://doi.org/10.1111/j.1600-6143.2009.02927.x.
23. Mourad G, Garrigue V, Squifflet JP, et al. Induction versus noninduction in renal transplant recipients with tacrolimus-based immunosuppression. Transplantation. 2001;72:1050–5.
24. Charpentier B, Rostaing L, Berthoux F, et al. A three-arm study comparing immediate tacrolimus therapy with antithymocyte globulin induction therapy followed by tacrolimus or cyclosporine A in adult renal transplant recipients. Transplantation. 2003;75:844–51.
25. Webster AC, Ruster LP, McGee R, Matheson SL, Higgins GY, Willis NS, Chapman JR, Craig JC. Interleukin 2 receptor antagonists for kidney transplant recipients. Cochrane Database Syst Rev. 2010, 2010;(1):CD003897. https://doi.org/10.1002/14651858.CD003897.pub3.
26. Brennan DC, Flavin K, Lowell JA, et al. A randomized, double-blinded comparison of thymoglobulin versus Atgam for induction immunosuppressive therapy in adult renal transplant recipients. Transplantation. 1999;67:1011–8.
27. Ciancio G, Burke GW, Gaynor JJ, Roth D, Kupin W, Rosen A, Cordovilla T, Tueros L, Herrada E, Miller J. A randomized trial of thymoglobulin vs. alemtuzumab (with lower dose maintenance immunosuppression) vs. daclizumab in renal transplantation at 24 months of follow-up. Clin Transpl. 2008;22:200–10.
28. Brennan DC, Schnitzler MA. Long-term results of rabbit antithymocyte globulin and basiliximab induction. N Engl J Med. 2008;359:1736–8.
29. Gonwa T, Johnson C, Ahsan N, et al. Randomized trial of tacrolimus + mycophenolate mofetil or azathioprine versus cyclosporine + mycophenolate mofetil after cadaveric kidney transplantation: results at three years. Transplantation. 2003;75:2048–53.
30. Krämer BK, European Tacrolimus vs Cyclosporin Microemulsion Renal Transplantation Study Group, Montagnino G, et al. Efficacy and safety of tacrolimus compared with cyclosporin A microemulsion in renal transplantation: 2 year follow-up results. Nephrol Dial Transplant. 2005;20:968–73.
31. Webster AC, Woodroffe RC, Taylor RS, Chapman JR, Craig JC. Tacrolimus versus ciclosporin as primary immunosuppression for kidney transplant recipients: meta-analysis and meta-regression of randomised trial data. BMJ. 2005;331(7520):810.
32. Guerra G, Ciancio G, Gaynor JJ, et al. Randomized trial of immunosuppressive regimens in renal transplantation. J Am Soc Nephrol. 2011;22:1758–68.
33. Vincenti F, Charpentier B, Vanrenterghem Y, et al. A phase III study of belatacept-based immunosuppression regimens versus cyclosporine in renal transplant recipients (BENEFIT study). Am J Transplant. 2010;10:535–46.
34. Vincenti F, Blancho G, Durrbach A, et al. Five-year safety and efficacy of belatacept in renal transplantation. J Am Soc Nephrol. 2010;21:1587–96.
35. Lebranchu Y, Halimi JM, Bock A, Chapman J, Dussol B, Fritsche L, Kliem V, Oppenheimer F, Pohanka E, Salvadori M, Soergel M, Tufveson G, MOST International Study Group. Delayed graft function: risk factors, consequences and parameters affecting outcome-results from MOST, a Multinational Observational Study. Transplant Proc. 2005;37(1):345–7.
36. Saidi RF, Elias N, Kawai T, Hertl M, Farrell ML, Goes N, Wong W, Hartono C, Fishman JA, Kotton CN, Tolkoff-Rubin N, Delmonico FL, Cosimi AB, Ko DS. Outcome of kidney transplantation using expanded criteria donors and donation after cardiac death kidneys: realities and costs. Am J Transplant. 2007;7(12):2769–74.
37. Naesens M, Kuypers DRJ, Sarwal M. Calcineurin inhibitor nephrotoxicity. Clin J Am Soc Nephrol. 2009;4:481–508.
38. Agena F, dos Santos Prado E, Souza PS, da Silva GV, FBC L, Mion D, Nahas WC, David-Neto E. Home blood pressure (BP) monitoring in kidney transplant recipients is more adequate to monitor BP than office BP. Nephrol Dial Transplant. 2011;26:3745–9.
39. Tait BD, Süsal C, Gebel HM, et al. Consensus guidelines on the testing and clinical management issues associated with HLA and non-HLA antibodies in transplantation. Transplantation. 2013;95:19–47.

40. Racusen LC. Protocol transplant biopsies in kidney allografts: why and when are they indicated? Clin J Am Soc Nephrol. 2006;1:144–7.
41. Wilkinson A. Protocol transplant biopsies: are they really needed? Clin J Am Soc Nephrol. 2006;1:130–7.
42. Henderson LK, Nankivell BJ, Chapman JR. Surveillance protocol kidney transplant biopsies: their evolving role in clinical practice. Am J Transplant. 2011;11(8):1570–5.
43. Owda AK, Abdallah AH, Haleem A, Hawas FA, Mousa D, Fedail H, Al-Sulaiman MH, Al-Khader AA. De novo diabetes mellitus in kidney allografts: nodular sclerosis and diffuse glomerulosclerosis leading to graft failure. Nephrol Dial Transplant. 1999;14:2004–7.
44. Ranghino A, Segoloni GP, Lasaponara F, Biancone L. Lymphatic disorders after renal transplantation: new insights for an old complication. Clin Kidney J. 2015;8:615–22.
45. Baliu C, Esforzado N, Campistol JM, Mascaró JM. Chronic lymphedema in renal transplant recipients under immunosuppression with sirolimus: presentation of 2 cases. JAMA Dermatol. 2014;150(9):1023–4.
46. Hamouda M, Sharma A, Halawa A. Urine leak after kidney transplant: a review of the literature. Exp Clin Transplant. 2018;16:90–5.
47. Bruno S. Transplant renal artery stenosis. J Am Soc Nephrol. 2004;15:134–41.
48. Roufosse C, Simmonds N, Clahsen-van Groningen M, et al. A 2018 reference guide to the Banff classification of renal allograft pathology. Transplantation. 2018;102:1795–814.
49. Haas M, Loupy A, Lefaucheur C, et al. The Banff 2017 kidney meeting report: revised diagnostic criteria for chronic active T cell-mediated rejection, antibody-mediated rejection, and prospects for integrative endpoints for next-generation clinical trials. Am J Transplant. 2018;18:293–307.
50. Vineyard GC, Fadem SZ, Dmochowski J, Carpenter CB, Wilson RE. Evaluation of corticosteroid therapy for acute renal allograft rejection. Surg Gynecol Obstet. 1974;138:225–9.
51. Hoitsma AJ, Reekers P, Kreeftenberg JG, van Lier HJ, Capel PJ, Koene RA. Treatment of acute rejection of cadaveric renal allografts with rabbit antithymocyte globulin. Transplantation. 1982;33:12–6.
52. Webster AC, Wu S, Tallapragada K, Park MY, Chapman JR, Carr SJ. Polyclonal and monoclonal antibodies for treating acute rejection episodes in kidney transplant recipients. Cochrane Database Syst Rev. 2017;7:CD004756. https://doi.org/10.1002/14651858.CD004756.pub4.
53. Djamali A, Kaufman DB, Ellis TM, Zhong W, Matas A, Samaniego M. Diagnosis and management of antibody-mediated rejection: current status and novel approaches. Am J Transplant. 2014;14:255–71.
54. Solez K, Colvin RB, Racusen LC, et al. Banff '05 meeting report: differential diagnosis of chronic allograft injury and elimination of chronic allograft nephropathy. Am J Transplant. 2007;7:518–26.
55. Cosio FG, Gloor JM, Sethi S, Stegall MD. Transplant glomerulopathy. Am J Transplant. 2008;8:492–6.
56. Solez K, Colvin RB, Racusen LC, et al. Banff 07 classification of renal allograft pathology: updates and future directions. Am J Transplant. 2008;8:753–60.
57. Carpenter CB. Long-term failure of renal transplants: adding insult to injury. Kidney Int Suppl. 1995;50:S40–4.
58. Butler JA, Roderick P, Mullee M, Mason JC, Peveler RC. Frequency and impact of nonadherence to immunosuppressants after renal transplantation: a systematic review. Transplantation. 2004;77:769–76.
59. Ramos E, Drachenberg CB, Wali R, Hirsch HH. The decade of polyomavirus BK-associated nephropathy: state of affairs. Transplantation. 2009;87:621–30.
60. Mengel M, Marwedel M, Radermacher J, Eden G, Schwarz A, Haller H, Kreipe H. Incidence of polyomavirus-nephropathy in renal allografts: influence of modern immunosuppressive drugs. Nephrol Dial Transplant. 2003;18:1190–6.

61. Dadhania D, Snopkowski C, Ding R, Muthukumar T, Chang C, Aull M, Lee J, Sharma VK, Kapur S, Suthanthiran M. Epidemiology of BK virus in renal allograft recipients: independent risk factors for BK virus replication. Transplantation. 2008;86:521–8.
62. Drachenberg CB, Papadimitriou JC. Polyomavirus-associated nephropathy: update in diagnosis. Transpl Infect Dis. 2006;8:68–75.
63. Wiseman AC. Polyomavirus nephropathy: a current perspective and clinical considerations. Am J Kidney Dis. 2009;54:131–42.
64. Sharma SG, Nickeleit V, Herlitz LC, de Gonzalez AK, Stokes MB, Singh HK, Markowitz GS, D'Agati VD. BK polyoma virus nephropathy in the native kidney. Nephrol Dial Transplant. 2001;28:620–31.
65. Awan AA, Niu J, Pan JS, Erickson KF, Mandayam S, Winkelmayer WC, Navaneethan SD, Ramanathan V. Trends in the causes of death among kidney transplant recipients in the United States (1996–2014). Am J Nephrol. 2018;48:472–81.
66. Gaston RS, Kasiske BL, Fieberg AM, Leduc R, Cosio FC, Gourishankar S, Halloran P, Hunsicker L, Rush D, Matas AJ. Use of cardioprotective medications in kidney transplant recipients. Am J Transplant. 2009;9:1811–5.
67. Holdaas H, Fellström B, Jardine AG, et al. Effect of fluvastatin on cardiac outcomes in renal transplant recipients: a multicentre, randomised, placebo-controlled trial. Lancet. 2003;361:2024–31.
68. Palmer SC, Navaneethan SD, Craig JC, Perkovic V, Johnson DW, Nigwekar SU, Hegbrant J, Strippoli GF. HMG CoA reductase inhibitors (statins) for kidney transplant recipients. Cochrane Database Syst Rev. 2014;1:CD005019. https://doi.org/10.1002/14651858. CD005019.pub4.
69. Wanner C, Tonelli M, Kidney Disease: Improving Global Outcomes Lipid Guideline Development Work Group Members. KDIGO clinical practice guideline for lipid management in CKD: summary of recommendation statements and clinical approach to the patient. Kidney Int. 2014;85:1303–9.
70. Whelton PK, Carey RM, Aronow WS, et al. 2017 ACC/AHA/AAPA/ABC/ACPM/AGS/APhA/ ASH/ASPC/NMA/PCNA guideline for the prevention, detection, evaluation, and management of high blood pressure in adults: a report of the American College of Cardiology/American Heart Association Task Force on Clinical Practice Guidelines. Hypertension. 2018;71(6):e13–e115. https://doi.org/10.1161/HYP.0000000000000065.
71. Porrini E, Moreno JM, Osuna A, et al. Prediabetes in patients receiving tacrolimus in the first year after kidney transplantation: a prospective and multicenter study. Transplantation. 2008;85:1133–8.
72. Heisel O, Heisel R, Balshaw R, Keown P. New onset diabetes mellitus in patients receiving calcineurin inhibitors: a systematic review and meta-analysis. Am J Transplant. 2004;4:583–95.
73. Kelly WD, Lillehei RC, Merkel FK, Idezuki Y, Goetz FC. Allotransplantation of the pancreas and duodenum along with the kidney in diabetic nephropathy. Surgery. 1967;61:827–37.
74. Gruessner RWG, Gruessner AC. The current state of pancreas transplantation. Nat Rev Endocrinol. 2013;9:555–62.
75. Gruessner RWG, Sutherland DER, Kandaswamy R, Gruessner AC. Over 500 solitary pancreas transplants in nonuremic patients with brittle diabetes mellitus. Transplantation. 2008;85:42–7.
76. Nathan DM, Fogel H, Norman D, Russell PS, Tolkoff-Rubin N, Delmonico FL, Auchincloss H, Camuso J, Cosimi AB. Long-term metabolic and quality of life results with pancreatic/renal transplantation in insulin-dependent diabetes mellitus. Transplantation. 1991;52:85–91.
77. Gruessner AC, Sutherland DER, Gruessner RWG. Long-term outcome after pancreas transplantation. Curr Opin Organ Transplant. 2012;17:100–5.
78. Gruessner RWG, Sutherland DER, Gruessner AC. Mortality assessment for pancreas transplants. Am J Transplant. 2004;4:2018–26.
79. Fioretto P, Steffes MW, Sutherland DE, Goetz FC, Mauer M. Reversal of lesions of diabetic nephropathy after pancreas transplantation. N Engl J Med. 1998;339:69–75.

80. Navarro X, Sutherland DE, Kennedy WR. Long-term effects of pancreatic transplantation on diabetic neuropathy. Ann Neurol. 1997;42:727–36.
81. Jukema JW, Smets YFC, van der Pijl JW, Zwinderman AH, Vliegen HW, Ringers J, Reiber JHC, Lemkes HHPJ, van der Wall EE, de Fijter JW. Impact of simultaneous pancreas and kidney transplantation on progression of coronary atherosclerosis in patients with end-stage renal failure due to type 1 diabetes. Diabetes Care. 2002;25:906–11.
82. Rogers J, Farney AC, Orlando G, Farooq U, Al-Shraideh Y, Stratta RJ. Pancreas transplantation with portal venous drainage with an emphasis on technical aspects. Clin Transpl. 2014;28:16–26.
83. El-Hennawy H, Stratta RJ, Smith F. Exocrine drainage in vascularized pancreas transplantation in the new millennium. World J Transplant. 2016;6:255–71.
84. Bloom RD, Olivares M, Rehman L, Raja RM, Yang S, Badosa F. Long-term pancreas allograft outcome in simultaneous pancreas-kidney transplantation: a comparison of enteric and bladder drainage. Transplantation. 1997;64:1689–95.
85. Dillman JR, Elsayes KM. Imaging of pancreas transplant. In: Elsayes KM, editor. Cross-sectional imaging of the abdomen and pelvis. New York: Springer; 2015.
86. Kandaswamy R, Stock PG, Gustafson SK, Skeans MA, Urban R, Fox A, Odorico JS, Israni AK, Snyder JJ, Kasiske BL. OPTN/SRTR 2017 annual data report: pancreas. Am J Transplant. 2019;19:124–83.
87. Bazerbachi F, Selzner M, Boehnert MU, Marquez MA, Norgate A, McGilvray ID, Schiff J, Cattral MS. Thymoglobulin versus basiliximab induction therapy for simultaneous kidney-pancreas transplantation: impact on rejection, graft function, and long-term outcome. Transplantation. 2011;92:1039–43.
88. Bechstein WO, Malaise J, Saudek F, et al. Efficacy and safety of tacrolimus compared with cyclosporine microemulsion in primary simultaneous pancreas-kidney transplantation: 1-year results of a large multicenter trial. Transplantation. 2004;77:1221–8.
89. Redfield RR, Kaufman DB, Odorico JS. Diagnosis and treatment of pancreas rejection. Curr Transplant Rep. 2015;2:169–75.
90. Dong M, Parsaik AK, Kremers W, et al. Acute pancreas allograft rejection is associated with increased risk of graft failure in pancreas transplantation. Am J Transplant. 2013;13:1019–25.
91. Niederhaus SV, Leverson GE, Lorentzen DF, Robillard DJ, Sollinger HW, Pirsch JD, Torrealba JR, Odorico JS. Acute cellular and antibody-mediated rejection of the pancreas allograft: incidence, risk factors and outcomes. Am J Transplant. 2013;13:2945–55.

Chapter 5
Primary Care of the Adult Liver Transplant Recipient

Lauren A. Beste and Anne M. Larson

Introduction

Chronic liver disease affects 30–35 million individuals in the United States (USA), 29 million in the European region, and an even greater number of persons worldwide [1]. The liver is the second most commonly transplanted solid organ in the USA, representing roughly one fifth of solid organ transplants since 1999 [2]. The demand for liver transplantation—up to 15,000 patients yearly—far exceeds the supply of 6000 to 6500 organs [3]. Contrasting with dialysis for kidney failure, no mechanical organ substitutes exist for liver failure. Excluding kidney transplants, the waiting list for liver transplant contains two times as many individuals as all other solid organ listings combined [3].

The most common indications for adult liver transplantation include chronic liver failure, hepatocellular carcinoma, and acute liver failure (most often due to toxic ingestion). The most common etiologies of chronic liver disease in the USA include hepatitis C virus infection (HCV), non-alcoholic steatohepatitis (NASH), and alcohol-related liver disease (ALD). HCV has historically been the leading indication for liver transplantation, but the advent of direct acting antiviral therapies has led to a decline in the proportion of transplants performed for HCV, from 23.9% in 2014 to 12.4% in 2017 [4]. Recent trends suggest that NASH disease has surpassed HCV as a cause for liver transplantation and shows no sign of slowing (Fig. 5.1) [5, 6].

L. A. Beste (✉)
Department of Medicine, Division of General Internal Medicine, University of Washington, Seattle, WA, USA

General Medicine Service, Veterans Affairs Puget Sound Health Care System, Seattle, WA, USA
e-mail: Lab25@uw.edu

A. M. Larson
Hepatology & Liver Transplantation, Division of Gastroenterology, University of Washington, Seattle, WA, USA
e-mail: amlarson@uw.edu

© Springer Nature Switzerland AG 2020
C. J. Wong (ed.), *Primary Care of the Solid Organ Transplant Recipient*,
https://doi.org/10.1007/978-3-030-50629-2_5

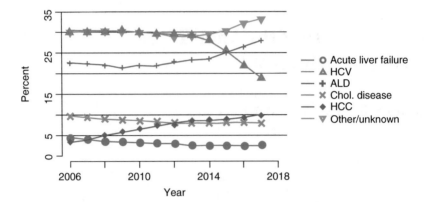

Fig. 5.1 Total liver transplants by diagnosis. ALD alcoholic liver disease, HCV hepatitis C virus, Chol cholestatic, HCC hepatocellular carcinoma; Other/unknown includes non-alcoholic steatohepatitis. (*Data from*: Scientific Registry of Transplant Recipients. Available at: https://srtr.transplant.hrsa. gov/annual_reports/2017/Liver.aspx#LI_50_tx_counts_diag_1_b64 Accessed July 1, 2019)

Survival after liver transplantation is generally excellent, with 1- and 5-year post-transplant survival at 90.4% and 75.9%, respectively, [4] while the rate of 10-year survival is over 50% [20]. Post-liver transplant complications are divided into acute (the first 3–6 months post-transplant) and chronic or long term. Liver transplant centers typically bear responsibility for managing the patient's immunosuppressive regimen and for addressing any hepatic or biliary complications that arise after liver transplantation [7]. Primary care providers (PCPs) should expect to manage the long-term metabolic side effects of immunosuppression, and to oversee preventive care such as vaccinations and cancer screenings. In addition, PCPs may be the first point of contact for patients when new symptoms arise.

Liver Transplant Anatomy

Deceased donor transplants comprise 95% of all liver transplants in the USA [4]:

- The donor liver is placed in the orthotopic position (same location as the native organ).
- Four surgical anastomoses must be created between the donor allograft and the recipient to implant the new liver: inferior vena cava/hepatic veins, hepatic artery, portal vein, and common bile duct (Fig. 5.2):
  - There are two predominant caval reconstructions: the conventional technique (caval replacement, in which the relevant portion of the recipient's inferior vena cava is resected and replaced with the donor portion; Fig. 5.3a) and the piggyback technique (Figs. 5.3b, c).

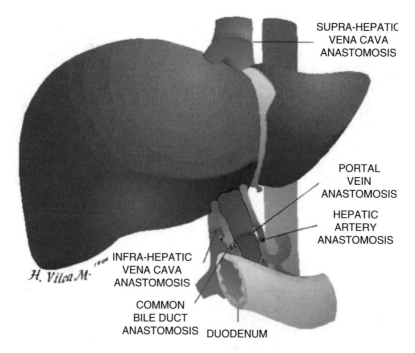

SUPRA-HEPATIC
VENA CAVA
ANASTOMOSIS

PORTAL
VEIN
ANASTOMOSIS

HEPATIC
ARTERY
ANASTOMOSIS

INFRA-HEPATIC
VENA CAVA
ANASTOMOSIS

H. Vilca M.

COMMON
BILE DUCT
ANASTOMOSIS   DUODENUM

Fig. 5.2 Anatomy and blood supply of the transplanted liver. (Reproduced with permission from: Berry et al. [47])

- The caval technique has largely been supplanted by the piggyback technique. The donor vena cava is closed inferiorly. The superior portion of the donor cava (including the hepatic veins) is anastomosed end-to-end to the recipient hepatic vein (Fig. 5.3b) or side-to-side (Fig. 5.3c) with the recipient vena cava. This technique reduces the need for veno-venous bypass.
- Both the donor and recipient gallbladder are removed at the time of surgery.
- In some settings, hepaticojejunostomy with Roux-en-Y reconstruction is necessary.
- Arterial or venous thromboses, stricture, or leakage from any of these anastomoses are a common source of early post-transplant complications.

Living donor liver transplants (i.e., transplanting a portion of a healthy person's liver) are performed less often due to risk to the donor, including death. Segmental living donor liver transplantation is occurring with increasing frequency, however, accounting for 401 liver transplants in 2018 [3]. The surgical anastomoses vary in this type of transplant depending on the hepatic segment used. This chapter focuses on transplantation from deceased donors in which the entire donor organ is implanted.

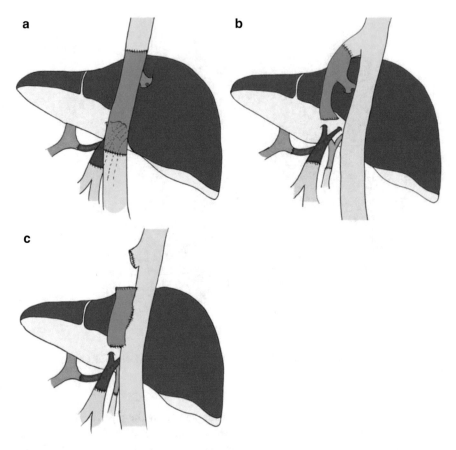

Fig. 5.3 Variations in caval reconstruction. (**a**) conventional technique. (**b**) piggyback technique with the superior portion of the donor cava anastomosed end-to-end to the recipient hepatic vein. (**c**) piggyback technique with the superior portion of the donor cava anastomosed side-to-side with the recipient vena cava (Reproduced with permission from: Chan et al. [48])

Early Post-transplant Period: 6–12 Months

Transplant recipients are closely monitored as inpatients during the immediate post-operative period for hemodynamic stability and acute complications. This management is carried out by a multidisciplinary team that includes surgeons, hepatologists, intensivists, pharmacists, dietitians, and nursing staff. In addition to the perioperative complications inherent in any surgery, such as bleeding, infection, or poor wound healing, liver transplant recipients have additional early risks. Very early post-transplant complications, within 3 months, include opportunistic infection, graft dysfunction, transplant-related surgical complications such as hepatic vascular thrombosis or biliary leaks, acute rejection, and other organ dysfunction (e.g., renal, pulmonary, neurologic) [8].

Typical Immunosuppressive Course

Transplant centers vary in their choice of immunosuppression in the first year post-transplant. Induction therapy is used during the first week post-liver transplant in some recipients, depending on the transplant center protocol. Induction therapies include antilymphocyte sera such as antithymocyte globulin or monoclonal antibodies (e.g. basiliximab) which act by blocking interleukin-2 receptors. Corticosteroids are often used immediately after liver transplantation and then tapered over the next 3–12 months.

Infections

Infection remains a significant risk in the setting of liver transplantation. Sources of infection include (a) the donor organ, (b) reactivation of prior infection in the recipient, and (c) de novo infection by exogenous or endogenous organisms. During the first month, infections are typically nosocomial. Viral infections (e.g., cytomegalovirus [CMV], Epstein-Barr virus [EBV]) predominate during the second to sixth month post-transplant, followed by fungal, bacterial, and parasitic infections [9]. Because of the risk of opportunistic infection, post-liver transplant patients routinely receive viral, bacterial, and fungal prophylaxis. Protocols vary by institution. In general, prophylaxis is provided for *pneumocystis jirovecii*. Prophylaxis is used against candida species and tailored by the center if endemic fungi are prominent (i.e., histoplasmosis, cryptococcus). CMV prophylaxis is typically given for seronegative recipients receiving CMV-positive livers, or those undergoing induction immunosuppression with a T-cell specific agent such as thymoglobulin [10, 11]. Acyclovir prophylaxis for herpes simplex is given if CMV prophylaxis is not used. The prophylactic agents are subsequently discontinued over the next 3–12 months, depending upon center protocol. After six months post-liver transplantation, infections are typically similar to those of the general population (see Chap. 8).

Graft Dysfunction

Primary nonfunction is one of the most serious immediate post-liver transplant complications, occurring in up to 10% of recipients. In this circumstance, the graft fails to function immediately following reperfusion, and the patient develops acute liver failure and must be urgently retransplanted. Additionally, subacute graft failure can develop in about 7.3% of liver transplant recipients by 6 months and 9.6% by 1 year and may require retransplantation [4]. Because early graft dysfunction may be asymptomatic, liver function is carefully monitored with frequent laboratory studies and imaging. Timing of studies varies, but, in general, laboratory testing ranges from weekly to every 3 months depending on how long has elapsed since transplant. Imaging is generally done every 3–6 months the first year—or for cause—then yearly. Protocol liver biopsies, used in the past to assess for rejection, are no longer performed. Factors associated with graft dysfunction include donation after cardiac death, donor macrovesicular steatosis, total ischemia time > 10 hours, reperfusion damage, older donor age (>60 years), and recurrent primary liver disease.

Vascular Complications

Post-transplant arterial complications include thrombosis, stenosis, pseudoaneurysm, and arterial rupture. Hepatic arterial pseudoaneurysms predispose to life-threatening hemorrhage and may require urgent endovascular or surgical intervention. Hepatic artery thrombosis (HAT) occurs in roughly 3–12% of liver transplant recipients and is a leading cause of early graft failure, requiring re-transplantation in up to 70% of cases [12]. The liver has a dual blood supply from both portal vein and hepatic artery, with only the hepatic artery carrying oxygenated blood. Even transient interruption of hepatic arterial flow may result in anoxic injury to the sensitive small bile ducts, especially if occurring within 4 weeks post-transplant ("early" HAT). The clinical consequences of HAT vary widely. Early HAT often leads to ischemia and necrosis of the allograft. Thrombolysis, thrombectomy, or surgical intervention may be attempted followed by anticoagulation; however, failure to recanalize the artery necessitates urgent retransplantation.

If thrombosis occurs later, it typically leads to biliary complications with preserved hepatic synthetic function. Complications of HAT include bile duct necrosis, intrahepatic bilomas, ischemic cholangiopathy, secondary biliary cirrhosis, and death unless corrected rapidly through surgical or interventional radiologic intervention. Therefore, most centers monitor laboratory results and routine duplex ultrasounds of the hepatic vessels in the early post-transplant setting (e.g., day 1 and day 5–7 post-transplant). Late hepatic artery thrombosis can present years after transplantation, although it may not require retransplantation if a collateral blood supply has developed. Late hepatic artery thrombosis is most often detected by routine duplex ultrasound or laboratory studies.

Portal vein thrombosis or stenosis occurs in up to 12% of liver recipients and is associated with increased risk of graft failure as well as increased mortality [12, 13]. Severe cases may result in portal hypertension with its subsequent complications of ascites and varices. The hepatic veins and inferior vena cava may also develop thromboses or stenoses, but this is less common.

Biliary Complications

Biliary complications develop in up to 30% of recipients and include bile leaks, bilomas (bile-filled fluid collections resulting from a biliary leak), strictures, and recurrent cholestatic liver disease [13]. They can be associated with hepatic arterial disease but may be related to technical aspects of the operation itself. Biliary complications may develop at any time post-transplant and often present with abnormal liver studies, fevers or abdominal pain. Abdominal imaging, magnetic resonance cholangiopancreatography (MRCP), and endoscopic retrograde cholangiopancreatography (ERCP) can all be helpful in determining the correct diagnosis. Strictures may be either anastomotic (80%) or non-anastomotic, with anastomotic strictures more often associated with biliary leakage. Hepatic arterial disease is causally associated with up to 53% of cases of refractory biliary disease, as hypoperfusion of the bile ducts leads to biliary strictures [14]. Additionally, biliary complications are associated with increased risk of infection.

Allograft Rejection

Early rejection is defined as development of acute cellular rejection (ACR) within the first year after liver transplantation. This type of rejection is cell-mediated and can frequently be reversed with appropriate immunosuppressive therapy. One or more episodes of ACR occur in 11.7%–26.9% of recipients, most commonly within the first 4–6 weeks post-liver transplantation [4, 15]. Patients are frequently asymptomatic but may rarely present with fever, malaise, or abdominal symptoms. Ongoing laboratory surveillance is performed regularly to identify early signs of hepatocellular injury. Timing of testing varies by center, but in general it is twice weekly for the first several weeks post-transplant, decreasing in frequency to every 3 months over the first year. Liver biopsy remains the gold standard for diagnosis if ACR is suspected. If confirmed, it is treated with high-dose corticosteroids followed by intensification of the patient's baseline immunosuppressive regimen. If corticosteroid-resistant ACR develops, T-cell directed therapies such as IL-2 inhibitors or antithymocyte globulin may be used. Acute rejection is associated with increased risk of graft failure (up to 10%), all-cause mortality, and transplant-related mortality [15].

Late Post-transplant Period

Survival and Cause of Death

Long-term survival continues to improve due to advancements in transplant technique and management. In addition to liver disease recurrence, long-term complications are generally associated with the use of immunosuppression: diabetes mellitus, systemic hypertension, dyslipidemia, obesity, de novo cancers, and nephrotoxicity. In the recipient who has survived 5 years or more after transplant, the primary causes of death are liver-related disease (27.3%), malignancy (21.1%), renal failure (10.2%), cardiovascular disease (8.6%), and infection (8.6%) [16]. It is anticipated that liver-related disease as a cause of post-transplant death will improve with the eradication of HCV infection.

Typical Immunosuppressive Course

In general, after the initial induction period, the backbone of maintenance immunosuppressive regimens includes the calcineurin inhibitor (CNI), tacrolimus, which has largely replaced cyclosporine. Because of the long-term toxicities of calcineurin inhibitors, antirejection regimens may include an antimetabolite medication to spare the dose of the calcineurin inhibitor. The antimetabolite, azathioprine, has almost universally been replaced by either mycophenolate mofetil or mycophenolic acid. If calcineurin inhibitors are contraindicated or intolerable side effects develop, alternative agents such as the mammalian target of rapamycin (mTOR) inhibitors (sirolimus or everolimus) can be substituted as second-line options. The most common immunosuppressive regimens in adult liver transplant recipients in the United States include tacrolimus, mycophenolate mofetil and corticosteroids, or tacrolimus plus mycophenolate mofetil [4]. It is now much more common to avoid use of long-term corticosteroids. Sample immunosuppressant drug targets are shown in Table 5.1. (See Chap. 3 for further discussion of mechanisms of action, side effects, and drug interactions. Metabolic complications are discussed in Chap. 11).

Evaluation of Liver Test Abnormalities

Any liver test abnormality in the post-liver transplant setting must be thoroughly evaluated. The testing performed will depend on the severity and type of abnormality. After the first post-transplant year, liver tests are typically monitored every 3 months or if new symptoms develop. Evaluation should be conducted in conjunction with the transplant center.

Table 5.1 Sample immunosuppressant trough targets[a] by time post-liver transplant

		Time post-liver transplant				
	Regimen	0–3 mo	3–6 mo	6–12 mo	12–24 mo	>24 mo
Tacrolimus level	Tacrolimus	5–8 ng/mL			5 ng/mL	3–5 ng/mL
	Tacrolimus-MMF (or AZA)-steroid	≤8 ng/mL			5 ng/mL	3–5 ng/mL
	Tacrolimus-sirolimus	5–8 ng/mL			5 ng/mL	3–5 ng/mL
Sirolimus level	Sirolimus-MMF-steroid	5–10 ng/mL				
	Sirolimus-tacrolimus	5–8 ng/mL			5 ng/mL	3–5 ng/mL
Cyclosporine level	CsA-MMF (or AZA)-steroid	150–200 ng/mL	150 ng/mL	100 ng/mL	80–100 ng/mL	60–80 ng/mL

[a]Immunosuppressive drug targets are individualized and generally managed by the patient's liver transplant center. The targets shown are for general information, not meant to guide clinical care. Abbreviations: *MMF* mycophenolate mofetil, *AZA* azathioprine, *CsA* cyclosporine, *ng/mL* nanograms per milliliter, *mo* month

In the asymptomatic patient with mildly elevated transaminases or bilirubin:

- If found on routine testing, the patient should be evaluated in person to confirm that he or she is asymptomatic, and to evaluate medication use, including new medications or supplements, as well as adherence to immunosuppressive medications, substance use (including alcohol), and for symptoms of recent infections.
- If truly asymptomatic and elevations in liver enzymes are mild, it may be reasonable to recheck liver tests in 1–2 weeks. If they normalize, further evaluation is unnecessary.
- Ongoing liver test abnormalities should be investigated with a duplex ultrasound to evaluate the liver, biliary tree, and the hepatic vessels. Additional testing may include immunosuppressive drug levels or tests for infection, such as hepatitis B virus (HBV), CMV, or EBV PCR.
- Any biliary abnormalities should prompt further evaluation of the biliary tree, such as magnetic resonance cholangiopancreatography or endoscopic retrograde cholangiopancreatography.
- Liver biopsy is often required to determine whether the test abnormality is secondary to rejection versus another cause. With appropriate immunosuppression management after transplant (Table 5.1), rejection episodes are generally minimized in the majority of patients.

Patients with severe transaminase or bilirubin elevation, or who are symptomatic, should immediately be referred for urgent evaluation either to the managing hepatologist or the emergency department, depending on the patient's clinical stability. If uncertain, then the hepatologist should be contacted to assist with triage and initial management.

Chronic Rejection

Chronic rejection can occur at any time post-liver transplantation, but generally presents more than 6 months after transplantation. Its pathogenesis remains unclear. This type of rejection leads to obliterative angiopathy and loss of the intrahepatic bile ducts (ductopenia). It presents predominantly with clinical and biochemical cholestasis. It is more common in patients with a history of steroid-refractory ACR and in patients with chronic viral hepatitis or autoimmune hepatitis (AIH) [17, 18]. Treatment remains difficult and retransplantation may be required.

Recurrence of Chronic Liver Disease

The underlying disease that resulted in liver failure may still be present after transplant. Recurrence can lead to significant morbidity and mortality following transplant and must be managed appropriately.

- Viral hepatitis: Viral hepatitis invariably returns after liver transplantation. In the past, recurrent HCV resulted in accelerated liver damage, cirrhosis, and rapid deterioration of the graft. With the advent of direct-acting antiviral (DAA) therapies, patients are either treated for HCV in anticipation of transplant or treated immediately afterwards. HCV treatment should only be carried out in collaboration with the transplant center since some DAAs may alter the levels of calcineurin inhibitors. HBV infection makes up less than 10% of US liver transplants, whereas it is the most common indication in Asia. Patients with HBV infection must remain virally suppressed indefinitely post-liver transplantation to prevent damage to the allograft. The combination of hepatitis B immune globulin at the time of transplantation plus chronic HBV antiviral medication prevents liver injury in nearly all liver transplant patients with chronic HBV.
- Nonalcoholic steatohepatitis: NASH is the fastest-growing etiology leading to liver transplantation, predicted to be the leading cause of liver transplantation by 2020–2030 (Fig. 5.1) [4, 14, 19]. Many comorbidities associated with NASH (e.g., obesity, diabetes, dyslipidemia, and hypertension) not only remain present post-transplant but may be exacerbated by antirejection drugs. Diabetes may result from corticosteroids or tacrolimus. CNIs can lead to systemic hypertension and sirolimus causes hyperlipidemia. Additionally, up to 70% of recipients will gain excessive weight over the first year post-transplant [20]. As a result, NASH frequently recurs post-transplant or can develop de novo [21]. Recurrent NASH may cause elevated liver tests and can lead to fibrosis; however, cirrhosis is uncommon in the first 5 years following liver transplantation. Primary care providers, therefore, have a critical role in helping to manage obesity and metabolic conditions post-liver transplantation to prevent recurrence or development of NASH.
- Autoimmune liver disease: The recurrence of autoimmune liver disease (primary sclerosing cholangitis [PSC], AIH, and primary biliary cholangitis [PBC]) varies from patient to patient. Recurrence of PSC has been reported in up to 50% of recipients by 5 years post-transplant, with graft loss seen in up to 25% [22, 23]. Patients with PSC and inflammatory bowel disease require annual colonoscopy after liver transplantation to screen for colon cancer. Recurrence of PBC develops in about 18% of liver transplant recipients and can be treated with ursodiol, similar to that used pre-transplant [19]. AIH recurs in 17–33% of patients post-transplant, with 6% requiring retransplantation [24]. Liver biopsy is often necessary to distinguish recurrent autoimmune liver disease from rejection.
- Hepatocellular carcinoma: Hepatocellular carcinoma (HCC) is a leading cause of liver transplantation. Patients with HCC must meet stringent criteria for the size and number of HCC lesions to be eligible for liver transplantation [25]. However, in many cases liver transplantation is an ideal choice to cure both HCC as well as underlying cirrhosis, if present. Patients with HCC who are transplanted within select criteria have been shown to have equivalent 5-year survival rates compare to liver transplant recipients overall [26]. Patients with a history of HCC must be screened carefully for recurrence after transplant, typically with multiphase CT or MRI of the liver every 6 months for at least 3 years. Post-

transplant HCC recurs in 6–18% of patients and may behave aggressively in the immunocompromised patient [27]. Management of post-transplant recurrent HCC requires a multidisciplinary approach.

- Alcohol-related liver disease: Patients transplanted for ALD have an overall survival similar to that of recipients without ALD [28]. To meet transplant eligibility requirements, all prospective liver transplant patients are closely screened for substance use disorders, insight into their drinking, psychosocial support, and typically must demonstrate a documented period of sobriety. Patients with ALD frequently lose the urge to drink while they have decompensated liver disease but are at risk for return to alcohol use post-transplant. In meta-analysis, the pooled prevalence of self-reported alcohol use after liver transplantation for those transplanted for ALD was 26.3% (95% CI 18–36.7%) over a median follow-up of 6 years [29]. The causes of death in ALD patients who return to heavy drinking tend to be liver-related [30]. All liver transplant recipients are recommended to undergo regular screening for alcohol misuse and to engage in behavioral health intervention and treatment to support sobriety, if indicated.

Late Surgical Complications

Biliary and vascular complications can develop at any time in the post-transplant period and are managed as discussed above. Incisional hernia may develop after liver transplantation. If repair is desired, surgeons typically recommend waiting approximately a year after transplantation to allow for abdominal wall healing, stable liver function, and reduced risk of infection. In the meantime, abdominal binders provide symptomatic management until surgery can be performed. Patients should be educated about the possibility of bowel incarceration.

Preventive Care for the Liver Transplant Recipient

Primary care providers are frequently the first point of contact for liver transplant recipients when new health concerns arise, especially if the patient resides far from their transplant center. Adult liver transplant recipients are most commonly between 50 and 64 years at the time of transplantation and may have non-hepatic comorbidities [4]. Among patients who survive more than 5 years after liver transplant, the most common causes of death include malignancy, cardiovascular disease, and renal failure. Close coordination with the transplant center is advised when considering new medications or liver-directed workup. A summary of clinical pearls for outpatient assessment of the liver transplant recipient is shown in Table 5.2, and typical testing intervals are shown in Table 5.3.

Table 5.2 Clinical pearls for the primary care provider—evaluating liver transplant recipients at outpatient clinic visits

Initial visit:
Review pre-transplant and initial post-transplant course:
Indication for transplant
Pre-transplant complications
Type of donor
Induction immunosuppression
Early complications (surgical complications, infection, rejection)
Symptoms, exam, medications, laboratory studies similar to follow-up visits
Follow-up visits:
Symptoms: Pain, symptoms of volume depletion or excess, side effects of medications, symptoms of infection, symptoms of liver dysfunction, including jaundice, confusion, bleeding
Exam: Blood pressure, heart, lung, abdomen exam, volume status
Medications: Current regimen, adherence, side effects, goal trough levels
Substance use: assess for alcohol and other substance use
Mental health screening: Screen for and treat depression and other mental health conditions
Laboratory and other studies: Adherence to routine surveillance schedule set forth by the transplant team; surveillance for rejection (see Table 5.3)
Surveillance: Adherence to surveillance for underlying conditions, if applicable (e.g., HCC, PSC) (see Table 5.3)
Metabolic complications: Assess and treat
Address obesity, diet, exercise, and other risk factors for NASH
Hypertension, dyslipidemia, diabetes, osteoporosis

See text for details, also see Chaps. 2, 10, 11 and 12

Immunosuppression Management

Liver transplant recipients remain on immunosuppression for the rest of their lives, with rare exception. Immunosuppressive medication adjustment is typically managed by the transplant center (sample trough target levels are described in Table 5.1) (see Chap. 3).

PCPs should be aware of drugs that may alter the levels of CNIs, and thus potentially provoke rejection or drug toxicity. Typical culprits include antiseizure medications (phenobarbital, phenytoin, carbamazepine) and anti-infectives (isoniazid, fluconazole). The use of vitamins and supplements should be assessed at every visit, as many will interact with calcineurin inhibitors (e.g., St. John's wort, kava kava, echinacea) [31]. Tobacco and cannabis use are specifically assessed in the pre-transplant setting, but may be associated with complications post-transplant. All patients should be queried regarding use of alcohol, tobacco, and recreational drugs (including all forms of cannabis) at each post-transplant visit. Liver transplant recipients should be advised to avoid any substance use, including tobacco and alcohol. Most programs recommend complete avoidance of cannabis as well. There is

Table 5.3 Typical post-liver transplant monitoring*

Test	Recommended frequency

Laboratory studies
  Liver panel with GGT and INR
  CBC/ differential
  Basic metabolic panel
  Immunosuppression trough levels
	Multiple times per week immediately post-transplant, ultimately every 3 months by year 1

Hemoglobin A1c	Every 3 months for first year, then annually
Lipid profile	Annually
Blood pressure	Every visit
24-hour urine protein OR urine protein-to-creatinine ratio	Annual to monitor for proteinuria, especially if treated with mTOR inhibitor
DEXA	Every 2–3 years if normal bone density Annually if low bone density or treated with steroids
Skin survey	Annually
Colonoscopy	Annually if history of inflammatory bowel disease Every 5–10 years if average risk
Cervical cancer screening	Annual Papanicolaou test (with HPV co-testing if ≥30 years old) for 3 years, then every 3 years if normal, at minimum through age 65
Liver biopsy	As indicated by transplant center. Routine protocol biopsies are no longer performed
Abdominal imaging	Yearly to assess vasculature and liver If history of HCC before transplant: Liver protocol CT or MRI q6 months for 3–5 years If recurrent cirrhosis: Liver ultrasound and alpha-fetoprotein every 6 months
Visit to transplant hepatologist	Every week for first 1–3 months, then every 3–12 months depending on stability and co-management setup

*Note testing varies by transplant center and by patient indications

very little data on the use and safety of edible or topical forms of cannabis in this setting. Patients who continue to use these substances against transplant center recommendations and require a second transplant may place their candidacy at risk.

Immunizations

Although this book focuses on the care of post-transplant recipients, it is worth noting that primary care providers should encourage potential liver transplant patients to undergo any necessary vaccinations in the pre-transplant setting since live virus vaccines are contraindicated post-liver transplant. Pre-transplant vaccinations include pneumococcus, hepatitis A virus, HBV, tetanus/diphtheria/pertussis, human papilloma virus, varicella virus, and herpes zoster.

Following transplant, inactivated virus vaccines may be given safely, the exception being the recombinant shingles (herpes zoster) vaccine, because of the potential for its immune response to precipitate rejection. The safety of the shingles vaccine is still being explored at this writing. All recipients should receive an annual influenza vaccination and repeat vaccinations for other diseases at appropriate intervals (e.g., pneumococcus). Vaccination guidelines are in place for the management of transplant recipients [32]. As vaccination recommendations change frequently, primary care providers should check the Centers for Disease Control and transplant guidelines regularly. (See Chap. 12 for further discussion of routine immunizations.)

Cancer Screening

As discussed in other chapters (Chaps. 10 and 12), liver transplant recipients have a dramatically elevated risk of skin cancer, solid organ tumors, and hematologic malignancy. Cancer may develop de novo or recur from prior disease. The incidence of de novo cancer is higher than that seen in the nontransplant population, increasing to 11–20% by 10 years post-transplant. Skin cancers – predominantly squamous and basal cell carcinomas – are the most common malignancy in this population. All liver transplant recipients should undergo annual skin survey, use sunscreen, and avoid sun exposure. Post-transplant lymphoproliferative disorder (PTLD) is associated with EBV. PTLD occurs in 1% of liver transplant recipients by post-transplant year 5 (roughly 2% for individuals without EBV antibodies) [4]. Screening for colon, prostate, and breast cancer is consistent with standard guidelines in most average-risk individuals with the exception of yearly colonoscopy for those with inflammatory bowel disease. Women on long-term immunosuppressive therapy are less likely to clear human papilloma virus (HPV) compared to average risk women, placing them at increased risk for cervical dysplasia and cancer. Women should receive annual cervical cancer screening via Papanicolaou test for 3 years (with HPV co-testing if ≥30 years old), then every 3 years if normal, at minimum through age 65. Surveillance for recurrent HCC is discussed above. Screening for malignancies in the liver transplant recipient is summarized in Table 5.3.

Fertility, Pregnancy, and Breast-Feeding

Liver failure is associated with reduced fertility and sexual dysfunction. Free testosterone levels improve in men and fertility returns in nearly all individuals by 1 year following transplant [33]. Sexual dysfunction may not resolve. Women who conceive after liver transplantation are at increased risk for obstetrical complications (up to 19%), including pregnancy-induced hypertension, pre-eclampsia, low birthweight, preterm delivery, and fetal demise although overall pregnancy outcomes are favorable [34–37].

All premenopausal liver transplant recipients who are at risk for conception should receive counseling to prevent unplanned pregnancy. Preferred contraceptive options include long-acting reversible contraceptives such as intrauterine devices or progesterone implants, barrier methods, progestin-only hormonal contraceptives, and tubal ligation. Combined hormonal contraceptives may be options in patients with stable allograft status and without contraindications such as uncontrolled hypertension or thromboembolic risks, though this should be discussed with the managing hepatologist prior to initiation [38]. Estrogen-containing contraceptives do not appear to significantly affect immunosuppression levels [10]. Emergency contraception appears to be safe in liver transplant recipients [38].

Liver transplant recipients who desire pregnancy should receive pre-conception counseling. Ideally, women should avoid pregnancy for 1–2 years post-transplant to ensure stable liver function and a consistent immunosuppressive regimen [38]. A higher proportion of women who conceive more than a year after transplantation have live births compared to those who conceive sooner (98% vs. 80%) [37]. All women who become pregnant after liver transplantation should be referred to a high-risk obstetrician or maternal-fetal-medicine specialist for management.

Immunosuppression must be continued and managed carefully during pregnancy. Medications with a category D status (known teratogen) should be avoided, particularly mycophenolate mofetil. Immunosuppressants that appear to be relatively safe in pregnancy at contemporary clinical dosing include corticosteroids, azathioprine, cyclosporine, and tacrolimus. Pregnancy is not associated with an increased risk for graft failure, but immunosuppression levels may fluctuate during pregnancy. Allograft function and CNI serum levels should be checked every 4 weeks until 32 weeks and then every 2 weeks until delivery [19]. Allograft function should be checked weekly for at least 1 month after delivery until stability is demonstrated.

Breastfeeding is not contraindicated in the liver transplant recipient. Although no immunosuppressants are labeled for use in lactation, there have been no infant adverse effects reported for breastfeeding with azathioprine, cyclosporine, or tacrolimus, despite trace amounts detectable in breastmilk [39]. Breastfeeding is not recommended with mycophenolate mofetil, everolimus, or sirolimus due to inadequate data on drug excretion in breastmilk [34]. Guidance can be sought though the LactMed database maintained by the National Institutes of Health [40].

Systemic Disease and Overall Health

Obesity and Nutrition

In 2017, 35.9% of liver transplant recipients were obese at the time of transplantation (BMI $\geq$30 kg/m^2) and 14.0% were severely obese (BMI $\geq$35 kg/m^2) [4]. As noted above, the rate of the metabolic syndrome (diabetes, hypertension, obesity, and dyslipidemia) increases after transplant [41]. Additionally, about 20% of lean transplant recipients will become obese by 2–3 years after liver transplantation. Patients should be counseled regarding dietary and lifestyle modifications. Those who are already obese may require referral to a behavioral weight-loss program or nutritionist. Bariatric surgery is not contraindicated in this setting, although the optimal timing and type of procedure is unknown.

Diabetes Mellitus

Diabetes in the post-liver transplant setting consists of pre-existing diabetes mellitus (DM) and new onset diabetes after transplant (NODAT). Insulin-requiring diabetes mellitus persists following transplant, and many patients who were on oral hypoglycemic medications pre-transplant may require transition to insulin. The prevalence of NODAT in the transplant recipient varies from 5% to 26% and may remit over time [14, 42]. Diabetes is negatively associated with all-cause mortality after transplant as well as mortality secondary to cardiovascular, infectious, and allograft-related events [41]. Similar to the non-transplant population, careful control of blood glucose likely decreases both morbidity and mortality. Both DM and NODAT adversely affect long-term survival following liver transplant. Management of post-transplant diabetes is similar to management of diabetes in the general population. Many experts recommend a hemoglobin A1c target of <7.0% as there appears to be no additional advantage to tighter glucose control [19].

Systemic Hypertension

Hypertension develops in the majority of recipients by 2–3 years post-transplant. The presence of hypertension in liver transplant recipients is associated with an increased risk of chronic kidney disease as well as both fatal and nonfatal cardiovascular events. Management is similar to the non-transplant setting. Lifestyle modifications with weight loss and sodium restriction should be encouraged. When treating hypertension, calcium channel blockers are preferred as the first line agent because these drugs counteract the vasoconstrictive effects of the CNIs [43]. Beta-blockers or thiazide diuretics can be added as second-line therapy. Angiotensin receptor blockers and angiotensin-converting enzyme inhibitors should be used cautiously or avoided altogether due to the risk of hyperkalemia and acute kidney injury in combination with calcineurin inhibitors [31].

Dyslipidemia

Dyslipidemia develops in up to 70% of liver transplant recipients [21, 44]. It is associated with an increase in cardiovascular morbidity and mortality. mTOR inhibitors are particularly implicated in causing markedly elevated triglyceride levels. For isolated hypertriglyceridemia, fish oil or fibric acid derivatives can be considered. Medication therapy should be considered if the low-density lipoprotein cholesterol level is >100 mg/dL, with or without elevated triglycerides. HMG-CoA reductase inhibitors are not contraindicated after liver transplantation if otherwise indicated. However, rosuvastatin and pravastatin are preferred due to lower risk of rhabdomyolysis caused by interaction with CNIs. If lipid control is suboptimal, the addition of ezetimibe to the statin can improve results [19].

Chronic Kidney Disease

The majority of liver transplant recipients will develop chronic kidney disease (CKD), with a prevalence of up to 80% [34]. Up to 10% will develop end-stage renal disease during the first 10 years post-transplant, necessitating hemodialysis. The etiology of CKD is multifactorial, including diabetes mellitus, calcineurin inhibitor use, hypertension, and perioperative acute kidney injury. Patients should have careful monitoring of their renal function. Many transplant centers require annual 24-hour urine collection for creatinine clearance and proteinuria. At minimum, a spot urine-protein-to-creatinine ratio should be evaluated at least once a year [45].

Infectious Disease

See Chap. 8 for further details. As noted above, recipients of liver transplantation are most at risk of infectious complications in the first 6 months following transplant. Pathogens seen during this time frame include opportunistic viruses (CMV, HSV, herpes zoster), fungi (*Aspergillus, Cryptococcus*), and bacteria (*Nocardia, Listeria*, mycobacteria). The use of prophylactic anti-infective medications minimizes the risk during this time period. Infectious risk declines after this, and the most common infections are then due to community-acquired pathogens.

Mental Health

Depression is common both before and after liver transplantation. Selective serotonin reuptake inhibitors may be used post-transplant, but side effects and drug interactions should be taken into consideration (see Chap. 3) [31].

Pain Management

Pain is a frequent complaint after liver transplant. Once liver function has been restored, a wide range of pain medications may be used as indicated. Acetaminophen is safe in doses up to 2000 mg per day. Non-steroidal anti-inflammatory drugs interact with calcineurin inhibitors and should be avoided or used with extreme caution to avoid nephrotoxicity [46]. Narcotic pain relievers are discouraged for chronic use in most patients due to tolerance concerns and an unfavorable side effect profile, but they will be metabolized normally by a well-functioning transplanted liver. Patients are frequently severely deconditioned prior to transplantation due to the muscle wasting that occurs in liver failure, as well as the effects of malnutrition and prolonged hospitalizations. Physical therapy and rehabilitation are often beneficial after transplantation to promote improvement in function as well as pain management.

Summary

Liver transplantation is a lifesaving and life-prolonging treatment for patients with liver failure. Long-term survival following transplant is outstanding and patients now routinely live beyond 10 years. Primary care providers are more likely than ever to have liver transplant recipients in their practice and are key to their overall management. In addition to close collaboration between the transplant center and the primary care provider, familiarity with common acute and chronic health issues in the liver transplant recipient is essential for all primary care providers who care for these patients.

References

1. Younossi ZM, Stepanova M, Afendy M, Fang Y, Younossi Y, Mir H, et al. Changes in the prevalence of the most common causes of chronic liver diseases in the United States from 1988 to 2008. Clin Gastroenterol Hepatol. 2011;9(6):524–30 e1; quiz e60.
2. United Network for Organ Sharing. "Transplant trends". Available at: https://unos.org/data/transplant-trends/. Accessed 8 May 2019.

3. Organ Procurement and Transplantation Network. "View Data Reports". Available at: https://optn.transplant.hrsa.gov/data/view-data-reports/nationaldata/. Accessed 13 May 2019.

4. Kim WR, Lake JR, Smith JM, Schladt DP, Skeans MA, Noreen SM, et al. OPTN/SRTR 2017 Annual Data Report: Liver. Am J Transplant. 2019;19(Suppl 2):184–283.

5. Cheung A, Levitsky J. Follow-up of the post-liver transplantation patient: a primer for the practicing gastroenterologist. Clin Liver Dis. 2017;21(4):793–813.

6. Parrish NF, Feurer ID, Matsuoka LK, Rega SA, Perri R, Alexopoulos SP. The changing face of liver transplantation in the United States: the effect of HCV antiviral eras on transplantation trends and outcomes. Transplant Direct. 2019;5(3):e427.

7. McCashland TM. Posttransplantation care: role of the primary care physician versus transplant center. Liver Transpl. 2001;7(11 Suppl 1):S2–12.

8. Kok B, Dong V, Karvellas CJ. Graft dysfunction and management in liver transplantation. Crit Care Clin. 2019;35(1):117–33.

9. Moreno R, Berenguer M. Post-liver transplantation medical complications. Ann Hepatol. 2006;5(2):77–85.

10. Kramer DJ, Siegal EM, Frogge SJ, Chadha MS. Perioperative management of the liver transplant recipient. Crit Care Clin. 2019;35(1):95–105.

11. Guenette A, Husain S. Infectious complications following solid organ transplantation. Crit Care Clin. 2019;35(1):151–68.

12. Duffy JP, Hong JC, Farmer DG, Ghobrial RM, Yersiz H, Hiatt JR, et al. Vascular complications of orthotopic liver transplantation: experience in more than 4,200 patients. J Am Coll Surg. 2009;208(5):896–903; discussion −5.

13. Chascsa DM, Vargas HE. The gastroenterologist's guide to management of the post-liver transplant patient. Am J Gastroenterol. 2018;113(6):819–28.

14. DaVee T, Geevarghese SK, Slaughter JC, Yachimski PS. Refractory anastomotic bile leaks after orthotopic liver transplantation are associated with hepatic artery disease. Gastrointest Endosc. 2017;85(5):984–92.

15. Levitsky J, Goldberg D, Smith AR, Mansfield SA, Gillespie BW, Merion RM, et al. Acute rejection increases risk of graft failure and death in recent liver transplant recipients. Clin Gastroenterol Hepatol. 2017;15(4):584–93. e2.

16. Watt KD, Pedersen RA, Kremers WK, Heimbach JK, Charlton MR. Evolution of causes and risk factors for mortality post-liver transplant: results of the NIDDK long-term follow-up study. Am J Transplant. 2010;10(6):1420–7.

17. Demetris AJ, Murase N, Lee RG, Randhawa P, Zeevi A, Pham S, et al. Chronic rejection. A general overview of histopathology and pathophysiology with emphasis on liver, heart and intestinal allografts. Ann Transplant. 1997;2(2):27–44.

18. Jain A, Demetris AJ, Kashyap R, Blakomer K, Ruppert K, Khan A, et al. Does tacrolimus offer virtual freedom from chronic rejection after primary liver transplantation? Risk and prognostic factors in 1,048 liver transplantations with a mean follow-up of 6 years. Liver Transpl. 2001;7(7):623–30.

19. Lucey MR, Terrault N, Ojo L, Hay JE, Neuberger J, Blumberg E, et al. Long-term management of the successful adult liver transplant: 2012 practice guideline by the American Association for the Study of Liver Diseases and the American Society of Transplantation. Liver Transpl. 2013;19(1):3–26.

20. Dureja P, Mellinger J, Agni R, Chang F, Avey G, Lucey M, et al. NAFLD recurrence in liver transplant recipients. Transplantation. 2011;91(6):684–9.

21. Watt KD, Charlton MR. Metabolic syndrome and liver transplantation: a review and guide to management. J Hepatol. 2010;53(1):199–206.

22. Steenstraten IC, Sebib Korkmaz K, Trivedi PJ, Inderson A, van Hoek B, Rodriguez Girondo MDM, et al. Systematic review with meta-analysis: risk factors for recurrent primary sclerosing cholangitis after liver transplantation. Aliment Pharmacol Ther. 2019;49(6):636–43.

23. Fosby B, Karlsen TH, Melum E. Recurrence and rejection in liver transplantation for primary sclerosing cholangitis. World J Gastroenterol. 2012;18(1):1–15.

24. Edmunds C, Ekong UD. Autoimmune liver disease post-liver transplantation: a summary and proposed areas for future research. Transplantation. 2016;100(3):515–24.
25. Organ Procurement and Transplantation Network. "Policies". Available at: https://optn.transplant.hrsa.gov/media/1200/optn_policies.pdf. Accessed 9 Jun 2019. p. 147–80.
26. Mazzaferro V, Regalia E, Doci R, Andreola S, Pulvirenti A, Bozzetti F, et al. Liver transplantation for the treatment of small hepatocellular carcinomas in patients with cirrhosis. N Engl J Med. 1996;334(11):693–9.
27. Au KP, Chok KSH. Multidisciplinary approach for post-liver transplant recurrence of hepatocellular carcinoma: a proposed management algorithm. World J Gastroenterol. 2018;24(45):5081–94.
28. Lucey MR. Liver transplantation in patients with alcoholic liver disease. Liver Transpl. 2011;17(7):751–9.
29. Kodali S, Kaif M, Tariq R, Singal AK. Alcohol relapse after liver transplantation for alcoholic cirrhosis-impact on liver graft and patient survival: a meta-analysis. Alcohol Alcohol. 2018;53(2):166–72.
30. Lucey MR. In patients with a first episode of severe alcoholic hepatitis non-responsive to medical therapy, early liver transplant increases 6-month survival. Evid Based Med. 2013;18(1):21–2.
31. Malat G, Culkin C. The ABCs of immunosuppression: a primer for primary care physicians. Med Clin North Am. 2016;100(3):505–18.
32. Danziger-Isakov L, Kumar D, Practice AICo. Vaccination of solid organ transplant candidates and recipients: Guidelines from the American society of transplantation infectious diseases community of practice. Clin Transplant. 2019;33:e13563.
33. Armenti VT, Daller JA, Constantinescu S, Silva P, Radomski JS, Moritz MJ, et al. Report from the National Transplantation Pregnancy Registry: outcomes of pregnancy after transplantation. Clin Transpl. 2006;57–70.
34. Sarkar M, Bramham K, Moritz MJ, Coscia L. Reproductive health in women following abdominal organ transplant. Am J Transplant. 2018;18(5):1068–76.
35. Coscia LA, Constantinescu S, Davison JM, Moritz MJ, Armenti VT. Immunosuppressive drugs and fetal outcome. Best Pract Res Clin Obstet Gynaecol. 2014;28(8):1174–87.
36. Prodromidou A, Kostakis ID, Machairas N, Garoufalia Z, Stamopoulos P, Paspala A, et al. Pregnancy outcomes after liver transplantation: a systematic review. Transplant Proc. 2019;51(2):446–9.
37. Kamarajah SK, Arntdz K, Bundred J, Gunson B, Haydon G, Thompson F. Outcomes of pregnancy in recipients of liver transplants. Clin Gastroenterol Hepatol. 2019;17(7):1398–404. e1.
38. Coscia LA, Davison JM, Moritz MJ, Armenti VT. Pregnancy after liver transplantation. In: Cataldo D, editor. Contemporary liver transplantation: the successful liver transplant program. Switzerland: Springer International Publishing; 2017.
39. Constantinescu S, Pai A, Coscia LA, Davison JM, Moritz MJ, Armenti VT. Breast-feeding after transplantation. Best Pract Res Clin Obstet Gynaecol. 2014;28(8):1163–73.
40. Database LDaL. Available at: https://toxnet.nlm.nih.gov/newtoxnet/lactmed.htm. Accessed 5 Jun 2019.
41. Parekh J, Corley DA, Feng S. Diabetes, hypertension and hyperlipidemia: prevalence over time and impact on long-term survival after liver transplantation. Am J Transplant. 2012;12(8):2181–7.
42. Kuo HT, Sampaio MS, Ye X, Reddy P, Martin P, Bunnapradist S. Risk factors for new-onset diabetes mellitus in adult liver transplant recipients, an analysis of the Organ Procurement and Transplant Network/United Network for Organ Sharing database. Transplantation. 2010;89(9):1134–40.
43. Galioto A, Semplicini A, Zanus G, Fasolato S, Sticca A, Boccagni P, et al. Nifedipine versus carvedilol in the treatment of de novo arterial hypertension after liver transplantation: results of a controlled clinical trial. Liver Transpl. 2008;14(7):1020–8.

44. Laish I, Braun M, Mor E, Sulkes J, Harif Y, Ben AZ. Metabolic syndrome in liver transplant recipients: prevalence, risk factors, and association with cardiovascular events. Liver Transpl. 2011;17(1):15–22.
45. Keane WF, Eknoyan G. Proteinuria, albuminuria, risk, assessment, detection, elimination (PARADE): a position paper of the National Kidney Foundation. Am J Kidney Dis. 1999;33(5):1004–10.
46. Benten D, Staufer K, Sterneck M. Orthotopic liver transplantation and what to do during follow-up: recommendations for the practitioner. Nat Clin Pract Gastroenterol Hepatol. 2009;6(1):23–36.
47. Berry PA, Melendez HV, Wendon JA. Postoperative care of the liver-transplant patient. In: O'Donnell JM, Nácul FE, editors. Surgical intensive care medicine. Boston: Springer; 2010.
48. Chan T, DeGiolamo K, Chartier-Plante S, Buczkowski AK. Comparison of three caval reconstruction techniques in orthotopic liver transplantation: a retrospective review. Am J Surg. 2017;2013(5):943–9.

Chapter 6
Primary Care of the Adult Heart Transplant Recipient

Vidang P. Nguyen, Andy Y. Lee, and Richard K. Cheng

Introduction

Heart failure is one of the most common causes of morbidity and mortality throughout the world. With an aging population and advances in treatment options including revascularization, neurohormonal blockade, and advanced device therapies, the prevalence of individuals living with heart failure is increasing [1]. In the United States, people over the age of 40 have a > 20% lifetime risk of developing heart failure [2]. Over 650,000 Americans are newly diagnosed with heart failure each year [3] with a worldwide prevalence of 26 million [4].

The New York Heart Association (NYHA) functional classification system describes patient symptoms: NYHA class I includes asymptomatic patients, with progressive limitation for NYHA class II and III. NYHA class IV includes patients with heart failure symptoms at rest who are unable to perform activities of daily living. In contrast to the NYHA classification, the American College of Cardiology (ACC) and American Heart Association (AHA) have described stages that outline structural changes of chronic heart failure [5]. ACC/AHA stage A and stage B heart failure include asymptomatic patients without and with structural heart changes, respectively. Stage C heart failure patients are those with symptoms of heart failure and stage D with refractory end-stage heart failure.

V. P. Nguyen
Cedars-Sinai Heart Institute, Cedars-Sinai Medical Center, Los Angeles, CA, USA

A. Y. Lee · R. K. Cheng (✉)
Department of Medicine, Division of Cardiology, University of Washington Medical Center, Seattle, WA, USA
e-mail: ayenlee@uw.edu; rkcheng@uw.edu

© Springer Nature Switzerland AG 2020
C. J. Wong (ed.), *Primary Care of the Solid Organ Transplant Recipient*,
https://doi.org/10.1007/978-3-030-50629-2_6

When patients with heart failure progress to stage D, specialist intervention is often required due to the high morbidity and mortality in this population. There is increasing use of mechanical circulatory support (MCS) devices such as the left ventricular assist device (LVAD). MCS devices have been used as both "destination therapy" (not eligible for heart transplantation) as well as "bridge-to-transplantation" (BTT) [6]. While successive generations of MCS devices have improved outcomes since the first LVAD was approved in 2004, the overall survival for heart transplantation exceeds that of destination therapy. Therefore, heart transplantation remains a critically important option for patients with stage D heart failure.

Heart transplantation was first made possible with the development of vascular anastomosis for the transplanted heart. Alexis Carrel and Charles Guthrie first described this technique in 1905 when they succeeded in transplanting a heart from one dog to another by connecting the donor's heart vessels to the recipient's carotid artery and jugular vein [7, 8]. Despite a successful anastomosis with adequate coronary artery perfusion, the heart was not able to provide circulatory assistance [9].

The surgical technique was continuously refined leading to the first orthotopic heart transplantation by Dr. Christiaan Barnard in 1967. With evolving surgical techniques and advances in immunosuppression, post-heart transplant survival has improved to approximately 90% at 1 year, with a median survival of greater than 15 years [10–12]. Heart transplantation volumes have grown in recent years with over 5000 transplantations performed worldwide in 2016 [13].

The increasing numbers of patients who have received heart transplantation, combined with improving survival, will lead to a growing population of heart transplant recipients expected to be at least partly evaluated and treated in the primary care setting.

Pre-transplant Course

While this chapter focuses on the treatment of post-heart transplant recipients, it is useful to review the patient's pre-transplant course.

Common Indications

Coronary artery disease is one of the most important contributors to heart failure, with highly prevalent population-attributable risk factors of hypertension, diabetes mellitus, obesity, and smoking. Therefore, it is no surprise that ischemic heart disease is the most common diagnosis in patients being evaluated for heart transplantation in developed countries. With improved revascularization techniques over the last several decades, the proportion of patients with ischemic cardiomyopathy being transplanted has decreased over time, whereas the non-ischemic cardiomyopathy (NICM), valvular cardiomyopathy, and restrictive cardiomyopathy (RCM) cohorts are increasing [10]. Patients with RCM and congenital heart disease (CHD) have a higher risk of death on the waitlist for heart transplantation as they typically do not benefit from MCS therapies [14]. As would be expected, the proportion of HF etiology varies by age group, with NICM being the most dominant diagnosis until age 60, after which ischemic cardiomyopathy becomes more common; this mirrors the findings of most large heart failure registries. In contrast, the diagnoses of RCM, CHD, hypertrophic cardiomyopathy, and myocarditis are more common among heart transplant recipients than the general heart failure population [10]. Following heart transplantation, there is a low likelihood of the underlying disease returning in the transplanted heart for most causes of heart failure. The risk is higher for certain diagnoses, such as giant cell myocarditis where one third of patients will have recurrence of the disease [15]. Even though quality of life and longevity are generally improved, there is an inherent trade-off to heart transplantation: replacing the symptoms and morbidity of chronic HF with the lifelong need for immunosuppression and its associated risks. Common indications for transplantation in North America are shown in Table 6.1.

Pre-transplant Workup and Treatment:
- Comprehensive cardiac evaluation is performed to identify potentially reversible causes prior to referral for heart transplantation. It is worthwhile reviewing a patient's indication, as well as his or her time on the waiting list, and any prior complications. Specific indications for heart transplantation include cardiogenic shock requiring inotropic therapy or MCS, refractory New York Heart Association (NYHA) functional class IV heart failure, end-stage congenital heart disease, poor cardiopulmonary exercise test (CPET) results, an anticipated one-year survival less than 80% due to progressive heart failure, refractory angina without options for further revascularization, or intractable life-threatening arrhythmias.
- Comorbid conditions that may be a barrier to heart transplantation are assessed thoroughly prior to transplantation, including cerebrovascular disease, peripheral vascular disease, chronic kidney disease (CKD), diabetes, obesity, cancer, and chronic infections.
- Mechanical circulatory support: LVAD as BTT may be a reasonable strategy for patients who are either anticipated to have a long wait time on the transplant list due to blood group and/or body type or as a "bridge-to-candidacy" for those who are not candidates at the time of evaluation, but have modifiable barriers that can

Table 6.1 Indications for heart transplantation in transplanted recipients 2009–2017 in North America [13]

Non-ischemic cardiomyopathy	49%
Ischemic cardiomyopathy	35%
Restrictive cardiomyopathy	4%
Retransplant	3%
Congenital heart disease	3%
Hypertrophic cardiomyopathy	3%
Valvular heart disease	2%
Other	1%

be overcome [16]. Despite a slightly higher 90-day post-transplant mortality, BTT LVAD patients have a similar 5-year conditional survival (conditional on 90-day survival), functional status, and quality of life in comparison to "de novo" primary heart transplant patients [17]. Review of the pre-transplant course should include whether the patient had MCS therapy prior to transplantation.

Anatomy

Early heart transplantations used the biatrial technique, consisting of a simple anastomosis at the mid-level of the left atrium and right atrium. The pulmonary artery and aorta were anastomosed above the semi-lunar valves. This surgical technique often led to long-term complications of tricuspid regurgitation and atrial arrhythmias due to distortion of the right atrial anatomy. It was replaced by the bicaval technique several years later, which preserves the donor right atrium by anastomosis of the superior and inferior vena cava (Fig. 6.1) [18].

Anastomoses (Bicaval Method):
- The donor left atrium is anastomosed to the recipient's pulmonary veins. In the most common method, the recipient's left and right paired pulmonary veins are

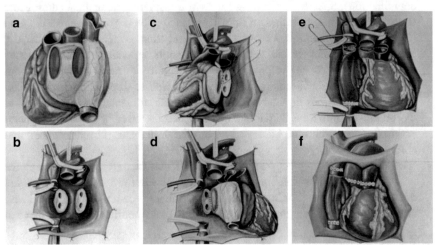

Fig. 6.1 Step-wise illustration of the bicaval orthotopic heart transplantation. (**a**) Donor heart (posterior view). The superior vena cava is divided above the azygos vein and the distal end is enlarged by cutting into the azygos vein stump. The pulmonary veins are joined on each side. (**b**) Recipient heart explanted. The vena cavae are transected circumferentially. The left atrium is completely removed, leaving only two left atrial cuffs, which include the ostia of the pulmonary veins. (**c**) Left pulmonary venous anastomosis to the corresponding orifice in the left atrium of the donor's heart. (**d**) Right pulmonary venous anastomosis. (**e**) The superior and inferior venae cavae are anastomosed in an end-to-end fashion. (**f**) Aorta and pulmonary artery reconstructed, and implantation of the cardiac allograft completed. (Adapted from Magliato and Trento [104]. Reprinted with permission)

left attached to a portion of the recipient left atrium—an atrial "cuff," to facilitate anastomosis to the donor left atrium. The donor left atrium pulmonary vein orifices are joined to create a matching left and right anastomosis for the atrial cuffs.

- The inferior and superior vena cavae are joined end-to-end between the donor and recipient.
- The donor aorta above the level of the coronary sinuses is anastomosed end-to-end to the recipient's ascending aorta.
- The donor main pulmonary artery is anastomosed end-to-end to the recipient's main pulmonary artery.

Certain patients who do not have favorable anatomy for a bicaval anastomosis may still require biatrial anastomosis. In extremely rare occasions, a heterotopic heart transplantation may be necessary, which involves preservation of the native heart and engraftment of the donor allograft in parallel to allow for biventricular support. This technique is considered in select situations when the donor is considered unstable or the recipient is rapidly deteriorating or has fixed pulmonary hypertension, and for this reason heterotopic heart transplantations carry a particularly high mortality when compared to orthotopic heart transplantation [19].

Denervation:
Because the native innervation of the heart muscle is transected at the time of cardiac transplant, the cardiac sympathetic and parasympathetic responses are lost. As the vagus nerve predominantly modulates the sinoatrial and atrioventricular node to slow native heart rate, parasympathetic activity is lost and the donor heart becomes persistently tachycardic at rest. Moreover, due to loss of sympathetic innervation, the donor heart rate is high at baseline and becomes reliant on circulating catecholamines in order to provide a sympathetic response, particularly during exertion. Therefore, heart transplant recipients frequently develop chronotropic incompetence and diminished exercise capacity. Due to this denervation, the ability to sense angina is lost, and patients may develop obstructive cardiac allograft vasculopathy without appreciable clinical symptoms after transplantation. Another impact of denervation is the loss of nocturnal decreases in blood pressure [20]. Interestingly, some recipients may reinnervate the donor heart, but this response is variable and unpredictable [21, 22]. In studies where this controversial phenomenon is described, reinnervation is not seen until at least 18 months post-transplant and increases with time. In addition, cardiac reinnervation is more likely to occur in young recipients who have an uncomplicated implantation surgery and low frequency of rejection [12].

Pericardium:
During heart transplantation surgery, the pericardium is left open and not typically reanastomosed. However, pericardial effusions are not uncommon post-transplant, especially during the acute post-operative period and as a result of early endomyocardial biopsies [23]. Chronic pericardial complications are uncommon, but there have been rare reports of constrictive pericarditis causing heart failure symptoms in heart transplant recipients in the late post-transplant period. This diagnosis may be

confounded by chronic graft rejection and thus the optimal management of these patients is uncertain [24].

Typical Anti-rejection Course

While anti-rejection medication therapy will typically be managed by the cardiologist or heart transplant specialist, it is important for primary care providers to understand treatments that the heart transplant recipient will likely be receiving. This section focuses on standard induction regimens and maintenance immunosuppression, with alternative regimens for special circumstances. Medications are discussed in Chap. 3. Almost all the medications used in heart transplantation are common to other solid organ transplants, with particular overlap with renal transplantation, with which many regimens are shared.

Induction

The purpose of induction for heart transplantation is to provide intense immunosuppression early after transplant, when the risk for rejection is the highest. The routine use of induction therapy with T-cell-depleting agents remains controversial among heart transplantation programs. Based on the International Society for Heart and Lung Transplantation (ISHLT) transplant registry data from 2018, approximately 50% of heart transplant recipients receive induction, with no difference in survival for induction compared to no induction [17]. Induction is associated with lower rates of acute rejection and thereby decreased risk of long-term cardiac allograft vasculopathy. Induction may also allow for a delay in loading with calcineurin inhibitors in patients with renal dysfunction. However, studies have suggested higher rates of infection and long-term malignancy after induction therapy due to this early depletion of T-cells and associated augmented immunosuppression [25–28].

The ISHLT guidelines suggest that induction can be useful for patients who are at (a) increased risk for rejection or (b) high risk for renal dysfunction in order to delay introduction of calcineurin inhibitors. However, the routine use of induction in all patients has not been shown to be superior to no induction, and no randomized trial has been completed at this time [29]. Overall, the use of induction immunosuppression varies by transplant center and may take into account individualized patient risk factors such as younger age, race, history of HLA mismatch, and history of long-term support on LVAD. Hence, a selective approach may yield the best risk/benefit ratio [30].

One common induction regimen is to routinely administer rabbit anti-thymocyte globulin (rATG) immediately after heart transplantation in uncomplicated cases. Rabbit ATG may be avoided in patients who have significant bleeding or an open chest due to concerns for potentially worsening instability or infection. In such cases, basiliximab, an IL-2 antagonist, may be used for induction. Epstein-Barr virus (EBV) mismatched patients (Donor+/Recipient−) will typically not receive induction due to increased risk for long-term post-transplant lymphoproliferative disorder (PTLD). Other protocols exist for induction that utilize rituximab or alemtuzumab but are less commonly used and are beyond the scope of this chapter.

Maintenance

The calcineurin inhibitors (CNIs), tacrolimus and cyclosporine, remain the cornerstone of maintenance immunosuppression in heart transplant recipients. Tacrolimus is associated with increased risk of diabetes mellitus, but less hypertension and dyslipidemia relative to cyclosporine (Table 6.2). Calcineurin inhibitors can result in long-term renal dysfunction. In the current era, tacrolimus is preferred over cyclosporine in heart transplant recipients due to lower rates of rejection [31, 32].

Antimetabolite agents are frequently utilized in combination with calcineurin inhibitors. These medications include azathioprine, mycophenolate mofetil (MMF) or mycophenolic acid (MPA). All antimetabolite agents can lead to significant myelosuppression and leukopenia. Mycophenolate formulations are preferred over

Table 6.2 Common side effects of immunosuppression

Drug	Side effects	Monitoring
Calcineurin inhibitors		
Tacrolimus (FK-506)	Nephrotoxicity, neurotoxicity, hyperkalemia, hypomagnesemia, hypertension, hyperglycemia, anorexia, alopecia, hemolytic uremic syndrome, hyperlipidemia	Basic metabolic panel, lipid panel, liver function tests, blood glucose, 12-hour trough FK levels
Cyclosporine (CSA)	Nephrotoxicity, neurotoxicity, hyperkalemia, hypomagnesemia, hypertension, hyperglycemia, hirsutism, hemolytic uremic syndrome, gum hyperplasia, hyperlipidemia	Basic metabolic panel, lipid panel, liver function tests, blood glucose, 12-hour trough CSA levels
Alkylating agents		
Cyclophosphamide	Leukopenia, anemia, thrombocytopenia, alopecia, hemorrhagic cystitis	Complete blood count
DNA synthesis blockade/anti-metabolites		
Azathioprine (AZA)	Leukopenia, anemia, thrombocytopenia, alopecia, nausea/vomiting, pancreatitis, hepatotoxicity	Baseline TPMT activity, complete blood count
Mycophenolate mofetil (MMF)	Leukopenia, anemia, thrombocytopenia, nausea/vomiting, diarrhea	Complete blood count, MPA levels
Mycophenolate sodium (MPA)	Leukopenia, anemia, thrombocytopenia. Lesser degree of nausea/vomiting and diarrhea compared to MMF	Complete blood count, MPA levels

(continued)

Table 6.2 (continued)

Drug	Side effects	Monitoring
Non-specific inhibitor of immune function		
Corticosteroids	Mood disturbance, hypertension, hyperglycemia, hallucinations, decreased wound healing, edema, moon facies, acne, increased appetite, weight gain, osteoporosis, cataracts	Lipid panel, blood glucose
mTOR inhibitors		
Sirolimus	Peripheral edema, hyperlipidemia, leukopenia, anemia, thrombocytopenia, mouth ulcers, decreased wound healing, dermatitis, joint pain, pleural effusions, proteinuria	Complete blood count, lipid panel, liver function test
Everolimus	Peripheral edema, hyperlipidemia, leukopenia, anemia, thrombocytopenia, mouth ulcers, decreased wound healing, dermatitis, joint pain, pleural effusions, proteinuria Black box warning: increased risk of mortality if used as de novo immunosuppression within the first 3 months of heart transplantation	Complete blood count, lipid panel, liver function test
Anti-lymphocyte polyclonal antibody		
Anti-thymocyte globulin (ATG)	Leukopenia, anemia, thrombocytopenia, infusion associated reactions—headache, fevers, chills, blood pressure changes, shortness of breath, rarely cytokine release syndrome	Complete blood count, CD3 count
Anti-HLA antibody modulator		
Immunoglobulin (IVIG)	Hypotension, shortness of breath, acute renal failure, possible anaphylaxis, chest tightness, tachycardia, headache, nausea, fever, chills, back pain	Administer in a monitored setting, epinephrine should be available

azathioprine as they are associated with better survival and lower rates of rejection [33]. Mycophenolate mofetil commonly causes nausea and/or diarrhea, and when patients cannot tolerate these gastrointestinal side effects, the MMF dose may be divided (e.g., changing from twice daily to a lower dose administered four times daily) or patients can be switched to MPA, an enteric-coated formulation that may be better tolerated. MMF is typically the initial form of mycophenolate chosen due to lower cost and greater availability. Although both mycophenolate and azathioprine can increase the risk for post-transplant malignancy, antimetabolite agents have remained one of the mainstay drugs in heart transplantation [34].

A standard maintenance immunosuppression regimen at time of discharge after heart transplantation commonly consists of tacrolimus, MMF, and prednisone. During the first year, patients are routinely tapered off prednisone starting at 1 month after heart transplantation with dose reductions after each endomyocardial biopsy (EMB). The majority of patients are able to discontinue corticosteroids after 6–12 months post-transplant. In patients with prior episodes of graft rejection or who develop antibodies against the donor graft, lifelong maintenance prednisone therapy should be considered.

A common long-term maintenance regimen consists of two complementary immunosuppression agents, typically tacrolimus and MMF. There are specific circumstances when alternative regimens besides the combination of tacrolimus and mycophenolate are utilized. Patients with renal dysfunction are sometimes switched to a calcineurin inhibitor-sparing regimen using either sirolimus or everolimus, antiproliferative agents in the mammalian target of rapamycin (mTOR) inhibitor class. Because sirolimus can potentiate the nephrotoxic effects of calcineurin inhibitors, a common regimen pairs sirolimus with MMF. Sirolimus can be associated with lower extremity edema, myelosuppression, dyslipidemia, oral ulcerations, and impaired wound healing [35]. Everolimus is less commonly used in the heart transplant population, partly because of a United States Food and Drug Administration (FDA) black box warning of increased mortality for patients started on high-dose everolimus as de novo immunosuppression within the first 3 months of heart transplantation. However, it appears to be safe in the longer-term setting [36]. Everolimus has a similar side effect profile to sirolimus, but they have not been directly compared in head to head trials. Since mTOR inhibitors can worsen proteinuria, both are contraindicated in the presence of significant baseline proteinuria.

For heart transplant recipients with cardiac allograft vasculopathy, transitioning to mTOR inhibitors can slow disease progression and decrease acute coronary events [35, 37, 38]. A nonrandomized, retrospective study demonstrated that conversion of CNI to sirolimus prior to 2 years after transplant was associated with attenuated CAV progression and improved survival compared to conversion after 2 years. However, the impact on pre-existing CAV disease remains unclear [39, 40]. Hence, the heart transplant specialist may transition patients who demonstrate evidence of early CAV on angiography to either a sirolimus/MMF regimen, with the additional benefit of protecting renal function, or a tacrolimus/sirolimus regimen for those at high risk for rejection. In addition to the benefits of preserving renal function and decreasing the risk of CAV, switching to mTOR inhibitors may decrease the risk for post-transplant de novo malignancy [41–43].

There is some evidence that select patients may be able to receive tacrolimus monotherapy [44]. Additional studies are needed to further assess the safety and potential candidates for tacrolimus monotherapy. Tacrolimus monotherapy can be considered in carefully selected patients at low risk for rejection after 1 year post-heart transplant who do not tolerate a second immunosuppressive agent.

Long-Term Dose Adjustments

Tacrolimus is dosed based on time since heart transplantation and routine monitoring consists of checking serum trough levels. Higher therapeutic targets are used early after transplantation and decreased over the first year to a long-term maintenance level. In patients with clinical rejection, relatively higher target levels are maintained compared to standard protocol. Conversely, the use of mycophenolic acid levels for dosing MMF or MPA remains controversial, and most centers do not adjust dosing of MMF or MPA based on serum levels although a high trough can indicate toxicity. Dose reductions are considered in patients who experience significant myelosuppression (see Chap. 3).

The Cylex Immuknow™ assay is a T-cell functional assay that is a marker of T-cell activation by measuring ATP release from activated CD4+ T-lymphocytes [45]. Limited data suggest that this assay may predict infectious risk in heart transplant recipients, although its association with rejection risk is inconclusive [46]. The Cylex™ assay can provide a target immunological response zone for minimizing infectious risk due to over-suppression of T-cells in heart transplant recipients, and some transplant centers titrate the MMF dose based on the Cylex™ assay [47]. For example, older patients who have a degree of immune senescence typically have low Cylex™ values and may require dose reduction of their immunosuppression.

Rejection

Pathophysiology

There are two classes of rejection in cardiac transplantation: acute cellular rejection (ACR) and antibody-mediated rejection (AMR) (Table 6.3). ACR is the more common form of rejection and is defined as a T-cell mediated immune response to donor cardiomyocytes with lymphocyte and macrophage infiltration leading to myocardial injury and eventual necrosis. AMR is a more obscure and indolent form of rejection as defined by graft dysfunction due to capillary injury related to antibody binding and complement activation [48]. The identification of AMR is transplant

Table 6.3 Summary of acute cellular rejection vs. antibody-mediated rejection

	Acute cellular rejection	Antibody-mediated rejection
Mechanism	T-cell-mediated reaction against donor cardiomyocytes Monocytes > PMNs	Antibody binding of donor HLA, leading to complement activation and endothelial injury PMNs > monocytes
Histology	Interstitial infiltration	Capillary inflammation, C4d positive staining
Time course	Acute	Indolent
Presentation	Graft dysfunction, heart failure and arrhythmias	Graft dysfunction, heart failure and arrhythmias
Monitoring	Endomyocardial biopsy, gene expression profiling	Donor-specific antibody (anti-HLA antibody) levels
Treatment	High dose corticosteroids, T-cell-depleting therapy (such as ATG)	IVIG, plasmapheresis, rituximab, bortezomib, steroids, ATG can be considered

center-dependent due to variations in histopathologic staining and laboratory diagnosis protocols. As a result, less is known regarding the true etiology and effective treatment for AMR.

Clinical Presentation

Although ACR and AMR differ at a histopathologic level, clinically they may be indiscernible except that ACR tends to be more acute in nature, whereas AMR is a more indolent process. Rejection typically occurs between 6 months and 1 year following heart transplantation and may largely be subclinical. Possible presenting symptoms include atrial or ventricular tachyarrhythmias and heart failure symptoms such as elevated jugular venous pressure, peripheral fluid retention, hypotension, peripheral hypoperfusion, orthopnea, paroxysmal nocturnal dyspnea, and presyncope or syncope. It is important to emphasize that angina is rare in this cohort of patients due to the lack of cardiac innervation, and rejection may in fact be clinically silent.

Evaluation

When there is clinical concern for allograft rejection, the patient should be urgently referred to their transplant center, and diagnostic testing should be performed immediately. The workup should include transthoracic echocardiography, electrocardiogram (ECG), cardiac enzyme testing, donor-specific antibody testing, and right heart catheterization with endomyocardial biopsy. There are newer strategies to the diagnosis of rejection which are in development, such as cell-free DNA (discussed in sect. Rejection Surveillance) and cardiac magnetic resonance imaging [49].

Rejection Surveillance

Cellular Rejection

Similar to induction use, a large degree of center-by-center variation exists in surveillance of allograft rejection. Surveillance methods include endomyocardial biopsy (EMB), as well as growing interest in the use of noninvasive methods to minimize risk and exposure associated with EMB.

- Endomyocardial biopsy: EMB remains the gold standard for rejection monitoring early after heart transplantation. The ISHLT guidelines for cellular rejection surveillance and an example protocol are shown in Table 6.4 [29].

Table 6.4 Endomyocardial biopsy guidelines for routine rejection surveillance

	ISHLT guidelines	Example EMB protocol (varies by center)
0–12 months	Periodic EMB	First month: 1 week, 2 weeks, 4 weeks Month 2–5: Monthly until 6 months Month 6–12: Every 2 months
1–5 years	Every 4–6 months in patients with risk factors for late rejection	Year 2: Every 3 months Year 3–5: Every 6 months
>5 years	Not well defined	No routine surveillance unless high risk with a recent history of rejection, in which case the schedule is individualized based on risk

- Gene expression profiling (GEP): Gene expression profiling can be considered as an alternative to EMB to monitor for ACR in appropriate low-risk patients at 2 months to 5 years post HTx. GEP (commercially available as Allomap®) is an FDA-approved, noninvasive alternative to EMB for monitoring for ACR in heart transplant recipients. The Allomap® test assesses gene expression by measuring RNA from peripheral blood mononuclear cells, with possible scores ranging from 0 to 40. Higher scores are correlated with histologic rejection. An Allomap® score below 30 has a negative predictive value of 99.6% for significant histologic rejection. Identification of genes that correlate with rejection was developed in the CARGO study (Cardiac Allograft Rejection Gene Expression Observation) which showed that such gene expression techniques could discriminate between no rejection versus moderate-to-severe rejection [50]. Trials of heart transplant recipients who are at low risk of rejection have shown that the use of GEP monitoring was noninferior to EMB for the development of rejection with hemodynamic compromise, graft dysfunction, death, or retransplantation [51]. Thus, GEP may be an option for noninvasive monitoring for cellular rejection that is non-inferior to EMB and, based on the trials' inclusion criteria, may be useful as soon as approximately 2 months after heart transplantation. Subsequent trials have sought to clarify whether the thresholds should change based on time interval post-transplant [52] or patient risk factors [53]. Additionally, GEP score-to-score variability is associated with future events of allograft dysfunction or death, and this risk is independent of the probability of rejection at the time of testing [54]. Since the Allomap® platform is based on GEP of leukocytes, other clinical events that impact the immune system can alter the score such as an acute infection. Hence, the assay is best used at steady-state on an outpatient basis.
- Cell-free DNA (cfDNA): There is growing interest in using cell-free DNA as a noninvasive test for monitoring for rejection. cfDNA is released from tissues in the presence of cell turnover or pathological cell death, which can result from myocardial injury in the case of heart transplant, ischemia, infarction, or any rejection. cfDNA testing can be used to detect donor-specific signatures by a novel method of comparing DNA variability, and in addition, cfDNA levels will increase in the setting of acute rejection [55, 56]. cfDNA levels have been found

to correlate to events of biopsy-based diagnosis of acute cellular rejection, and in a subset of patients, cfDNA was also increased in the setting of antibody-mediated rejection [57]. Although approved for use in renal transplantation, the use of cfDNA for monitoring in heart transplant recipients is not yet FDA-approved and is an area of active research [5].

- Cardiac imaging: The use of cardiac imaging to monitor for rejection is discussed later in this chapter and often viewed as a complementary modality, but does not replace EMB or GEP.

Antibody-Mediated Rejection

In the contemporary era, antibody-mediated rejection is increasingly recognized as an important contributor to adverse outcomes after heart transplantation. Antibody-mediated rejection develops when recipient antibodies are directed against donor HLA antigens on the endothelium, resulting in complement activation, an inflammatory response, and tissue injury. Antibody-mediated rejection is confirmed pathologically by intravascular macrophages and positive staining for C4d/C3d, which indicates complement activation [58].

Donor-specific antibodies (DSAs): Independent from a pathologic diagnosis of antibody-mediated rejection, the presence of circulating donor-specific antibodies is associated with allograft injury, antibody-mediated rejection, cardiac allograft vasculopathy, and decreased survival [58, 59]. Testing for donor-specific antibodies is performed by checking the recipient's blood for antibodies against HLA antigens that are known to be part of the donor's HLA profile. Despite consensus on the importance of monitoring these anti-HLA antibodies, additional work is necessary to determine the optimal monitoring schedule and to clarify indications to treat if donor-specific antibodies are found. A consensus conference from ISHLT recommended that donor-specific antibodies should be routinely tested at 2 weeks, then 1, 3, 6, and 12 months post-transplant, annually and when antibody-mediated rejection is suspected [48]. An American Heart Association consensus statement recommends checking for donor-specific antibodies at 3, 6, and 12 months and annually or in accordance with the transplant center's surveillance protocol. This statement also recommends staining for C4d and C3d on the EMB sample during the first 90 days after heart transplantation or when AMR is suspected, and it is reasonable to perform immunopathologic assessment for AMR at months 3, 6, and 12 [58]. Additionally, it is reasonable to not only screen for DSAs as part of routine post heart transplant follow-up at time intervals based on the ISHLT and AHA recommendations, but also to consider screening more frequently for patients that are at increased risk for AMR (history of allosensitization, multiparity, multiple blood transfusions, history of LVAD).

Overall Rejection Surveillance Strategies

The overall surveillance methods will vary by transplant center and individual patient factors. As described above, the transplant center will monitor for both acute cellular rejection as well as antibody-mediated rejection. In some cases, patients may be able to transition to noninvasive testing alone; for example, a patient whose Allomap® scores are stable and correlate well with endomyocardial biopsy results, and who have higher risk of complications from biopsies may be able to be monitored with noninvasive surveillance alone. However, patients with variable Allomap® scores and positive donor-specific antibodies will likely need to continue routine endomyocardial biopsies. Additionally, Allomap® is used as a screening tool and is not confirmatory for acute cellular rejection; for patients with a change in their Allomap® score from baseline, they still require further evaluation with a biopsy for confirmation. Allomap® only screens for cellular rejection and does not detect antibody-mediated rejection. For the primary care provider, reviewing the transplant team's documentation is useful to make sure that the patient is following the recommended surveillance protocol.

Graft Function Surveillance

In addition to evaluating the heart transplant recipient for rejection, the transplant team routinely monitors for overall donor allograft function by echocardiography and right heart catheterization. The surveillance frequency is protocolized according to time lapsed following transplantation. As such, the intervals of surveillance may differ depending on whether complications arose at different time periods.

Impact of Timing

The interval of time between heart transplantation and onset of graft dysfunction may make a particular diagnosis more likely (Fig. 6.2). For example, because the first year following heart transplantation is the highest risk period for rejection, right heart catheterization is frequently performed in conjunction with EMB to assess graft hemodynamics to guide dose reductions in immunosuppression. Imaging assessment of graft function does not replace invasive surveillance for rejection given the lack of strong correlation between echocardiographic data and evidence of rejection on EMB [60]. However, any graft dysfunction as defined by ventricular dysfunction or abnormal hemodynamics may suggest pathology including rejection. Likewise, an ECG is useful to detect arrhythmias such as atrial fibrillation, atrial flutter, or premature atrial contractions, which may reflect graft dysfunction and/or possible rejection as well [61]. However, a screening ECG is not sensitive for graft dysfunction or rejection.

Fig. 6.2 Overview of the most common causes of death depending on the time from heart transplantation

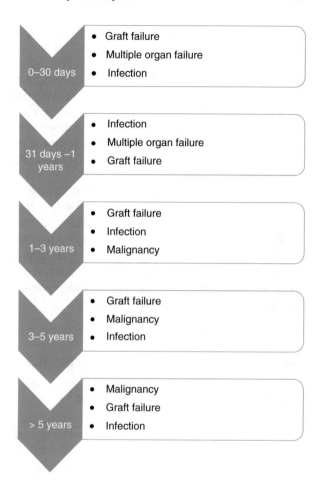

| 0–30 days | • Graft failure • Multiple organ failure • Infection |

| 31 days –1 years | • Infection • Multiple organ failure • Graft failure |

| 1–3 years | • Graft failure • Infection • Malignancy |

| 3–5 years | • Graft failure • Malignancy • Infection |

| > 5 years | • Malignancy • Graft failure • Infection |

Echocardiograms and coronary angiograms are routinely performed to ensure stable graft function. In particular, CAV is an independent etiology of graft dysfunction [62]. Both noninvasive and invasive methods are vital for the detection of CAV and carry treatment implications that will be discussed later. Most donor organs are from healthy donors free of major comorbidities. However, with the continued expansion of the donor population, more grafts may be from older donors with comorbidities. More donor hearts may therefore be predisposed to graft dysfunction or CAV and monitoring may need to be intensified for the recipient.

Cardiac Imaging and Biomarkers

Echocardiography has been the primary noninvasive imaging modality for cardiologists in the last several decades and its utility applies to heart transplant recipients as well. Advanced techniques within echocardiography, including stress echocardiography, diastolic function measurements, and myocardial strain, adds further value in the assessment of graft function, and abnormal results may increase suspicion for acute allograft rejection [63–65]. Some centers will perform a limited echocardiogram with every EMB for graft surveillance. At the authors' transplant center, echocardiograms are obtained 1 week after transplant, repeated prior to discharge, then at 1 year and yearly thereafter, and additionally as needed if there are clinical changes or concern for rejection or graft dysfunction. An echocardiogram can be a useful adjunct test in cases suspicious for rejection, but does not replace endomyocardial biopsy, which allows for pathological assessment.

Although data suggest that cardiac magnetic resonance imaging (CMR) is a useful tool for cases of rejection, not many programs have utilized CMR. Currently, EMB remains the gold standard for suspected rejection [49]. Overall, guideline-driven protocols for graft function surveillance are lacking, and many centers rely on their noninvasive laboratory expertise to develop a protocol suitable for their needs. Per the ISHLT guidelines, the use of echocardiography or cardiac biomarkers (BNP, troponin-I) in place of performing endomyocardial biopsy for routine rejection monitoring is not recommended [29].

Complications Specific to Heart Transplantation

Cardiac Allograft Vasculopathy (CAV)

- Background: CAV is a complication unique to heart transplantation involving obstruction of the coronary arteries of the allograft. Although it may appear similar to coronary artery disease, its mechanistically different pathophysiology dictates a unique diagnostic and treatment approach. With recent improvements in immunosuppression strategies and therapies to extend life after heart transplant, CAV is becoming increasingly recognized, with 46.8% of patients having CAV 10 years after heart transplant, independently contributing to about 1–2% of deaths [66].
- Pathophysiology: CAV is a complex process that is driven in part by immunological factors. At the time of heart implantation, the donor heart sheds HLA antigens and heat shock proteins that lead to activation of T-cells within the recipient. Donor arrest, ischemic time, and reperfusion trigger an inflammatory process within the endothelial cell layers of the graft and ultimately lead to smooth muscle proliferation, lipid deposition, and thrombosis [67]. This process is indolent in nature, and in contrast to atherosclerotic coronary artery disease, CAV leads to diffuse narrowing of large epicardial coronary vessels and "pruning" of the distal vessels and smaller coronary arteries. Histologically, CAV involves thickening of the intima whereas typical coronary atherosclerosis disrupts the intima (Figs. 6.3 and 6.4).

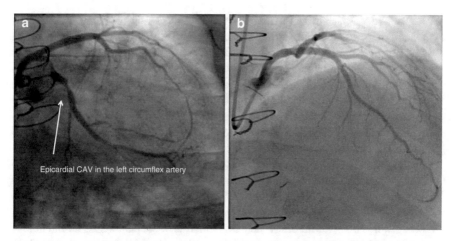

Epicardial CAV in the left circumflex artery

Fig. 6.3 (**a**) Coronary angiogram in the right anterior oblique (RAO) caudal view demonstrates epicardial CAV involving the left circumflex artery. (**b**) An RAO cranial view of the same patient, which shows the left anterior descending artery free of obstructive disease. These angiographic findings are from a heart transplant recipient who presented with dyspnea on exertion and fatigue. His echocardiogram showed hypokinesis of the lateral wall

Fig. 6.4 Intravascular ultrasound of the same patient's left anterior descending artery (LAD), showing 3 mm of CAV at the level of the LAD just distal to the take-off of the diagonal branch

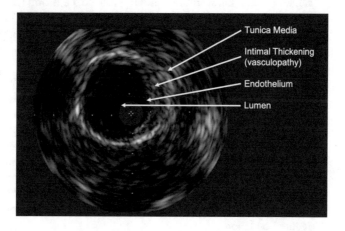

Tunica Media

Intimal Thickening (vasculopathy)

Endothelium

Lumen

- Monitoring: Because of these histological differences, transplant centers may elect to monitor for CAV not only angiographically but also with intravascular ultrasound (IVUS). IVUS has the advantage of assessing both the luminal diameter and cross-sectional area as well as the ability to perform virtual histology of the vessel including intimal and adventitial thickness and in certain circumstances differentiation between donor atherosclerosis and CAV.
- Prognostic significance: Depending on the findings at the time of coronary angiogram or IVUS, CAV may be graded for management implications and prognostic value [68, 69]. Increased vessel thickness and luminal narrowing is associated with higher risk of needing retransplantation and mortality. The typical time-course for CAV is variable but more common at later time periods after transplantation, while earlier onset CAV carries a worse prognosis [70].

- Risk factors: Risk factors associated with CAV include older age, CMV mismatch, diabetes, hypertension, dyslipidemia, and any prior episodes of rejection despite successful treatment. Thus, early prevention of any rejection episode is crucial and early intervention is indicated to prevent the longstanding effects on the allograft endothelium. Although some of these risk factors overlap with those related to coronary atherosclerosis, it is important to understand that CAV is an immunologically-mediated process possibly related to a mismatch of HLA subtypes; moreover, donor-specific antibodies, when present, are often associated with CAV and carry a worse prognosis [71, 72]. Once CAV has developed, treatment is often ineffective and thus, prevention is key.
- Non-invasive imaging: In addition to coronary angiography and IVUS, noninvasive methods such as stress echocardiography, CMR, and coronary computed tomography angiography (CCTA) have been shown to have utility. Preferences for specific choice of modality vary between transplant centers. Although noninvasive stress testing is not considered the gold standard for the detection of CAV, their application in the monitoring of CAV progression is still beneficial as CAV may occur subclinically [68]. More recently, multi-detector gated CCTA allows for accurate imaging of the coronary macrovasculature and may be useful for the detection of CAV in appropriate patients [73]. However, more work is needed to refine the imaging resolution and to produce a uniform CAV diagnosis with this noninvasive method. Positron emission tomography (PET) based stress testing can provide incremental information by estimating coronary flow reserve of the vasculature, which can reflect not only macrovascular disease but microvascular disease.
- Guidelines: The ISHLT guidelines assign a class I recommendation to perform coronary angiography either annually or biannually for the first 3–5 years after heart transplantation. Non-invasive stress testing with imaging is an option in patients who are unable to tolerate invasive coronary angiography (Class IIa-B recommendation). As the utility of CCTA continues to improve, it may eventually become a reasonable option in patients who have normal heart rates, as tachycardia can distort CCTA acquisition (Class IIb-C recommendation). Certain centers may elect to perform initial coronary angiography at 4–6 weeks posttransplant with or without IVUS to evaluate for donor CAD (Class IIa-B recommendation).
- Prevention: The 2010 ISHLT guidelines recommend cardiovascular risk factor modification and statin therapy for the prevention of CAV. Pravastatin is the best-studied medication for post-transplant patients and is preferred in terms of safety and drug-drug interactions. There is limited data on high-intensity statin use in this cohort and thus should be considered on a case-by-case basis with the clinician and transplant pharmacist.
- Treatment: CAV is treated by modifying the anti-rejection regimen by replacing one of the immunosuppression medications with a proliferation signal inhibitor such as sirolimus or everolimus (Class IIa-B recommendation). With obstructive CAV, percutaneous coronary intervention (PCI) or coronary artery bypass graft-

ing (CABG) may be performed as palliation, although the only definitive treatment for severe CAV is retransplantation (Class IIa-C recommendation). PCI for CAV may be done with bare-metal or drug-eluting stents and typically requires a year of dual anti-platelet therapy. Repeat coronary angiography should be performed 6 months after PCI to assess stent patency and exclude progression of disease [29]. Although evidence supports the use of statin drugs to prevent CAV, it is less certain whether intensifying statin therapy after CAV develops is effective. Once CAV develops, switching to mTOR inhibitors is considered to slow CAV progression, however these patients may still develop graft failure over time.

De Novo Coronary Atherosclerosis

In addition to CAV, there is a possibility of developing new onset atherosclerotic coronary artery disease (CAD).

Pre-existing coronary artery disease in the donor is unlikely, as donor hearts with pre-existing CAD are typically not accepted for transplantation. However, with increasing efforts to expand the donor pool, the use of older donors will likely increase the prevalence of donor atherosclerosis. Potential heart donors with risk factors for CAD such as diabetes, hypertension, male gender, tobacco use, and adult age should ideally have a coronary angiogram to screen for CAD prior to accepting the organ. Transplant centers may elect to perform coronary angiography 4–6 weeks following heart transplantation to screen for donor coronary atherosclerosis if not performed prior to transplantation.

More commonly, de novo coronary atherosclerosis may occur similar to the general population. As discussed above, donor atherosclerosis may be distinguished from CAV by intravascular imaging techniques such as IVUS and optical coherence tomography (OCT). In general, statins, which have been shown to decrease progression of CAV, should also limit the progression of existing coronary atherosclerosis. Pravastatin and rosuvastatin are preferred over other statins in heart transplant recipients due to a lower risk of interactions with other medications. Consistent with recommendations for the general population, lifestyle modification and tobacco cessation are of the utmost importance in limiting the progression of heart disease. Pharmacologic management of hyperlipidemia consists of statin therapy as discussed in other areas of this chapter, and ezetimibe and PCSK-9 inhibitors have demonstrated safety in this population as well [74, 75].

Arrhythmias

Monitoring the electrical activity of the donor graft is vital for detecting any potential pathology associated with graft function. Possible types of cardiac arrhythmias include atrial and ventricular arrhythmias.

- Supraventricular tachycardias (SVTs) may include regular, narrow complex rhythms including atrial flutter, atrioventricular reentrant tachycardia (AVRT) or atrioventricular nodal reentrant tachycardia (AVNRT). These re-entrant rhythms are often related to myocardial scar near the suture-line as a result of cardiac surgery or native pathways within the donor graft. Electrophysiologists may manage persistent arrhythmias with either antiarrhythmic medical therapy or catheter ablation [76].
- The occurrence of atrial fibrillation following cardiac transplantation is less common than re-entrant rhythms since donors tend to be young without substantial atrial fibrosis. When atrial fibrillation does occur, there is an association with allograft rejection—therefore, any new onset atrial fibrillation must prompt further work up by the transplant cardiologist [61]. In the event that a non-heart transplant center is responsible for treating a heart transplant recipient for rapid ventricular rates in the acute setting, beta-blockers and nondihydropyridine calcium channel blockers are permissible but must be used with caution. In particular, there is upregulation of beta-adrenergic receptors in the donor allograft due to chronic lack of innervation, which may predispose to particular sensitivity to beta-blockade. Depending on the temporality of the atrial arrhythmia, antiarrhythmic medications may be used for a limited duration. Digoxin and atropine are not effective given their chronotropic effects being mediated by the parasympathetic nervous system in a denervated heart.
- Atrial bradyarrhythmias may be a cause for concern, as denervation of the heart normally leads to higher resting heart rates as discussed previously. For this reason, bradyarrhythmias require prompt cardiology consultation. In the acute post-heart transplant period, sinus node dysfunction such as sinus bradycardia, sinus arrhythmia, or sino-atrial block may occur. Sinus node dysfunction is due to a combination of cardiac denervation, ischemia at the time of organ procurement, myocardial edema along the conduction system, and surgical technique (in particular with patients receiving a biatrial anastomosis) [77]. Most atrial bradyarrhythmias are self-resolving and are treated medically in the early post-heart transplant period with chronotropic agents such as isoproterenol, theophylline, or terbutaline. However, if atrial bradyarrhythmias persist without evidence of recovery, a permanent pacemaker may be indicated for advanced conduction disease. Fortunately, permanent pacemaker implantation does not impact long-term outcomes [78]. As the bicaval anastomosis is increasingly favored over the biatrial anastomosis, the incidence of heart transplant recipients requiring a permanent pacemaker is low.

Valvular Disease

Valvular heart disease is seldom seen in the heart transplant recipient due to careful donor selection in which donor hearts with significant valve dysfunction are not procured. The most common post-heart transplant valve dysfunction is tricuspid regurgitation, which is frequently iatrogenic as a complication from EMB or damage during the time of surgery. New right-sided heart failure symptoms in a heart transplant recipient following routine EMB should prompt a referral for urgent echocardiogram and follow up with their heart transplant physician. Prior case studies suggest that tricuspid valve repair or replacement is feasible and may be beneficial if severe tricuspid regurgitation occurs [79].

Complications and Clinical Pearls

At outpatient primary care visits, primary care providers can assist with evaluation of the heart transplant recipient's graft function, adherence to medications, and preventive health measures, in addition to managing comorbidities. At each outpatient visit, the following should be assessed (Table 6.5):

Table 6.5 *Clinical pearls for the primary care provider—evaluation of the heart transplant recipient at outpatient clinic visits* (see text for details; also see Chap. 2 for discussion of general history-taking)

Initial visit:
Review pre-transplant and initial post-transplant course:
Indication for transplant, type of induction immunosuppression
Early complications (surgical complications, infection, rejection)
Symptoms, exam, medications, laboratory studies, metabolic complications, and general preventive health similar to follow-up visits
Follow-up visits:
Dyspnea, angina, edema, dizziness, palpitations, syncope; localizing symptoms of infection or fever
Symptoms:
Exam: Heart rate (may have high resting heart rate—determine the baseline), blood pressure, cardiovascular (higher than usual resting heart rate, or tachyarrhythmias should be evaluated further), lungs, abdomen, volume status
Medications:
Review immunosuppressive medication regimen, adherence, side effects, goal trough levels
Review opportunistic infection prophylaxis, if prescribed
Aspirin and statin unless contraindicated
Endocarditis prophylaxis
Laboratory and other studies:
Adherence to surveillance schedule set forth by the transplant team; surveillance for rejection (endomyocardial biopsy, gene expression profiling (ACR), donor-specific antibodies (AMR))
Surveillance for graft function
Renal function, complete blood count (monitor for cytopenia)
Metabolic complications:
Assess and treat if present, including hypomagnesemia, gout, osteopenia or osteoporosis, diabetes, hypertension, chronic kidney disease
General preventive health:
Immunizations, skin exams, other routine screening

- History: At the initial visit, the pre-transplant history and post-transplant course should be reviewed. Patients should be asked about cardiac and pulmonary symptoms, adherence to medications, and ensure that they understand the surveillance schedule developed by their transplant cardiologist. Knowledge of common side effects of anti-rejection medications can assist in asking about adherence. Symptoms of infection or malignancy should be asked.
- Examination: As with all patients, vital signs and clinical stability should be assessed. As noted above, the denervated heart will have a higher than normal resting heart rate. Chest exam will show scars from the median sternotomy, smaller scars at the site of prior chest tubes or mediastinal drains. In most cases, cardiac implantable electronic devices (CIED) such as implantable pacemakers or cardioverter-defibrillators are removed at the time of surgery. However, in cases of significant device fibrosis, the leads may be left behind. For heart transplant recipients who need an MRI, it is important to determine if they have any retained wires from prior CIED devices. New cardiac murmurs, signs of volume overload, or a new S3 gallop, should be evaluated expediently by the transplant team.
- Medications: In addition to asking about adherence, the medication list should be reviewed for aspirin and statin therapy, both of which should be present unless there are contraindications or intolerances. Look for medications that may have been prescribed by other providers for potential drug-drug interactions with the anti-rejection medications. In most cases, heart transplant recipients should not take over-the-counter supplements unless approved by their transplant team.
- Laboratory and other studies: While the primary care provider will likely not be ordering the routine surveillance blood tests, echocardiograms, and biopsies, tests performed by the transplant team should be reviewed.
- Assess and treat metabolic complications: Diabetes, hypertension, chronic kidney disease, osteopenia, and osteoporosis are common. For more details, see Chap. 11.

Prevention and Treatment of Infections

In the early period after transplantation, common complications and morbidity are driven by graft dysfunction, rejection and infection. Long-term immunosuppression puts the recipient at a higher risk for infection [80], and the risk of death from infection is higher in older patients due to age-related senescence of the immune system [81, 82].

All age-appropriate vaccines are administered, including vaccines against pneumococcal pneumonia, tetanus, hepatitis A and hepatitis B, although live vaccines are contraindicated and the recombinant herpes zoster vaccine is not recommended because of concern that its immune response may increase the risk of rejection. Heart transplant recipients should avoid exposure to known sick contacts (see Chaps. 8 and 12).

Cardiovascular disease:

The underlying disease process and clinical course for CAV were described earlier in this chapter.

- HMG CoA reductase inhibitors (statins): Statins should be prescribed for all heart transplant recipients for primary prevention regardless of baseline lipid profile. Both pravastatin and simvastatin have been shown to decrease the risk of CAV if started soon after heart transplantation [83]. In addition, pravastatin has the additional benefit of inhibiting natural killer cells to reduce the inflammatory process [84]. Because of drug interactions with calcineurin inhibitors, simvastatin is not recommended first-line, although patients who have been taking it along with their immunosuppressant medications without problem may continue it. Pravastatin and rosuvastatin (if a higher potency statin is indicated) are preferred statins in most solid organ transplant recipients because of a lower risk of drug-drug interactions.
- Aspirin: Aspirin is also prescribed for all heart transplant recipients.
- Symptoms of heart disease should be assessed at each visit.
  - CAV may present with very vague or atypical symptoms. Therefore, it is essential to have a high level of suspicion for CAV in heart transplant recipients who present with new-onset shortness of breath, angina, or malaise.
  - Heart failure symptoms or signs should be discussed urgently with the transplant team, as the patient may be having graft dysfunction.
  - As noted above, the resting heart rate may be elevated due to lack of vagus stimulation. If the heart rate is elevated over baseline, however, an ECG should be obtained to look for both worsening sinus tachycardia as well as other arrhythmias, both of which can be associated with rejection
- As discussed previously, CAV and rejection may be asymptomatic, resulting in the need for surveillance even without symptoms.

Chronic Kidney Disease

Due to CNI-associated nephrotoxicity and pre-transplant cardiorenal syndrome in many cases, CKD is common in patients after heart transplantation and is seen in two thirds of patients 10 years after transplantation. After a decade, 10% of patients will either require dialysis or consideration for renal transplantation [85]. The development of CKD is associated with non-modifiable risk factors, such as age, gender, and time since transplant as well as modifiable risk factors, including diabetes and hypertension [86, 87]. While the transplant cardiologist will tailor the immunosuppression regimen if needed because of the onset or worsening of CKD, the primary care provider can collaborate in the management of hypertension, diabetes, and other comorbidities that affect renal function. All heart transplant recipients should avoid any use of non-steroidal anti-inflammatory medications.

Cancer

Malignancy is the fourth most common cause of death after transplantation and occurs in the setting of chronic immunosuppression [13]. Skin malignancies are the most common cancer followed by lymphoma, and any history of pre-transplant malignancy increases the risk of malignancy after transplant [88]. Male gender and recipient age > 50 years may also be associated with an increased risk of cancer [89]. Heart transplant recipients should receive an annual dermatology examination. The risk of malignancy may potentially be mitigated by varying the immunosuppression regimen. Emerging data show that conversion to sirolimus is associated with decreased risk for de novo malignancies and post-transplant lymphoproliferative disorders, with improved long-term survival; however, routine use is limited by medication intolerance due to side effects. Sirolimus is not used as first-line therapy as it impairs wound healing immediately post-transplant, and there has been mixed data suggesting a possible increased risk for rejection compared to CNI's [43] (see Chap. 10).

Hypertension

Due to abnormal cardiorenal neuroendocrine reflexes, heart transplant recipients have a decreased natriuretic and diuretic response and therefore have particularly salt-sensitive hypertension [90]. In addition, blood pressure is often elevated due to the impact of calcineurin inhibitors and glucocorticoids. Cyclosporine and tacrolimus are associated with an especially high incidence of hypertension after transplantation [91]. Although glucocorticoids are weaned over time, long-term calcineurin inhibitor therapy is expected. Treatment of hypertension is especially important because both calcineurin inhibitors and systemic hypertension can contribute to the development of chronic kidney disease [92]. The author group typically favors treating hypertension with respect to comorbidities: i.e., ACE-inhibitor (ACEi) or ARB in patients with diabetes or CKD, thiazide diuretics for patients with a tendency to retain volume. Amlodipine or hydralazine is considered for patients who are intolerant or do not benefit from those therapies. There are data suggesting that ACEi/ARB or dihydropyridine calcium channel blockers may protect against CNI-induced vasoconstriction, so these medications may be considered preferentially. Beta blockers are uncommonly used after heart transplantation, but when used for hypertension, a nonselective agent such as carvedilol is preferred. Caution must be exercised with patients early-post heart transplant with beta-blockers as many patients are dependent on their higher heart rate and can be very sensitive to beta-blockers from upregulation of their beta-receptors due to relying on circulating catecholamines driven by donor heart denervation. It is important to avoid agents that may be implicated in drug-drug interactions such as diltiazem which is a CYP3A4 inhibitor (see Chap. 11).

Diabetes

Due to glucocorticoid therapy, heart transplant recipients are at risk for hyperglycemia and diabetes. Although diabetes may resolve over time as patients are weaned off their steroids, calcineurin inhibitors may cause ongoing post-transplant diabetes (PTDM). The risk of developing PTDM parallels the degree of pre-transplant glucose intolerance and confers an increased long-term mortality risk in heart transplant recipients [93, 94]. However, with improved PTDM management, this mortality risk can be mitigated [95]. For primary care providers, strict glucose control should be considered, even if insulin therapy is required. Treatment of PTDM mirrors that of non-transplant cardiac patients and includes insulin, glipizide, glinides, thiazolidinediones if graft function is normal, and metformin if tolerated by the renal function. (See Chap. 11).

Infectious Endocarditis Prophylaxis

Compared to the general population, heart transplant recipients have a higher incidence of infective endocarditis (IE) [96]. Although the risk of dental procedures is not well known, infective endocarditis in the transplanted heart can have devastating effects and is associated with increased mortality. Based on the 2007 AHA guidelines, heart transplant recipients should receive infective endocarditis prophylaxis for all dental procedures that involve manipulation of dental tissues [97]. A suggested regimen is amoxicillin 2000 mg given orally 1 hour prior to dental procedures.

Pregnancy

Pregnancy is generally not encouraged in women of child-bearing age after heart transplantation. Nevertheless, if a patient desires pregnancy, she should discuss with her heart transplant specialist about her individualized risks, and in most cases, perinatal care should be coordinated by a multidisciplinary team of providers, including a transplant cardiologist, maternal fetal medicine specialist, neonatologist, psychologist, and social worker [98]. Throughout pregnancy and in the immediate post-partum period, the patient should be closely monitored for graft dysfunction and rejection. We recommend close monitoring of the left ventricular function. As most immunosuppressive therapy regimens have some degree of teratogenic potential, certain changes can be made to increase the chance of successful pregnancy [99]. Given the rare occurrence of pregnancy in this population, no official guidelines exist on this topic. Mycophenolate should be stopped and the patient can often be maintained on tacrolimus monotherapy.

Activity and Exercise

As with other patients who undergo open-heart surgery, there are strict sternotomy precautions following discharge from the hospital. During this early recovery period, patients are most likely primarily cared for by the transplant team. Following heart transplantation, patients are referred to cardiac rehabilitation on discharge. Although rehabilitation has not been shown to improve quality of life at 1 year, exercise-based cardiac rehabilitation does improve exercise capacity in the recovery period [100]. Due to the issues of denervation and chronotropic incompetence, patients should warm up prior to physical activity to stimulate catecholamine circulation and increase their heart rate. Abrupt transition from stop-to-start may not be well tolerated due to the lack of normal sympathetic innervation. When the heart transplant recipient returns to primary care, the primary care provider should review the transplant team's recommendations for activity level for a given patient.

Diet

Most end-stage heart disease patients experience cardiac cachexia prior to heart transplantation, and as patients recover from their surgery, this condition typically reverses with improved functional status [101]. Dedicated dietary counseling may improve metabolic derangements and should be considered [102]. For prevention of infection, heart transplant recipients should not consume raw meats or raw fish. Any meat from a deli should be microwaved prior to consumption. Early after transplant, patients must follow a carbohydrate-managed diet while they are on high-dose glucocorticoids, and although the glucocorticoid dose is typically weaned over time, risk of diabetes persists and patients should still have a heart healthy diet without excessive carbohydrates. Many patients require additional dietary modifications if they develop chronic kidney disease. Salt should be avoided in the presence of fluid retention and hypertension.

Case Studies

1. A 40-year-old man underwent heart transplant 6 months ago and now presents to the primary care setting with diarrhea. He had end-stage heart failure due to familial cardiomyopathy, and was bridged with LVAD prior to transplantation. His initial course was complicated by early graft dysfunction, but this improved several days after surgery. He was discharged to home and has had regular follow-up with the transplant team. His routine surveillance for rejection has been negative. He is CMV D+/R−. He now has frequent episodes of watery diarrhea,

up to eight episodes per day, without abdominal pain, melena, hematochezia, nausea, or emesis. His weight has been stable. He has no chest pain, dyspnea, or fever. On examination he is afebrile with a normal blood pressure and a heart rate of 90 which is baseline for him since transplantation. His cardiac, pulmonary, and abdominal exams are normal.

How should this patient be managed?

In a heart transplant recipient who presents with diarrhea, it is important to exclude infection. If the patient is stable, a serum cytomegalovirus (CMV) DNA quantification test should be sent, as well as a stool enteric pathogen panel. Stool pathogen panels vary by laboratory—for acute diarrhea, a standard bacterial panel should be tested; if recent antibiotics or hospitalization, then *Clostridium difficile* PCR should be tested. Testing for parasitic infections should strongly be considered for chronic diarrhea, especially in endemic regions or if there are any exposures to susceptible food or water sources. Diagnosis of CMV colitis is confirmed on pathology—therefore consultation with a gastroenterologist may be needed to perform a colonoscopy. The transplant team should be alerted to this workup, and if testing is negative, they may consider reassessing his medications, as mycophenolate mofetil and magnesium oxide are common causes of diarrhea in transplant recipients. Unstable patients should be transferred to an acute care setting such as the emergency department in case volume resuscitation or a more rapid workup and treatment are needed.

In his case, the infectious studies are negative. He is switched from MMF to MPA and his magnesium supplementation is changed to a slow-release formulation. In addition, he is prescribed loperamide as needed and supplemental fiber. On a follow-up phone call several days later, the patient notes his stools are much improved (see also Chap. 9).

2. A 69-year-old man with history of ischemic cardiomyopathy undergoes heart transplantation. He received rATG induction and was started on a standard regimen of tacrolimus, MMF, and prednisone. His initial course was notable for leukopenia thought to be secondary to the rATG induction. He required temporarily holding and then dose reduction of his mycophenolate mofetil; additionally, valganciclovir was stopped, sulfamethoxazole/trimethoprim was switched to dapsone, and his counts recovered. Eight months later, he presents to primary care and asks to review his most recent labs. He had been seen in urgent care for a respiratory infection and had a CBC drawn. His respiratory symptoms have since resolved.

The primary care provider reviews his transplant course to date, notable for no rejection episodes and good graft function. His laboratory studies show a white blood cell count of 1300/µl and an absolute neutrophil count of 700/µl.

How should this patient be managed?

There are many potential causes of cytopenias in the heart transplant recipient. Leukopenias may be caused by several factors. rATG induction is a common cause of leukopenia in patients early post-HTx. The primary care provider is likely not involved closely in care at that point in time, but if there are episodes of rejection requiring additional rATG, then PCPs should be aware that recurrent leukopenia can occur.

In addition, other routine post-transplant medications that can result in neutropenia include MMF, prophylactic valganciclovir, and sulfamethoxazole/trimethoprim. The medication list should be reviewed for the presence of any non-transplant medications that may cause cytopenias themselves or have drug interactions with the transplant medications. In a stable patient, the CBC should be repeated. If persistent or severe leukopenia is seen, then the PCP should discuss this urgently with the transplant team. The PCP should not adjust any transplant medications without consultation.

In this case, the patient's MMF was held, but he continued to have recurrent leukopenia when rechallenged. Based on the TICTAC study and his advanced age, his transplant team transitioned him to tacrolimus monotherapy, which in turn increases his baseline risk for rejection. He does well on monotherapy without any clinical rejection. If there were concern for rejection on monotherapy going forward, an alternative regimen would be tacrolimus in combination with sirolimus with close monitoring of renal function, diabetes, and wound healing. Conversely, azathioprine would not be a good option as it is also myelosuppressive.

Case #3

A 40-year-old woman with a history of non-ischemic cardiomyopathy underwent heart transplantation. Her post-transplant course was unremarkable.

One year later, she presents with progressive dyspnea on exertion and fatigue. She denies any lower extremity edema, abdominal bloating, palpitations, presyncope or syncope. She has consistently taken all her anti-rejection medications. Her examination shows normal lung and heart exam, no peripheral edema, or elevated jugular venous pressure.

How should this patient be managed?

An ECG should be obtained in clinic. A routine chest X-ray and laboratory studies to look for anemia should be obtained. If the patient is unstable or develops progressive shortness of breath, then more urgent in evaluation in an emergency setting should be facilitated. This patient's presentation is concerning for cardiac allograft vasculopathy given her symptoms without any signs of heart failure. As she is clinically stable, an expedited outpatient workup may be performed. The transplant cardiologist should be contacted.

In this case, an urgent echocardiogram is obtained and shows new hypokinesis of the lateral wall. She undergoes urgent cardiac catheterization and is found to have left circumflex disease consistent with CAV. Unfortunately, despite percutaneous coronary intervention, she develops progressive, diffuse coronary vasculopathy and ultimately undergoes retransplantation.

Conclusion

Survival following heart transplantation continues to improve over time [13]. The median survival is expected to be 15 years in the current era [103]. Following heart transplantation, most patients experience a significant improvement in their quality of life. However, close monitoring for complications and preventive healthcare remains essential to maintain this quality of life. Primary care providers can contribute greatly in the assessment and management of the health of heart transplant recipients as they partner with the transplant team.

Acknowledgments We would like to thank Beatrice S. Wong, PharmD, for reviewing the accuracy of information in this chapter. We would also like to thank the University of Washington Heart Transplant Team, including the physicians, coordinators, and allied staff, for their collaborative care for our patients.

References

1. Metra M, Teerlink JR. Heart failure. Lancet (London, England). 2017;390(10106):1981–95.
2. Djoussé L, Driver JA, Gaziano JM. Relation between modifiable lifestyle factors and lifetime risk of heart failure. JAMA. 2009;302(4):394–400.
3. Curtis LH, Whellan DJ, Hammill BG, Hernandez AF, Anstrom KJ, Shea AM, et al. Incidence and prevalence of heart failure in elderly persons, 1994-2003. JAMA Intern Med. 2008;168(4):418–24.
4. Ambrosy AP, Fonarow GC, Butler J, Chioncel O, Greene SJ, Vaduganathan M, et al. The global health and economic burden of hospitalizations for heart failure: lessons learned from hospitalized heart failure registries. J Am Coll Cardiol. 2014;63(12):1123–33.
5. Yancy CW, Jessup M, Bozkurt B, Butler J, Casey DE Jr, Drazner MH, et al. 2013 ACCF/ AHA guideline for the management of heart failure: a report of the American College of Cardiology Foundation/American Heart Association Task Force on practice guidelines. Circulation. 2013;128(16):e240–327.
6. Ciarka A, Edwards L, Nilsson J, Stehlik J, Lund LH. Trends in the use of mechanical circulatory support as a bridge to heart transplantation across different age groups. Int J Cardiol. 2017;231:225–7.
7. Krau SD. The evolution of heart transplantation. Crit Care Nurs Clin North Am. 2000;12(1):1–9.
8. Hardy JD. Landmark perspective. Transplantation of blood vessels, organs, and limbs. JAMA. 1983;250(7):954–7.
9. DiBardino DJ. The history and development of cardiac transplantation. Tex Heart Inst J. 1999;26(3):198–205.
10. Lund LH, Edwards LB, Dipchand AI, Goldfarb S, Kucheryavaya AY, Levvey BJ, et al. The Registry of the International Society for Heart and Lung Transplantation: thirty-third adult heart transplantation report-2016; focus theme: primary diagnostic indications for transplant. J Heart Lung Transplant. 2016;35(10):1158–69.
11. McKellar S. Clinical firsts—Christiaan Barnard's heart transplantations. N Engl J Med. 2017;377(23):2211–3.
12. Bengel FM, Ueberfuhr P, Hesse T, Schiepel N, Ziegler SI, Scholz S, et al. Clinical determinants of ventricular sympathetic reinnervation after orthotopic heart transplantation. Circulation. 2002;106(7):831–5.
13. Khush KK, Cherikh WS, Chambers DC, Goldfarb S, Hayes D Jr, Kucheryavaya AY, et al. The International Thoracic Organ Transplant Registry of the International Society for Heart

and Lung Transplantation: thirty-fifth adult heart transplantation report-2018; focus theme: multiorgan transplantation. J Heart Lung Transplant. 2018;37(10):1155–68.

14. Hsich EM, Rogers JG, McNamara DM, Taylor DO, Starling RC, Blackstone EH, et al. Does survival on the heart transplant waiting list depend on the underlying heart disease? JACC Heart Fail. 2016;4(9):689–97.

15. Kandolin R, Lehtonen J, Salmenkivi K, Raisanen-Sokolowski A, Lommi J, Kupari M. Diagnosis, treatment, and outcome of giant-cell myocarditis in the era of combined immunosuppression. Circ Heart Fail. 2013;6(1):15–22.

16. Zimpfer D, Zrunek P, Sandner S, Schima H, Grimm M, Zuckermann A, et al. Post-transplant survival after lowering fixed pulmonary hypertension using left ventricular assist devices☆. Eur J Cardiothorac Surg. 2007;31(4):698–702.

17. Suarez-Pierre A, Zhou X, Fraser CD 3rd, Grimm JC, Crawford TC, Lui C, et al. Survival and functional status after bridge-to-transplant with a left ventricular assist device. ASAIO J. 2018;65:661.

18. Badano LP, Miglioranza MH, Edvardsen T, Colafranceschi AS, Muraru D, Bacal F, et al. European Association of Cardiovascular Imaging/Cardiovascular Imaging Department of the Brazilian Society of Cardiology recommendations for the use of cardiac imaging to assess and follow patients after heart transplantation. Eur Heart J Cardiovasc Imaging. 2015;16(9):919–48.

19. Sekela ME, Smart FW, Noon GP, Young JB. Attenuation of waiting time mortality with heterotropic heart transplantation. Ann Thorac Surg. 1992;54(3):547–51.

20. Braith RW, Wood CE, Limacher MC, Pollock ML, Lowenthal DT, Phillips MI, et al. Abnormal neuroendocrine responses during exercise in heart transplant recipients. Circulation. 1992;86(5):1453–63.

21. Bengel FM, Ueberfuhr P, Ziegler SI, Nekolla S, Reichart B, Schwaiger M. Serial assessment of sympathetic reinnervation after orthotopic heart transplantation. A longitudinal study using PET and C-11 hydroxyephedrine. Circulation. 1999;99(14):1866–71.

22. Bernardi L, Valenti C, Wdowczyck-Szulc J, Frey AW, Rinaldi M, Spadacini G, et al. Influence of type of surgery on the occurrence of parasympathetic reinnervation after cardiac transplantation. Circulation. 1998;97(14):1368–74.

23. Hauptman PJ, Couper GS, Aranki SF, Kartashov A, Mudge GH Jr, Loh E. Pericardial effusions after cardiac transplantation. J Am Coll Cardiol. 1994;23(7):1625–9.

24. Bansal R, Perez L, Razzouk A, Wang N, Bailey L. Pericardial constriction after cardiac transplantation. J Heart Lung Transplant. 2010;29(3):371–7.

25. Swinnen LJ, Costanzo-Nordin MR, Fisher SG, O'Sullivan EJ, Johnson MR, Heroux AL, et al. Increased incidence of lymphoproliferative disorder after immunosuppression with the monoclonal antibody OKT3 in cardiac-transplant recipients. N Engl J Med. 1990;323(25):1723–8.

26. Prieto M, Lake KD, Pritzker MR, Jorgensen CR, Arom KV, Love KR, et al. OKT3 induction and steroid-free maintenance immunosuppression for treatment of high-risk heart transplant recipients. J Heart Lung Transplant. 1991;10(6):901–11.

27. Beniaminovitz A, Itescu S, Lietz K, Donovan M, Burke EM, Groff BD, et al. Prevention of rejection in cardiac transplantation by blockade of the interleukin-2 receptor with a monoclonal antibody. N Engl J Med. 2000;342(9):613–9.

28. Penninga L, Moller CH, Gustafsson F, Gluud C, Steinbruchel DA. Immunosuppressive T-cell antibody induction for heart transplant recipients. Cochrane Database Syst Rev. 2013;(12):CD008842.

29. Costanzo MR, Dipchand A, Starling R, Anderson A, Chan M, Desai S, et al. The International Society of Heart and Lung Transplantation Guidelines for the care of heart transplant recipients. J Heart Lung Transplant. 2010;29(8):914–56.

30. Higgins R, Kirklin JK, Brown RN, Rayburn BK, Wagoner L, Oren R, et al. To induce or not to induce: do patients at greatest risk for fatal rejection benefit from cytolytic induction therapy? J Heart Lung Transplant. 2005;24(4):392–400.

31. Grimm M, Rinaldi M, Yonan NA, Arpesella G, Arizon Del Prado JM, Pulpon LA, et al. Superior prevention of acute rejection by tacrolimus vs. cyclosporine in heart transplant recipients--a large European trial. Am J Transplant. 2006;6(6):1387–97.
32. Kobashigawa JA, Miller LW, Russell SD, Ewald GA, Zucker MJ, Goldberg LR, et al. Tacrolimus with mycophenolate mofetil (MMF) or sirolimus vs. cyclosporine with MMF in cardiac transplant patients: 1-year report. Am J Transplant. 2006;6(6):1377–86.
33. Kobashigawa J, Miller L, Renlund D, Mentzer R, Alderman E, Bourge R, et al. A randomized active-controlled trial of mycophenolate mofetil in heart transplant recipients. Mycophenolate Mofetil Investigators. Transplantation. 1998;66(4):507–15.
34. Youn JC, Stehlik J, Wilk AR, Cherikh W, Kim IC, Park GH, et al. Temporal trends of De Novo malignancy development after heart transplantation. J Am Coll Cardiol. 2018;71(1):40–9.
35. Keogh A, Richardson M, Ruygrok P, Spratt P, Galbraith A, O'Driscoll G, et al. Sirolimus in de novo heart transplant recipients reduces acute rejection and prevents coronary artery disease at 2 years: a randomized clinical trial. Circulation. 2004;110(17):2694–700.
36. Potena L, Pellegrini C, Grigioni F, Amarelli C, Livi U, Maccherini M, et al. Optimizing the safety profile of Everolimus by delayed initiation in De Novo heart transplant recipients: results of the prospective randomized study EVERHEART. Transplantation. 2018;102(3):493–501.
37. Eisen HJ, Tuzcu EM, Dorent R, Kobashigawa J, Mancini D, Valantine-von Kaeppler HA, et al. Everolimus for the prevention of allograft rejection and vasculopathy in cardiac-transplant recipients. N Engl J Med. 2003;349(9):847–58.
38. Raichlin E, Bae JH, Khalpey Z, Edwards BS, Kremers WK, Clavell AL, et al. Conversion to sirolimus as primary immunosuppression attenuates the progression of allograft vasculopathy after cardiac transplantation. Circulation. 2007;116(23):2726–33.
39. Asleh R, Briasoulis A, Kremers WK, Adigun R, Boilson BA, Pereira NL, et al. Long-term sirolimus for primary immunosuppression in heart transplant recipients. J Am Coll Cardiol. 2018;71(6):636–50.
40. Gullestad L, Eiskjaer H, Gustafsson F, Riise GC, Karason K, Dellgren G, et al. Long-term outcomes of thoracic transplant recipients following conversion to everolimus with reduced calcineurin inhibitor in a multicenter, open-label, randomized trial. Transpl Int. 2016;29(7):819–29.
41. Kauffman HM, Cherikh WS, Cheng Y, Hanto DW, Kahan BD. Maintenance immunosuppression with target-of-rapamycin inhibitors is associated with a reduced incidence of de novo malignancies. Transplantation. 2005;80(7):883–9.
42. Campistol JM, Eris J, Oberbauer R, Friend P, Hutchison B, Morales JM, et al. Sirolimus therapy after early cyclosporine withdrawal reduces the risk for cancer in adult renal transplantation. J Am Soc Nephrol. 2006;17(2):581–9.
43. Asleh R, Clavell AL, Pereira NL, Smith B, Briasoulis A, Alnsasra H, et al. Incidence of malignancies in patients treated with sirolimus following heart transplantation. J Am Coll Cardiol. 2019;73(21):2676–88.
44. Baran DA, Zucker MJ, Arroyo LH, Camacho M, Goldschmidt ME, Nicholls SJ, et al. A prospective, randomized trial of single-drug versus dual-drug immunosuppression in heart transplantation: the tacrolimus in combination, tacrolimus alone compared (TICTAC) trial. Circ Heart Fail. 2011;4(2):129–37.
45. Zeevi A, Lunz J. Cylex ImmuKnow cell function assay. Methods Mol Biol (Clifton, NJ). 2013;1034:343–51.
46. Kobashigawa JA, Kiyosaki KK, Patel JK, Kittleson MM, Kubak BM, Davis SN, et al. Benefit of immune monitoring in heart transplant patients using ATP production in activated lymphocytes. J Heart Lung Transplant. 2010;29(5):504–8.
47. Kowalski RJ, Post DR, Mannon RB, Sebastian A, Wright HI, Sigle G, et al. Assessing relative risks of infection and rejection: a meta-analysis using an immune function assay. Transplantation. 2006;82(5):663–8.
48. Kobashigawa J, Crespo-Leiro MG, Ensminger SM, Reichenspurner H, Angelini A, Berry G, et al. Report from a consensus conference on antibody-mediated rejection in heart transplantation. J Heart Lung Transplant. 2011;30(3):252–69.

49. Dolan RS, Rahsepar AA, Blaisdell J, Suwa K, Ghafourian K, Wilcox JE, et al. Multiparametric cardiac magnetic resonance imaging can detect acute cardiac allograft rejection after heart transplantation. J Am Coll Cardiol Img. 2019;12:1632.
50. Deng MC, Eisen HJ, Mehra MR, Billingham M, Marboe CC, Berry G, et al. Noninvasive discrimination of rejection in cardiac allograft recipients using gene expression profiling. Am J Transplant. 2006;6(1):150–60.
51. Pham MX, Teuteberg JJ, Kfoury AG, Starling RC, Deng MC, Cappola TP, et al. Gene-expression profiling for rejection surveillance after cardiac transplantation. N Engl J Med. 2010;362(20):1890–900.
52. Starling RC, Pham M, Valantine H, Miller L, Eisen H, Rodriguez ER, et al. Molecular testing in the management of cardiac transplant recipients: initial clinical experience. J Heart Lung Transplant. 2006;25(12):1389–95.
53. Crespo-Leiro MG, Stypmann J, Schulz U, Zuckermann A, Mohacsi P, Bara C, et al. Clinical usefulness of gene-expression profile to rule out acute rejection after heart transplantation: CARGO II. Eur Heart J. 2016;37(33):2591–601.
54. Deng MC, Elashoff B, Pham MX, Teuteberg JJ, Kfoury AG, Starling RC, et al. Utility of gene expression profiling score variability to predict clinical events in heart transplant recipients. Transplantation. 2014;97(6):708–14.
55. Snyder TM, Khush KK, Valantine HA, Quake SR. Universal noninvasive detection of solid organ transplant rejection. Proc Natl Acad Sci U S A. 2011;108(15):6229–34.
56. De Vlaminck I, Valantine HA, Snyder TM, Strehl C, Cohen G, Luikart H, et al. Circulating cell-free DNA enables noninvasive diagnosis of heart transplant rejection. Sci Transl Med. 2014;6(241):241ra77.
57. Khush KK, Patel J, Pinney S, Kao A, Alharethi R, DePasquale E, et al. Noninvasive detection of graft injury after heart transplant using donor-derived cell-free DNA: a prospective multicenter study. Am J Transplant. 2019;19:2889.
58. Colvin MM, Cook JL, Chang P, Francis G, Hsu DT, Kiernan MS, et al. Antibody-mediated rejection in cardiac transplantation: emerging knowledge in diagnosis and management: a scientific statement from the American Heart Association. Circulation. 2015;131(18):1608–39.
59. Tambur AR, Pamboukian SV, Costanzo MR, Herrera ND, Dunlap S, Montpetit M, et al. The presence of HLA-directed antibodies after heart transplantation is associated with poor allograft outcome. Transplantation. 2005;80(8):1019–25.
60. Rosenthal DN, Chin C, Nishimura K, Perry SB, Robbins RC, Reitz B, et al. Identifying cardiac transplant rejection in children: diagnostic utility of echocardiography, right heart catheterization and endomyocardial biopsy data. J Heart Lung Transplant. 2004;23(3):323–9.
61. Cohn WE, Gregoric ID, Radovancevic B, Wolf RK, Frazier OH. Atrial fibrillation after cardiac transplantation: experience in 498 consecutive cases. Ann Thorac Surg. 2008;85(1):56–8.
62. Chih S, Chong AY, Mielniczuk LM, Bhatt DL, Beanlands RS. Allograft vasculopathy: the Achilles' heel of heart transplantation. J Am Coll Cardiol. 2016;68(1):80–91.
63. Chirakarnjanakorn S, Starling RC, Popovic ZB, Griffin BP, Desai MY. Dobutamine stress echocardiography during follow-up surveillance in heart transplant patients: diagnostic accuracy and predictors of outcomes. J Heart Lung Transplant. 2015;34(5):710–7.
64. Mena C, Wencker D, Krumholz HM, McNamara RL. Detection of heart transplant rejection in adults by echocardiographic diastolic indices: a systematic review of the literature. J Am Soc Echocardiogr. 2006;19(10):1295–300.
65. Clemmensen TS, Eiskjaer H, Logstrup BB, Ilkjaer LB, Poulsen SH. Left ventricular global longitudinal strain predicts major adverse cardiac events and all-cause mortality in heart transplant patients. J Heart Lung Transplant. 2017;36(5):567–76.
66. Khush KK, Cherikh WS, Chambers DC, Harhay MO, Hayes D Jr, Hsich E, et al. The International Thoracic Organ Transplant Registry of the International Society for Heart and Lung Transplantation: thirty-sixth adult heart transplantation report - 2019; focus theme: donor and recipient size match. J Heart Lung Transplant. 2019;38(10):1056–66.

67. Valantine H. Cardiac allograft vasculopathy after heart transplantation: risk factors and management. J Heart Lung Transplant. 2004;23(5 Suppl):S187–93.
68. Mehra MR, Crespo-Leiro MG, Dipchand A, Ensminger SM, Hiemann NE, Kobashigawa JA, et al. International Society for Heart and Lung Transplantation working formulation of a standardized nomenclature for cardiac allograft vasculopathy-2010. J Heart Lung Transplant. 2010;29(7):717–27.
69. St Goar FG, Pinto FJ, Alderman EL, Valantine HA, Schroeder JS, Gao SZ, et al. Intracoronary ultrasound in cardiac transplant recipients. In vivo evidence of "angiographically silent" intimal thickening. Circulation. 1992;85(3):979–87.
70. Gao SZ, Hunt SA, Schroeder JS, Alderman EL, Hill IR, Stinson EB. Early development of accelerated graft coronary artery disease: risk factors and course. J Am Coll Cardiol. 1996;28(3):673–9.
71. Tran A, Fixler D, Huang R, Meza T, Lacelle C, Das BB. Donor-specific HLA alloantibodies: impact on cardiac allograft vasculopathy, rejection, and survival after pediatric heart transplantation. J Heart Lung Transplant. 2016;35(1):87–91.
72. Costanzo-Nordin MR. Cardiac allograft vasculopathy: relationship with acute cellular rejection and histocompatibility. J Heart Lung Transplant. 1992;11(3 Pt 2):S90–103.
73. Wever-Pinzon O, Romero J, Kelesidis I, Wever-Pinzon J, Manrique C, Budge D, et al. Coronary computed tomography angiography for the detection of cardiac allograft vasculopathy: a meta-analysis of prospective trials. J Am Coll Cardiol. 2014;63(19):1992–2004.
74. Moayedi Y, Kozuszko S, Knowles JW, Chih S, Oro G, Lee R, et al. Safety and efficacy of PCSK9 inhibitors after heart transplantation. Can J Cardiol. 2019;35(1):104e1–3.
75. Quarta CC, Potena L, Grigioni F, Scalone A, Magnani G, Coccolo F, et al. Safety and efficacy of ezetimibe with low doses of simvastatin in heart transplant recipients. J Heart Lung Transplant. 2008;27(6):685–8.
76. Vaseghi M, Boyle NG, Kedia R, Patel JK, Cesario DA, Wiener I, et al. Supraventricular tachycardia after orthotopic cardiac transplantation. J Am Coll Cardiol. 2008;51(23):2241–9.
77. DiBiase A, Tse TM, Schnittger I, Wexler L, Stinson EB, Valantine HA. Frequency and mechanism of bradycardia in cardiac transplant recipients and need for pacemakers. Am J Cardiol. 1991;67(16):1385–9.
78. Cantillon DJ, Tarakji KG, Hu T, Hsu A, Smedira NG, Starling RC, et al. Long-term outcomes and clinical predictors for pacemaker-requiring bradyarrhythmias after cardiac transplantation: analysis of the UNOS/OPTN cardiac transplant database. Heart Rhythm. 2010;7(11):1567–71.
79. Filsoufi F, Salzberg SP, Anderson CA, Couper GS, Cohn LH, Adams DH. Optimal surgical management of severe tricuspid regurgitation in cardiac transplant patients. J Heart Lung Transplant. 2006;25(3):289–93.
80. Cisneros JM, Muñoz P, Torre-Cisneros J, Gurgui M, Rodriguez-Hernandez MJ, Aguado JM, et al. Pneumonia after heart transplantation: a multiinstitutional study. Clin Infect Dis. 1998;27(2):324–31.
81. John R, Lietz K, Schuster M. Older recipient age is associated with reduced alloreactivity and graft rejection after cardiac transplantation. J Heart Lung Transplant. 2001;20:212.
82. Wever-Pinzon O, Edwards LB, Taylor DO, Kfoury AG, Drakos SG, Selzman CH, et al. Association of recipient age and causes of heart transplant mortality: implications for personalization of post-transplant management—an analysis of the International Society for Heart and Lung Transplantation Registry. J Heart Lung Transplant. 2017;36(4):407–17.
83. Wenke K, Meiser B, Thiery J, Nagel D, von Scheidt W, Steinbeck G, et al. Simvastatin reduces graft vessel disease and mortality after heart transplantation: a four-year randomized trial. Circulation. 1997;96(5):1398–402.
84. Kobashigawa JA, Katznelson S, Laks H, Johnson JA, Yeatman L, Wang XM, et al. Effect of pravastatin on outcomes after cardiac transplantation. N Engl J Med. 1995;333(10):621–7.
85. McCartney SL, Patel C, Del Rio JM. Long-term outcomes and management of the heart transplant recipient. Best Pract Res Clin Anaesthesiol. 2017;31(2):237–48.

86. Gonzalez-Vilchez F, Arizon JM, Segovia J, Almenar L, Crespo-Leiro MG, Palomo J, et al. Chronic renal dysfunction in maintenance heart transplant patients: the ICEBERG study. Transplant Proc. 2014;46(1):14–20.
87. Lachance K, White M, de Denus S. Risk factors for chronic renal insufficiency following cardiac transplantation. Ann Transplant. 2015;20:576–87.
88. Yoosabai A, Mehta A, Kang W, Chaiwatcharayut W, Sampaio M, Huang E, et al. Pretransplant malignancy as a risk factor for posttransplant malignancy after heart transplantation. Transplantation. 2015;99(2):345–50.
89. Van Keer J, Droogne W, Van Cleemput J, Voros G, Rega F, Meyns B, et al. Cancer after heart transplantation: a 25-year single-center perspective. Transplant Proc. 2016;48(6):2172–7.
90. Braith RW, Mills RM Jr, Wilcox CS, Davis GL, Wood CE. Breakdown of blood pressure and body fluid homeostasis in heart transplant recipients. J Am Coll Cardiol. 1996;27(2):375–83.
91. Ozdogan E, Banner N, Fitzgerald M, Musumeci F, Khaghani A, Yacoub M. Factors influencing the development of hypertension after heart transplantation. J Heart Transplant. 1990;9(5):548–53.
92. Morath C, Opelz G, Dohler B, Zeier M, Susal C. Influence of blood pressure and calcineurin inhibitors on kidney function after heart or liver transplantation. Transplantation. 2018;102(5):845–52.
93. Nieuwenhuis MG, Kirkels JH. Predictability and other aspects of post-transplant diabetes mellitus in heart transplant recipients. J Heart Lung Transplant. 2001;20(7):703–8.
94. Jenssen T, Hartmann A. Post-transplant diabetes mellitus in patients with solid organ transplants. Nat Rev Endocrinol. 2019;15(3):172–88.
95. Klingenberg R, Gleissner C, Koch A, Schnabel PA, Sack FU, Zimmermann R, et al. Impact of pre-operative diabetes mellitus upon early and late survival after heart transplantation: a possible era effect. J Heart Lung Transplant. 2005;24(9):1239–46.
96. Sherman-Weber S, Axelrod P, Suh B, Rubin S, Beltramo D, Manacchio J, et al. Infective endocarditis following orthotopic heart transplantation: 10 cases and a review of the literature. Transpl Infect Dis. 2004;6(4):165–70.
97. Wilson W, Taubert KA, Gewitz M, Lockhart PB, Baddour LM, Levison M, et al. Prevention of infective endocarditis: guidelines from the American Heart Association: a guideline from the American Heart Association Rheumatic Fever, Endocarditis, and Kawasaki Disease Committee, Council on Cardiovascular Disease in the Young, and the Council on Clinical Cardiology, Council on Cardiovascular Surgery and Anesthesia, and the Quality of Care and Outcomes Research Interdisciplinary Working Group. Circulation. 2007;116(15):1736–54.
98. Abdalla M, Mancini DM. Management of pregnancy in the post-cardiac transplant patient. Semin Perinatol. 2014;38(5):318–25.
99. Baran DA. Pregnancy after heart transplant: not for the faint of heart. Transplant Int. 2018. https://doi.org/10.1111/tri.13151.
100. Anderson L, Nguyen TT, Dall CH, Burgess L, Bridges C, Taylor RS. Exercise-based cardiac rehabilitation in heart transplant recipients. Cochrane Database Syst Rev. 2017;4:Cd012264.
101. Amarelli C, Buonocore M, Romano G, Maiello C, De Santo LS. Nutritional issues in heart transplant candidates and recipients. Front Biosci (Elite edition). 2012;4:662–8.
102. Zeltzer SM, Taylor DO, Tang WH. Long-term dietary habits and interventions in solid-organ transplantation. J Heart Lung Transplant. 2015;34(11):1357–65.
103. Stehlik J, Kobashigawa J, Hunt SA, Reichenspurner H, Kirklin JK. Honoring 50 years of clinical heart transplantation in circulation: in-depth state-of-the-art review. Circulation. 2018;137(1):71–87.
104. Magliato KE, Trento A. Heart transplantation – surgical results. Heart Fail Rev. 2001;6:213–9.

Chapter 7
Primary Care of the Adult Lung Transplant Recipient

Erika D. Lease

Introduction

Lung transplantation has become an increasingly frequent treatment for patients with a variety of end-stage lung diseases. In 2016, there were over 4600 lung transplants worldwide reported to the registry for the International Society for Heart and Lung Transplantation (ISHLT) with nearly 2600 of those performed in North America [1]. The registry data also shows that the face of the lung transplant recipient has been changing over time. In 1987 the median age of lung transplant recipients was 43 years and in 2017 this had risen to 59 years, with the largest increase in lung transplants performed proportionally occurring in patients older than 65 years. As of 2016, as reported to the ISHLT, idiopathic pulmonary fibrosis (IPF) is the most common indication for lung transplantation in ~30%, followed by chronic obstructive pulmonary disease (COPD) in ~25%, and cystic fibrosis (CF) in ~15%. This propensity for lung transplantation in patients with IPF is increased in the United States as reported to the Scientific Registry of Transplant Recipients (SRTR). Between July 1, 2018, and June 30, 2019, over half of patients undergoing lung transplantation in the United States had a diagnosis of IPF, approximately one-quarter with COPD, and 10% with CF. [2]

Survival after lung transplantation has improved but is still limited as compared to other solid organ transplant recipients. In the most recent era defined as 2009 to June 2016, the median life expectancy for a lung transplant recipient is 6.5 years [1]. This survival is improved from a median of 4.3 years during the era of 1990–1998. For patients who survive the first year after a lung transplant, the median survival improves to 8.6 years in the most recent era for which data is available, 1999–2008. Survival following lung transplantation varies based on underlying lung disease,

E. D. Lease (✉)
Department of Medicine, Division of Pulmonary, Critical Care, and Sleep Medicine,
University of Washington, Seattle, WA, USA
e-mail: edlease@u.washington.edu

© Springer Nature Switzerland AG 2020
C. J. Wong (ed.), *Primary Care of the Solid Organ Transplant Recipient*,
https://doi.org/10.1007/978-3-030-50629-2_7

ranging from an overall median survival of 5.2 years for patients with IPF to a median survival of 9.5 years for patients with CF. For patients who survive the first year after a lung transplant, the median survival ranges from 7.2 years for patients with IPF to 12.2 years for patients with CF. There are many longer living lung transplant survivors, however. The longest living post-lung transplant and post-heart-lung transplant survivors at the author's center will be 27 years and 30 years post-transplant in early 2020 respectively.

Chronic lung allograft dysfunction (CLAD) is a significant contributor to morbidity and mortality after lung transplantation, occurring in 40% of patients by 5 years post-transplant [1]. It is the leading cause of death after the first year, being reported as the cause of death in approximately 25–30% of patients. CLAD is one of the primary reason lung transplant recipients require such intensive monitoring for the remainder of their life following lung transplantation.

With increased rates of transplantation and improving survival, it is increasingly likely that the primary care provider will assist in caring for recipients of a lung transplant.

Lung Transplant Anatomy

Lung transplantation is performed in the orthotopic position. There are various surgical techniques. The most common approach for a bilateral lung transplant is through bilateral anterior thoracotomies with transverse sternotomy (the "clamshell" incision in the front of the chest), or, if a unilateral transplant, a posterolateral thoracotomy incision. This chapter does not cover heart-lung transplantation or living-related lobar lung transplantation.

Anastomoses (Fig. 7.1)

- Pulmonary artery: The donor pulmonary artery is anastomosed to the corresponding recipient's pulmonary artery.
- Pulmonary veins: There are different techniques to anastomose the pulmonary veins and may depend on the anatomic variant found during surgery. When two or more distinct pulmonary veins are present, one common method is to join the recipient's pulmonary veins as a single insertion to the left atrium. This technique allows for a single anastomosis rather than joining each pulmonary vein individually.
- Bronchial arteries: The recipient bronchial arteries are ligated and generally not anastomosed.
- Airway: The donor and recipient bronchi are anastomosed at the level of the mainstem bronchi.

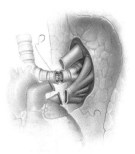
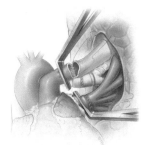
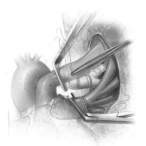

Bronchial anastomosis

Pulmonary vein anastomosis (red) completed; pulmonary artery (blue) anastomosis being performed

Pulmonary artery anastomosis (blue) being completed.

Fig. 7.1 Lung transplantation anatomy. (Note: Anastomoses for a single lung transplant are shown for educational purposes; techniques and anatomy may vary.) (Figure reprinted with permission from Siguenza et al. [3]).

- Pleura: During bilateral lung transplantation via the clamshell approach, there is disruption of the individual pleural spaces resulting in interpleural communication (i.e., connection between the right and left pleural spaces). This is pertinent in the case of post-transplant pleural complications such as pneumothorax or empyema in which there may be extension to the contralateral pleural space.
- Lymphatics: Normally, lymphatic vessels from the lungs drain into the thoracic duct. After lung transplantation there is no lymphatic vessel anastomosis and therefore disruption of normal lymphatic drainage. There is likely lymphangiogenesis to a certain extent with development of collateral lymphatic drainage within several weeks following the transplant surgery; however, this has not been fully elucidated.

Immunosuppression in the Lung Transplant Recipient

Immunosuppression following lung transplantation can be divided into induction and maintenance immunosuppression.

Induction

Induction immunosuppression is used in the immediate perioperative and postoperative periods. It is intended to deplete circulating T cells with the purpose of reducing acute cellular rejection (ACR) immediately following lung transplantation, particularly until maintenance immunosuppression has reached full effect.

The use of induction immunosuppression appears to be increasing with time with 76% of lung transplant recipients receiving induction immunosuppressive agents in 2016. The most commonly used agent is an interleukin-2 receptor (IL-2R) antagonist such as basiliximab, reported to be used in ~65% of all lung transplant recipients [1]. Other induction immunosuppression regimens include polyclonal or monoclonal T-cell antibody treatments, such as anti-thymocyte globulin (ATG) or muromonab-CD3 (OKT3) [1].

Maintenance

Maintenance immunosuppression is used for the remainder of the patient's life after lung transplantation. Significant improvements in immunosuppressive agents have been made since the beginnings of solid organ transplantation; however, the optimal post-transplant maintenance immunosuppression regimen in lung transplant recipients remains unclear. In data reported from 2016, at 1 year post-lung transplant, the vast majority of lung transplant recipients received the calcineurin inhibitor tacrolimus (93%), mycophenolate mofetil or mycophenolic acid (83%), and prednisone [1]. In contrast, at 1 year post-transplant, only 5% of lung transplant recipients received the calcineurin inhibitor cyclosporine, 7% received a mammalian target of rapamycin (mTOR) inhibitor such as sirolimus or everolimus, and 9% received azathioprine. In the 2018 ISHLT annual registry report, unadjusted data showed statistically significant lower rates of ACR within the first year post-transplant in patients who receive maintenance immunosuppression therapy with tacrolimus plus mycophenolate mofetil or mycophenolic acid [1]. There was no difference found between tacrolimus plus azathioprine and cyclosporine plus mycophenolate mofetil or mycophenolic acid, but there was a statistically significantly increased risk for ACR in patients receiving cyclosporine plus azathioprine [1].

Regardless of the maintenance immunosuppression regimen used, optimization of the prescribed regimen should be assured by adherence, avoidance of interacting medications or foods, and close monitoring of drug trough levels when available. Medication nonadherence is a complicating factor in lung transplant recipients as with all patients. One single-center study found an average individual medication timing adherence (± 30 minutes from prescribed timing) of 98.1%, although the range was 31.2–100% [4]. Overall, medication adherence, defined as having an individual timing-adherence score of ≥80%, was seen in 92.3% of recipients. However, over 14% of patients missed one or more 24 hour period of medication, with over 40% in the non-adherent group (an individual timing-adherence score of ≤80%) missing one or more 24 hour period of medication. Instruction and emphasis on the importance of taking immunosuppressant medication regularly and at the prescribed time are important factors to assure adequate immunosuppression levels. Primary care providers can assist by evaluating adherence at each outpatient visit.

In general, many lung transplant recipients will remain on at least a three-drug immunosuppression regimen for the remainder of their life post-transplant unless there are side effects or complications requiring a reduction in immunosuppression. In patients with CLAD, it is common to see patients prescribed four maintenance immunosuppressive agents.

See Chap. 3 for more discussion of immunosuppressive medications and side effects.

Post-Transplant Surveillance and Monitoring for Complications

Recipients of a lung transplant require intensive, life-long monitoring for the assessment, evaluation, and management of both allograft and non-allograft transplant-related complications. While every lung transplant center has an individualized follow-up plan/schedule, most centers request that patients undergo formal spirometry at least several times a year and be seen by the lung transplant team at least 1–2 times a year. In addition, lung transplant centers will require laboratory testing generally every 1–3 months to measure immunosuppressive drug levels and monitor for transplant-related complications such as chronic kidney disease (CKD), diabetes mellitus (DM), cytopenias, and other issues as needed. In addition, post-lung transplant monitoring may include home spirometry measurements as well as periodic surveillance bronchoscopy as discussed below.

Monitoring/Spirometry

As a decline in forced expiratory volume in 1 second (FEV_1) is often the first sign of acute rejection and/or CLAD, close monitoring of spirometry is essential for early identification [5]. Lung transplant recipients are encouraged to utilize home spirometers to monitor lung function parameters such as the FEV_1 and the forced expiratory capacity (FVC). Monitoring of daily home spirometry has been shown to improve detection of a sustained decline for 3 days or more of FEV_1 by $\geq 20\%$ from the lung transplant recipient's baseline best FEV_1 by an average of 276 days earlier than without daily home monitoring [6]. Despite this significantly earlier detection, no studies have demonstrated a benefit in survival with home spirometry monitoring, although several studies have shown a non-statistically significant positive trend for freedom from bronchiolitis obliterans syndrome (BOS) and reduced rates of re-transplantation [7].

Monitoring/Surveillance Bronchoscopy

Despite being commonly performed, there is little data to support the utilization of surveillance screening for ACR via bronchoscopy and transbronchial biopsy (TBBX) [8]. The intention of surveillance monitoring by TBBX is to attempt to identify subclinical ACR before the onset of symptoms or graft dysfunction and to intervene therapeutically with the belief that early and prompt treatment of ACR is beneficial for improving outcomes and decreasing the risk of CLAD in lung transplant recipients. However, there is no definitive evidence that earlier identification of these abnormalities in an asymptomatic patient with preserved lung function alters the treatment course or overall outcome in lung transplant recipients. Bronchoscopy can result in many complications including, but not limited to, pneumothorax, bleeding, and complications of sedation; therefore, further studies are needed to determine if there is a benefit in performing surveillance bronchoscopy with TBBX in lung transplant recipients and if the benefit outweighs the procedural risks.

Post-Lung Transplant Pulmonary Complications

General Issues

There are a myriad of pulmonary issues that may arise after a lung transplant, and while many times these issues are benign, subtle findings may herald a much more concerning complication or trigger lung function decline. As such, the lung transplant team should be notified to help direct evaluation and management for any lung transplant recipient who presents with respiratory symptoms or signs including, but not limited to, decline in spirometry, decline in oxygenation by pulse oximetry, dyspnea, cough, decreased exercise tolerance, respiratory viral symptoms, or new/worsened edema. Empiric corticosteroids and/or antibiotics for respiratory symptoms should be avoided unless directed by the lung transplant team as they may greatly impact the ability to diagnose lung transplant complications, particularly acute rejection, if a patient develops significant worsening of symptoms. In addition, many post-lung transplant recipients are colonized with bacteria that will not respond to the typical empiric antibiotics given for conditions such as community-acquired pneumonia or may already be prescribed azithromycin as an anti-inflammatory agent in the setting of CLAD. Finally, due to the disrupted lymphatic drainage after lung transplantation, lung transplant recipients are highly susceptible to pulmonary edema with the administration of large-volume intravenous (IV) fluids. IV fluids should not be administered to a lung transplant recipient outside of the acute setting such as sepsis or other severe, life-threatening hypotension or blood loss, without a discussion with the lung transplant team (see Table 7.1).

Patients who present with new respiratory symptoms or a decline in spirometry despite the presence or absence of symptoms should undergo formal evaluation for diagnosis. Possible etiologies include, but are not limited to, acute cellular or antibody-mediated rejection, infection, anastomotic and/or airway stenoses, or the onset of CLAD. Testing by the lung transplant team will generally include formal spirometry, computed tomography (CT) scan of the chest with inspiratory and expiratory images, testing for donor-specific antibodies (DSA) as part of the diagnosis of antibody-mediated rejection, as well as bronchoscopy to evaluate for anastomotic

Table 7.1 Clinical pearls for the primary care provider—evaluation of a lung transplant recipient with respiratory symptoms (see text for details)

Discuss new respiratory symptoms with the transplant team, especially if:
  Decline in baseline spirometry, particularly FEV_1 or $FEF_{25-75\%}$
  Dyspnea
  Cough
  Decreased exercise tolerance
  Edema (new or worsening)
Discuss with the transplant team first if considering the following treatments:
  Antibiotics (for a respiratory infection)
    Avoid empiric antibiotics unless directed by the transplant team
    If antibiotics are required, discuss choice with transplant team because of potential drug-resistant organisms and drug interactions
    Additional testing may be indicated (e.g., radiographic chest imaging, extended-spectrum respiratory viral panel, sputum sample, bronchoscopy)
  Corticosteroids for wheezing or respiratory symptoms
    Avoid empiric corticosteroids in lung transplant recipients—discuss with transplant team first
    Can complicate workup for acute rejection
  IV fluids
    Avoid IV fluids unless emergently required (risk of pulmonary edema)
Transfer to acute care setting (e.g., Emergency Department) if unstable and alert the transplant team so they may be in contact with the Emergency Department providers to help direct evaluation and management
Alert the transplant team even in cases of mild respiratory viral infections
  Associated with development of acute cellular rejection and chronic lung allograft dysfunction
  May require more frequent monitoring

and/or airway stenoses and to obtain specimens via bronchoalveolar lavage (BAL) and transbronchial biopsies (TBBX). Additional evaluation and testing may be warranted depending on the clinical presentation.

Acute Rejection

Acute cellular rejection (ACR) and antibody-mediated (humoral) rejection (AMR) are two forms of acute rejection seen following lung transplantation.

- Symptoms: Most lung transplant recipients with ACR or AMR present with minimal to no symptoms and are generally identified due to a decline in home or formal spirometry. If symptoms are present, they most commonly include dyspnea and/or cough. At times, lung transplant recipients may present with more acute respiratory failure ranging from mild hypoxia to acute respiratory distress syndrome (ARDS). Importantly, there is no clear distinction in symptoms that differentiate between acute rejection and other post-lung transplant complications such as infection.

- Exam findings: Physical exam findings in acute rejection are generally absent or nonspecific. Patients presenting with advanced or fulminant acute rejection may show mild to severe hypoxia on O_2 saturation monitoring, evidence of increased work of breathing, and nonspecific findings on pulmonary examination.
- Evaluation: Evaluation for acute rejection should be directed by the transplant team and may include formal spirometry, chest radiographic imaging, testing for donor specific antibodies, and bronchoscopy. Because infection may present similarly, broad infectious testing will often be performed in the setting of a decline in spirometry or new respiratory symptoms, including an extended-spectrum respiratory viral panel, respiratory cultures, and other testing. It is important to note that respiratory infection may trigger acute rejection, further limiting the ability to clinically differentiate post-lung transplant complications without additional testing. An evaluation may occur in the inpatient or the outpatient setting, depending on the severity of the patient's presentation as well as the ability to expeditiously obtain the necessary testing.
- Treatment: The management of ACR and AMR is complex and may be individualized based on the unique situation of each patient but is guided by early diagnosis and prompt treatment that includes augmentation of immunosuppression among a variety of additional medical strategies. Treatment of ACR and AMR is important not only because of the risk of acute graft loss during the rejection episode but also because acute rejection is associated with the subsequent development of CLAD.

Airway Complications

Airway-related complications after lung transplantation have been reported to range from 2% to 18% and are felt to be related to donor bronchial ischemia [9]. Airway dehiscence occurs at the surgical anastomotic sites while airway stenosis and/or malacia can occur at the surgical anastomotic sites as well as the more distal airways. The airway-related complications often present with a decline in spirometry with or without dyspnea or evidence of unilateral large airway noise on physical exam. As with the evaluation of any decline of spirometry or new respiratory symptoms in a lung transplant recipient, evaluation for the concern of airway-related complications should be dictated by the transplant team. Management may include monitoring, balloon dilation, stent placement, ablative therapies, or surgical intervention. While many airway complications occur early post-lung transplant, a proportion of patients may have persistent issues that require management for years.

Infections

Respiratory viruses, both symptomatic and asymptomatic, have been found to possibly play a role in the development of ACR [10]. In addition, respiratory viral infections when present concurrently with ACR may cause more severe lung dysfunction and a slower short-term recovery [11]. Perhaps more importantly, however, respiratory viruses have been associated with the subsequent development of CLAD [9, 12]. Fisher et al. found an adjusted hazard ratio of 1.9 (1.1–3.5, $p = 0.03$) for CLAD following the diagnosis of an upper or lower respiratory tract viral infection. The association of the development of CLAD following a respiratory viral infection was stronger the earlier after the respiratory viral infection but persisted for 12 months following the diagnosis (HR 4.8 (1.9–11.6), $P < 0.01$; 3.4 (1.5–7.5), $P < 0.01$; and 2.4 (1.2–5.0), $P = 0.02$ in multivariate analysis for 3, 6, and 12 months following respiratory viral infection, respectively). As such, even mild respiratory viral infections in lung transplant recipients should prompt review by the lung transplant team with close monitoring for the development of worsening symptoms or decline in lung function. An extended-spectrum respiratory viral panel by nasal swab can be helpful even in the setting of mild upper respiratory infection in order to potentially identify the causative virus, provide treatment if warranted, and depending on the causative viral infection determine the need for closer follow-up to monitor for post-respiratory viral complications (i.e., acute rejection, development of CLAD, etc.). If additional evaluation or treatment is being considered due to clinical symptoms or findings, it is reasonable to contact the transplant team for guidance as to the most appropriate evaluation and/or treatment based on the individual patient's clinical transplant history.

Transplant centers vary widely with respect to antiviral prophylaxis for cytomegalovirus (CMV) but are generally driven by the donor and recipient serostatus, tolerance of the medication, and the recipient's post-transplant CMV history. CMV seronegative recipients (R) of a CMV seropositive donor (D) organ (CMV D+/R−) are at the highest risk of CMV reactivation. However, any lung transplant recipient may experience CMV reactivation regardless of donor or recipient serostatus with the exception of CMV seronegative recipients of a seronegative donor organ (CMV D−/R−) who are at risk of developing primary CMV infection. Valganciclovir is generally the agent used for CMV prophylaxis with the duration dependent on the specific transplant center protocol, which can range from 3 months to indefinite prophylaxis. Acyclovir may be used for early postoperative HSV or VZV prophylaxis in CMV D−/R− lung transplants or later post-transplant in any recipient with recurrent HSV or VZV reactivation.

Overall, it is important to recognize the increased risk for any pulmonary or non-pulmonary infection in a lung transplant recipient. Given the range of infectious complications and the complexity of managing infections in the setting of immunosuppression, it is reasonable to contact the transplant team to alert them to any infection in a lung transplant recipient, so they may provide insight into atypical infectious etiologies as well as preferred treatment and treatment duration. The transplant team may also elect to adjust immunosuppression in the setting of active or recurrent infections. While lung transplant recipients may present with "typical" infections as in the general population, they may also present with what appears to be a "typical" infection but, in fact, is something much more serious (for example, gram-negative or fungal cellulitis). Delayed or inadequate treatment of an infection can have dire consequences, thus early involvement of the transplant team may be beneficial to assist the primary care provider managing an infection in a lung transplant recipient (see also Chap. 8).

The COVID-19/SARS-CoV-2 pandemic that began in 2020 may pose particular risk to lung transplant recipients. At the time of this book's publication, data regarding this infection's presentation and outcomes in lung transplant recipients continues to evolve. Evaluation and management should be directed by the transplant pulmonologist and take into consideration local epidemiology and public health guidelines. Lung transplant recipients are in a high risk category and should avoid potential exposures to SARS-CoV-2.

Gastroesophageal Reflux Disease

Gastroesophageal reflux disease (GERD) irrespective of symptoms or acid content appears to have the potential for a significant impact on post-lung transplant graft function likely due to the predisposition to aspiration of gastroesophageal reflux contents and the subsequent injury that occurs. Several studies in lung transplant recipients have found that GERD diagnosed by 24-hour pH study or 24-hour pH-impedance study is associated with an earlier onset of ACR, higher rate of ACR, and multiple episodes of ACR [13, 14]. In addition, one study found that anti-reflux surgery performed either pre-transplant or within the first 6 months following lung transplantation resulted in a decreased risk of ACR in the first year [15].

Several studies have shown that the occurrence of GERD increases after lung transplantation and may increase with time following transplant surgery [16–18]. Although no studies have found a causative link between GERD and CLAD, several studies have evaluated the impact of post-transplant fundoplication surgery and the development or progression of CLAD. Lung transplant recipients who undergo early post-transplant fundoplication for documented GERD have been found to have a better FEV_1 at 1-year post-transplant, higher peak FEV_1, and longer survival [19, 20]. Evaluation and management of GERD are therefore critical in lung transplant recipients that present with graft dysfunction particularly if no immunologic etiology is found.

Many lung transplant centers will prescribe life-long proton-pump inhibitors (PPIs) for all lung transplant recipients regardless of a diagnosis of GERD or GERD symptoms given the concern that even episodic acidic reflux with microaspiration may result in lung allograft injury. The primary care provider should contact the transplant team if there is concern for side effects relating to the use of PPIs so that there may be a discussion about the risk-benefit ratio in the setting of lung transplantation.

Chronic Lung Allograft Dysfunction (CLAD)

CLAD is the leading cause of death after the first year following lung transplantation, being reported as the primary cause of death in approximately 25–30% of lung transplant recipients [1]. CLAD is a clinical diagnosis based purely on a sustained decline of $\geq 20\%$ in FEV_1 from a lung transplant recipient's baseline best FEV_1

without another clinical explanation [19]. Frequently, lung transplant recipients are diagnosed with CLAD solely by a sustained decline in spirometry and remain asymptomatic with no functional limitations. CLAD is divided into two phenotypes: obstructive CLAD, previously termed bronchiolitis obliterans syndrome (BOS), and restrictive CLAD, also referred to as restrictive allograft syndrome (RAS). CLAD may be progressive either due to an ongoing process resulting in continuing allograft injury or due to a series of independent injuries. Over time, lung transplant recipients may develop end-stage obstructive or restrictive lung disease with manifestations of dyspnea with exertion, chronic hypoxia requiring supplemental oxygen, and a decline in functional status.

If a lung transplant recipient manifests a sustained decline of $\geq 10\%$ in FEV_1 from their baseline best FEV_1, the lung transplant team will determine the appropriate evaluation and management. As CLAD is a clinical diagnosis, bronchoscopy with transbronchial biopsies is primarily helpful to exclude ACR, infection, and/or airway stenosis as the cause of decreased spirometry. Chest CT may show air-trapping or areas of fibrosis; however, these findings are supportive of the diagnosis of CLAD, not diagnostic in isolation.

Unfortunately, there are no true treatments for CLAD; thus the effort is focused on preserving the remaining lung function and treating contributing factors and pulmonary complications (i.e., rejection, infection, etc.) as soon as possible. Azithromycin may be used for its anti-inflammatory properties as a means to mitigate ongoing lung function decline due to inflammation but not to reverse allograft injury that has already occurred.

Primary Care of the Lung Transplant Recipient

General Issues

Following transplantation, medical management of the lung transplant recipient is vital for maintaining the health of the allograft and to promote an overall successful outcome after a lung transplant surgery. A large number of non-pulmonary complications that may arise following lung transplantation are related to immunosuppressant effects and/or toxicities. Non-pulmonary complications include, but are not limited to, renal dysfunction, hematologic abnormalities, gastrointestinal complications, neurologic sequelae, oncologic manifestations, and metabolic derangements. While monitoring lung allograft function following transplantation is critical to overall survival, monitoring for the subsequent non-pulmonary complications is also important to avoid increased morbidity and mortality in lung transplant recipients.

Given the range of non-pulmonary complications following lung transplantation, any new medical diagnoses should be discussed with the lung transplant team to assure that no changes in the post-lung transplant medication regimen are warranted. In addition, new medications prescribed for non-pulmonary medical issues should also be discussed with the lung transplant team to assure that no potential interactions exist between the new medication and the immunosuppressive medications in particular. For example, diltiazem and the azoles, such as fluconazole, have significant interactions with the calcineurin inhibitors, tacrolimus and cyclosporine, resulting in decreased metabolism of these medications. The doses of the calcineurin inhibitors will need to be reduced in the setting of administration of diltiazem or the azoles in order to prevent toxic levels resulting in renal failure or severe neurologic issues (see Chap. 3).

General age-related health maintenance and screening for lung transplant recipients should not be different from the general population outside of the known issues

Table 7.2 Clinical pearls for the primary care provider—evaluation of the lung transplant recipient at outpatient clinic visits (see text for details, also see Chap. 2 for discussion of general history-taking)

Initial visit:
Review pre-transplant and initial post-transplant course:
Indication for transplant
Single vs bilateral lung transplant
EBV and CMV serostatus
Type of induction immunosuppression
Complications (surgical complications, infection, rejection)

Symptoms, exam, medications, laboratory studies, metabolic complications, and general preventive health similar to follow-up visits

Follow-up visits:
Symptoms:
Inquire about dyspnea, cough, symptoms of infection, malignancy, or medication side effects

Habits:
Ask about tobacco, marijuana, and other use

Exam:
Should have expected surgical scars from incision, drains, etc.
Complete exam for abnormal respiratory findings

Medications:
Review immunosuppressive medication regimen, adherence, side effects
Review infectious prophylaxis
Review other possible medications intended to treat or prevent post-transplant complications (PPIs, azithromycin, magnesium supplementation, calcium/vitamin D supplementation, statin, among others)

Laboratory and other studies:
Adherence to surveillance schedule set forth by the transplant team

Surveillance for graft function
Home spirometry
Formal spirometry
Bronchoscopy (if done)

Metabolic complications:
Assess and treat, in conjunction with the transplant team, if present, including hypomagnesemia, gout, osteopenia or osteoporosis, diabetes, hypertension, chronic kidney disease

General preventive health:
Review immunizations, skin exams including history of skin cancer, other routine screening

relating to the side effects and complications of post-lung transplant medications (see Chap. 12). Patients are strongly recommended to stay up to date; however, their immunosuppressed state may worsen or complicate management of routine age-related medical diagnoses.

At the initial visit, the patient's history should be reviewed (Table 7.2).

- The pre-transplant course should be reviewed. In some cases, patients have had a prolonged course on the waiting list and may have suffered from complications, hospitalizations, and frailty.
- The indication for transplantation should be clearly identified.
  - In some cases, the disease may continue to affect other organ systems—for example, a patient with cystic fibrosis may have a well-functioning bilateral lung transplant without complications but still have pancreatic disease, sinusitis, and episodes of distal intestinal obstruction syndrome (DIOS). The primary care provider may be actively involved in managing these other conditions.
- Single lung transplant recipients may continue to have disease and complications in the native lung. For example, a patient with a single lung transplant for COPD is still at risk for cancer and pneumothorax in the native lung.
- The initial transplant postoperative course should be reviewed for complications, rejection episodes, and opportunistic infections.

At all visits (initial and follow-up), the primary care provider should review the following (Table 7.2):

- Symptoms: Patients should be asked about symptoms of allograft dysfunction, including dyspnea or cough. Symptoms of infection and malignancy should also be addressed, as well as potential side effects of immunosuppressant or infection prophylaxis medications.
- Adherence: As noted above, nonadherence is common and should be discussed. Knowing the common side effects will help the PCP direct questions, as side effects are a potential factor in nonadherence (see Chap. 3).
- Habits: Smoking relapse can occur in patients after lung transplantation. Primary care providers should actively inquire about smoking and treat aggressively if needed. Other inhaled substances are also strongly discouraged, including vaping marijuana. The transplant team should be made aware if a patient is smoking or inhaling any substance so that they may be able to counsel the patient appropriately from a lung transplant perspective.
- Exam: In addition to any other physical examination as indicated, lung transplant recipients should be assessed for abnormal respiratory findings, including oxygenation. Examination should show expected surgical scars and a well-functioning lung allograft should be clear to auscultation. The extremities should be assessed for edema and cyanosis. Lung transplant recipients should be monitored for excessive weight gain and, if present, managed aggressively.
- Laboratory and surveillance: The lung transplant recipient will have frequent, life-long laboratory monitoring as dictated by the transplant team. It is helpful to review the transplant team's documentation and reinforce the surveillance sched-

ule with the patient, especially if the patient is past due for routine surveillance. The patient should be encouraged to perform life-long home spirometry and the data should be reviewed for changes. If a decrease in home spirometry is present, the transplant team should be alerted regardless of the presence or absence of respiratory symptoms. Abnormal lab tests may require follow-up by the PCP (e.g., hyperglycemia).

- Manage complications: It is important to continue to screen for medical complications and treat them as they arise. Patients with good allograft function might see their lung transplant team twice yearly, but their PCP more often to manage diabetes, hypertension, and other conditions. (Complications are discussed in more detail below and also more generally in Chaps. 10 and 11).
- Preventive health: Primary care providers should continue to conduct routine age-appropriate health screening and immunizations. Note that live virus immunizations are contraindicated due to immunosuppression, and the recombinant shingles vaccine is currently not recommended, pending further evaluation in the transplant population. Vaccine recommendations change frequently and the PCP should review current guidelines and, if in doubt, contact the transplant center (See Chap. 12).

Renal, Cardiovascular, and Metabolic Complications Post-Lung Transplant

While these complications are discussed elsewhere in this book, it is important to recognize the frequency with which non-pulmonary renal, cardiovascular, and metabolic complications occur following lung transplantation. Patients with pre-transplant risk factors for these non-pulmonary issues, such as patients with cystic fibrosis, may have significant worsening of these conditions following lung transplantation and the administration of immunosuppressive medications. Careful monitoring is necessary to prevent long-term sequelae and morbidity due to these complications.

Renal disease is a common and an increasingly recognized complication following lung transplantation. According to data collected by the ISHLT, at 1 year following lung transplantation, nearly 6% of recipients meet the criteria for severe renal dysfunction (creatinine >2.5 mg/dL) and nearly 1.3% require dialysis. By 5-years post-transplant, over 16% of recipients meet the criteria for severe renal dysfunction with an additional 3% requiring dialysis and 0.6% having undergone renal transplantation [1]. If a lung transplant recipient develops proteinuria or a rising creatinine, in addition to the standard workup for acute or chronic kidney disease, the transplant team should be notified. In some cases, the patient's immunosuppression regimen may be reassessed and/or modified. If the renal disease is progressive, a nephrologist familiar with the care of transplant recipients should be involved.

Several cardiovascular and metabolic alterations can occur following lung transplantation, most commonly due to side effects related to the immunosuppressive medications. Hypertension, hypercholesterolemia, diabetes mellitus, and osteoporosis are all potential complications in lung transplant recipients. Several studies have evaluated the prevalence of these cardiovascular and metabolic alterations. Hypertension has been found to be present in 45% of lung transplant recipients at 1-year post-transplant, 65% by 3-year post-transplant, and 67% by 5-year post-transplant [21]. Similarly, hypercholesterolemia is present in 16% of lung transplant recipients at 1-year post-transplant, 33% by 3-year post-transplant, and 48% by 5-year post-transplant [22]. The estimated prevalence of diabetes mellitus following lung transplantation has varied among studies with 6–23% by 1-year post-transplant and 7–39% by 3-year post-transplant [21, 23, 24]. The prevalence of metabolic syndrome is also increased with 24% of lung transplant recipients meeting the criteria by 1-year post-transplant.

Loss of bone mineral density also is a common complication following lung transplantation, although many patients have preexisting bone mineral density alterations prior to transplant. Wang et al. found that 36% of lung transplant candidates had osteopenia based on bone mineral density testing and 31% had osteoporosis [25]. This increased prevalence is likely due to the common use of corticosteroids in advanced lung disease management, a known risk factor for loss of bone mineral density. Significant bone loss is common following lung transplantation, again primarily to the use of corticosteroids as a mainstay of the transplant immunosuppressive regimen. As such, prevention of bone loss with post-transplant administration of calcium and vitamin D, as well as appropriate monitoring for bone loss and treatment when needed, is essential to reduce the risk of fracture.

For further discussion not specific to lung transplant recipients, see Chap. 11.

Malignancy

Malignancy following lung transplantation is common and increases with time after transplant. According to the ISHLT, over 11% of deaths between years 1 and 5 post-lung transplant and over 17% after 5-years post-lung transplant are attributable to malignancy. In addition, post-transplant lymphoproliferative disorder (PTLD) is responsible for 2% of deaths following the first 30 days after transplant [1].

Skin cancer accounts for the majority of malignancy following lung transplantation, with squamous cell carcinoma (SCC) predominating over basal cell carcinoma (BCC) [26]. Lung and heart transplant recipients are more likely to develop skin cancer than other solid organ transplant recipients, likely due to the increased overall intensity of immunosuppression required. Immunosuppression alone is not the only post-transplant medication contributing to the development of skin cancer, however. Exposure to voriconazole, an anti-fungal medication used frequently after lung transplantation, has also been found to significantly impact the occurrence of skin cancer. A retrospective study of over 300 lung transplant recipients found a

2.6-fold increased risk for SCC in patients who had any exposure to voriconazole with a cumulative effect showing a 5.6% increase in risk for every 60-day exposure [27].

Post-transplant lymphoproliferative disorder (PTLD) is a broad category that contains several distinct processes and is characterized by the proliferation of immune cells in the setting of post-transplant immunosuppression. A review of the United Network of Sharing database, a database of solid organ transplants performed in the United States, found the incidence of PTLD in lung transplant recipients to be 3.7% [28]. Other studies have reported higher incidences with ranges of 6.2–9.4% [29]. PTLD is more common in lung transplant recipients, occurring twice as frequently as in other solid organ transplant recipients [28]. EBV serostatus is the most important risk factor for the development of PTLD, with an EBV seropositive donor organ transplanted into an EBV seronegative recipient having the highest risk. Lung transplant recipients in this category have a 20-fold increased risk of developing PTLD than lung transplant recipients who are seropositive prior to transplantation [28]. As PTLD may present at any time post-transplant and in a variety of locations (i.e., pulmonary, GI, CNS, bone marrow, etc.), patients may possibly present to primary care providers with symptoms of malignancy. Therefore, primary care providers must be aware of this condition and have a high degree of suspicion in order to diagnose it accurately in a timely fashion.

Colon cancer has been found to be generally increased in patients with CF. In a recent review of the US Cystic Fibrosis Foundation Registry during the years 1990 to 2009, the standardized incidence ratio (SIR), defined as the number of observed cases of colon cancer divided by the number of expected cases of colon cancer, was 6.2 in all patients with CF. [30] In patients with CF who underwent organ transplantation, the SIR for colon cancer was 30.1. Screening recommendations for colon cancer in lung transplant recipients with CF have been published with recommendations for both pre- and post-transplant screening initiation and intervals [31].

Short telomere syndromes have been associated with the development of IPF and other interstitial pneumonias and have been shown to be a critical factor driving myelodysplastic syndrome (MDS) and leukemia. Patients with telomeropathies who undergo lung transplantation should be monitored closely for the development of myelodysplasia and other associated hematologic disorders. [32, 33] Consideration should be taken for lung transplant recipients with short telomere syndromes to be proactively followed by hematologist-oncologists who are familiar with the evaluation and management of hematologic disorders associated with telomeropathies.

Lung cancer also appears to occur more frequently following lung transplantation. Several studies have shown an increased risk of lung cancer, particularly in the native lung in COPD and IPF recipients of a single lung transplant [34–36]. These patients have been found to have prevalence of native lung cancer ranging from 1.5% to 8.9% [35]. Although there are no current guidelines for screening for lung cancer in lung transplant recipients, consideration should be given to using current lung screening guidelines in patients who may be at high risk such as recipients of single lung transplants due to COPD and IPF. Screening and evaluation for lung cancer in lung transplant recipients should be a joint effort between the lung transplant team and the primary care provider.

(See also Chap. 10).

Conclusions

Lung transplantation has become an increasingly frequent treatment for patients with a variety of end-stage lung diseases. Survival after lung transplantation has improved over time but is still limited as compared to other solid organ transplant recipients. There are a myriad of pulmonary issues that may arise after a lung transplant as well as a large number of non-pulmonary complications frequently related to immunosuppressant effects and/or toxicities. Non-pulmonary complications include, but are not limited to, renal dysfunction, hematologic abnormalities, gastrointestinal complications, neurologic sequelae, oncologic manifestations, and metabolic derangements. For these reasons, following a lung transplant recipients require intensive, life-long monitoring for the assessment, evaluation, and management of both allograft and non-allograft transplant-related complications.

References

1. Chambers DC, Cherikh WS, Goldfarb SB, et al. The international thoracic organ transplant registry of the international society for heart and lung transplantation: thirty-fifth adult lung and heart-lung transplant report-2018. J Heart Lung Transplant. 2018;37(10):1169–83.
2. Data from www. srtr.org.
3. Matilla Siguenza JR, Aigner C, Klepetko W. Lung transplantation. In: Dienemann HC, et al., editors. Chest surgery, Springer Surgery Atlas Series, 497. New York: © Springer-Verlag Berlin Heidelberg; 2015. https://doi.org/10.1007/978-3-642-12044-2_48.
4. Bosma OH, Vermeulen KM, Verschuuren EA, Erasmus ME, van der Bij W. Adherence to immunosuppression in adult lung transplant recipients: prevalence and risk factors. J Heart Lung Transplant. 2011;30:1275–80.
5. Bjotuft O, Johansen B, Boe J, Foerster A, Holter E, Geiran O. Daily home spirometry facilitates early detection of rejection in single lung transplant recipients with emphysema. Eur Respir J. 1993;6:705–8.
6. Finkelstein SM, Snyder M, Stibbe CE, Lindgren B, Sabati N, Killoren T, et al. Staging of bronchiolitis obliterans syndrome using home spirometry. Chest. 1999;116:120–6.
7. Robson KS, West AJ. Improving survival outcomes in lung transplant recipients through early detection of bronchiolitis obliterans: daily home spirometry versus standard pulmonary function testing. Can J Respir Ther. 2014;50(1):17–22.
8. Glanville AR. The role of surveillance bronchoscopy post–lung transplantation. Semin Respir Crit Care Med. 2013;34:414–20.
9. Crespo MM, McCarthy DP, Hopkins PM, Clark SC, Budev M, Bermudez CA, Benden C, Eghtesady P, Lease ED, Leard L, D'Cunha J, Wigfield CH, Cypel M, Diamond JM, Yun JJ, Yarmus L, Machuzak M, Klepetko W, Verleden G, Hoetzenecker K, Dellgren G, Mulligan M. ISHLT Consensus Statement on adult and pediatric airway complications after lung transplantation: definitions, grading system, and therapeutics. J Heart Lung Transplant. 2018;37:548–63.

150   E. D. Lease

10. Kumar D, Husain S, Hong Chen M, Moussa G, Himsworth D, Manuel O, et al. Study evaluating the clinical impact of community-acquired respiratory viruses in lung transplant recipients. Transplantation. 2010;89:1028–33.
11. Soccal PM, Aubert J-D, Bridevaux P-O, Garbino J, Thomas Y, Rochat T, et al. Upper and lower respiratory tract viral infections and acute graft rejection in lung transplant recipients. Clin Infect Dis. 2010;51:163–70.
12. Fisher CE, Preiksaitis CM, Lease ED, Edelman J, Kirby KA, Leisenring WM, Raghu G, Boeckh M, Limaye AP. Symptomatic respiratory virus infection and chronic lung allograft dysfunction. Clin Infect Dis. 2016;62(3):313–9.
13. Lo WK, Burakoff R, Goldberg HJ, Feldman N, Chan WW. Pre-transplant impedance measures of reflux are associated with early allograft injury after lung transplantation. J Heart Lung Transplant. 2015;34:26–35.
14. Shah N, Force SD, Mitchell PO, Lin E, Lawrence EC, Easley K, et al. Gastroesophageal reflux disease is associated with an increased rate of acute rejection in lung transplant allografts. Transplant Proc. 2010;42:2702–6.
15. Lo WK, Goldberg HJ, Wee J, Fisichella PM, Chan WW. Both pre-transplant and early post-transplant antireflux surgery prevent development of early allograft injury after lung transplantation. J Gastrointest Surg. 2016;20:111–8.
16. D'Ovidio F, Mura M, Ridsdale R, Takahashi H, Waddell TK, Hutcheon M, et al. The effect of reflux and bile acid aspiration on the lung allograft and its surfactant and innate immunity molecules SP-A and SP-D. Am J Transplant. 2006;6:1930–8.
17. Young LR, Hadjiliadis D, Davis RD, Palmer SM. Lung transplantation exacerbates gastroesophageal reflux disease. Chest. 2003;124:1689–93.
18. Hadjiliadis D, Duane Davis R, Steele MP, Messier RH, Lau CL, Eubanks SS, et al. Gastroesophageal reflux disease in lung transplant recipients. Clin Transpl. 2003;17:363–8.
19. Hartwig MG, Anderson DJ, Onaitis MW, Reddy S, Snyder LD, et al. Fundoplication after lung transplantation prevents the allograft dysfunction associated with reflux. Ann Thorac Surg. 2011;92(2):462–8.
20. Cantu E III, Appel JZ III, Hartwig MG, Woreta H, Green C, et al. J. Maxwell Chamberlain Memorial Paper. Early fundoplication prevents chronic allograft dysfunction in patients with gastroesophageal reflux disease. Ann Thorac Surg. 2004;78(4):1142–51.
21. Verleden GM, Glanville AR, Lease ED, Fisher AJ, Calbrese F, et al. Chronic lung allograft dysfunction: definition, diagnostic criteria, and approaches to treatment – a consensus report from the Pulmonary Council of the ISHLT. J Heart Lung Transplant. 2019;38(5):493–503.
22. Silverborn M, Jeppsson A, Mårtensson G, Nilsson F. New-onset cardiovascular risk factors in lung transplant recipients. J Heart Lung Transplant. 2005;24:1536–43.
23. Ollech JE, Kramer MR, Peled N, Ollech A, Amital A, et al. Post-transplant diabetes mellitus in lung transplant recipients: incidence and risk factors. Eur J Cardiothorac Surg. 2008;33(5):844–8.
24. Savioli G, Surbone S, Giovi I, Salinaro F, Preti P, et al. Early development of metabolic syndrome in patients subjected to lung transplantation. Clin Transpl. 2013;27(3):E237–43.
25. Wang TKM, O'Sullivan S, Gamble GD, Ruygrok PN. Bone density in heart or lung transplant recipients – a longitudinal study. Transplant Proc. 2013;45:2357–65.
26. Robbins HY, Arcasoy SM. Malignancies following lung transplantation. Clin Chest Med. 2011;32:343–55.
27. Singer JP, Boker A, Metchnikoff C, Binstock M, Boettger R, Golden JA, et al. High cumulative dose exposure to voriconazole is associated with cutaneous squamous cell carcinoma in lung transplant recipients. J Heart Lung Transplant. 2012;31:694–9.
28. Dharnidharka VR, Tejani AH, Ho PL, Harmon WE. Post-transplant lymphoproliferative disorder in the United States: young Caucasian males are at highest risk. Am J Transplant. 2002;2(10):993–8.

29. Aris RM, Maia DM, Neuringer IP, Gott K, Kiley S, Gertis K, et al. Post-transplantation lymphoproliferative disorder in the Epstein-Barr virus-naïve lung transplant recipient. Am J Respir Crit Care Med. 1996;154(6 Pt 1):1712–7.
30. Maisonneuve P, Marshall BC, Knapp EA, Lowenfels AB. Cancer risk in cystic fibrosis: a 20-year nationwide study from the United States. J Natl Cancer Inst. 2013;105(2):122–9.
31. Hadjiliadis D, Khoruts A, Zauber AG, Hempstead SE, Maisonneuve P, Lowenfels AB, Cystic Fibrosis Colorectal Cancer Screening Task Force. Cystic fibrosis colorectal cancer screening consensus recommendations. Gastroenterology. 2018;154(3):736–45.
32. Colla S, Ong DS, Ogoti Y, Marchesini M, Mistry NA, Clise-Dwyer K, Ang SA, Storti P, Viale A, Giuliani N, Ruisaard K, Ganan Gomez I, Bristow CA, Estecio M, Weksberg DC, Ho YW, Hu B, Genovese G, Pettazzoni P, Multani AS, Jiang S, Hua S, Ryan MC, Carugo A, Nezi L, Wei Y, Yang H, D'Anca M, Zhang L, Gaddis S, Gong T, Horner JW, Heffernan TP, Jones P, Cooper LJ, Liang H, Kantarjian H, Wang YA, Chin L, Bueso-Ramos C, Garcia-Manero G, De Pinho RA. Telomere dysfunction drives aberrant hematopoietic differentiation and myelodysplastic syndrome. Cancer Cell. 2015;27(5):644–57.
33. Townsley DM, Dumitriu B, Young NS. Bone marrow failure and the telomeropathies. Blood. 2014;124(18):2775–83.
34. Grewal AS, Padera RF, Boukedes S, Divo M, Rosas IO, Camp PC, et al. Prevalence and outcome of lung cancer in lung transplant recipients. Respir Med. 2015;109(3):427–33.
35. Olland AB, Falcoz PE, Santelmo N, Kessler R, Massard G. Primary lung cancer in lung transplant recipients. Ann Thorac Surg. 2014;98(1):362–71.
36. Belli EV, Landolfo K, Keller C, Thomas M, Odell J. Lung cancer following lung transplant: single institution 10 year experience. Lung Cancer. 2013;81(3):451–4.

Chapter 8
Infections in the Adult Solid Organ Transplant Recipient

Gabrielle N. Berger and Genevieve L. Pagalilauan

Introduction

There is a clear mortality benefit from solid organ transplantation with an average of 4.3 years of life gained per organ transplant [1]. Solid organ transplantation necessitates immunosuppression that is intense immediately following transplantation and, in most cases, decreases over time. Improvements in immunosuppression management have reduced the incidence of acute rejection and improved graft survival. However, infection remains a significant risk for all solid organ transplant recipients and can shorten life expectancy as well as shorten the life of the graft [2]. The nature of such infections varies depending on time since transplantation, degree of immunosuppression, type of transplant, unique donor and recipient characteristics, and environmental exposures. This chapter reviews both common and serious infections, as well as explores diagnostic and therapeutic considerations in this unique population. Given the complexities of this population including the potential for unusual pathogenic organisms, increased risk for rapid evolution of infections, and the need to still consider antimicrobial stewardship, consultation with a transplant infectious disease specialist should be considered when treating infections in solid organ transplant recipients.

Timeline of Immunosuppression and Related Infection Risk

The time elapsed since solid organ transplantation affects the susceptibility to infection. Infectious risks can be divided into the early, intermediate, and late post-transplant periods (See Table 8.1).

G. N. Berger (✉) · G. L. Pagalilauan
Department of Medicine, Division of General Internal Medicine, University of Washington, Seattle, WA, USA
e-mail: gberger@uw.edu; jadepag@uw.edu

© Springer Nature Switzerland AG 2020
C. J. Wong (ed.), *Primary Care of the Solid Organ Transplant Recipient*,
https://doi.org/10.1007/978-3-030-50629-2_8

Table 8.1 Timeline for infection risk post solid organ transplant [2, 3]

Timeline	<1 month	1–6 months	>6 months
Types of infection	Nosocomial, surgical, donor, or recipient pre-existing infections	Latent infections, opportunistic infections assuming standard prophylaxis for CMV, HBV, PJP	Community-acquired infections

Organisms	Bacteria:
	  MRSA
	  VRE
	  Carbepenem-resistant *Klebsiella* pneumonia (CRKP)
	  Carbepenem-resistant enterobacteriacae (CRE)
	  Clostridioides difficile (Cdiff)
	  Pseudomonas
	  Burkholderia (lung transplant)
	Fungal:
	  Candida (including non-albicans)
	  Aspergillus (recipient)
	Viral (less common, from donor)
	  HSV
	  HIV
	  West Nile
	  Lymphocytic choriomeningitis virus (LCMV)
		Viral:
		  HCV
		  Adenovirus
		  Influenza
		  BK virus
		Bacterial:
		  Cdiff
		  M. tuberculosis
			Viral:
			  CMV (colitis, retinitis)
			  HBV, HCV (hepatitis)
			  HSV (encephalitis)
			Bacteria:
			  Community-acquired pneumonia and UTIs
			  Nocardia
			Fungal:
			  Aspergillus
			  Atypical molds

Routes of infection	Catheters Ventilator Extracorporeal membrane oxygenation (ECMO) Surgical wounds/ anastomoses		

MRSA methicillin-resistant *Staphylococcus aureus*, *VRE* vancomycin-resistant enterococcus, *HCV* hepatitis C virus, *M. tuberculosis* mycobacterium tuberculosis, *CMV* cytomegalovirus, *HBV* hepatitis B virus, *HSV* herpes simplex virus, *HIV* human immunodeficiency virus

The early post-transplant period (0–1 month)

This period confers increased risk for nosocomial infections and immediate donor-borne infection transmission with patients being cared for in intensive care unit (ICU) and hospital settings. Surgical complications such as wound infections, anastomotic leaks, as well as ICU-related illness including central venous catheter infections, urinary catheter infections, and ventilator-associated pneumonias are common. Donors are screened for viral hepatitis, human immunodeficiency virus

(HIV), herpes simplex virus (HSV), as well as with bacterial and fungal blood and urine cultures in most cases. However, donor-derived infections do occur, and while they are likely at low rates, the exact incidence is unknown due to limited reporting data. Donor-derived infections may result from variation in donor infection screening protocols as well as the limited time window in which to assess potential donors [4]. While primary care providers are most likely not involved in the care of solid organ transplant recipients during this early period, it can be helpful to review the patient's early transplant course for a history of prior infectious complications.

The intermediate post-transplant period (1–6 months, up to 12 months)

This period is characterized by maximal effects of immunosuppression dosing. These medications suppress both T- and B-cell immunity and increase the risk for opportunistic infections similar to the risk in patients with HIV. Prophylaxis against cytomegalovirus (CMV) includes valganciclovir or ganciclovir for 3–12 months depending on CMV status and type of transplant [5]. Those who are CMV-negative for both donor and recipient (D−/R−) and therefore not receiving CMV prophylaxis should be considered for antiviral prophylaxis against HSV and VZV. Antiviral therapy to prevent HSV reactivation is recommended in solid organ transplant recipients who are HSV seropositive (and not receiving CMV prophylaxis) for at least 1 month post-transplant [6]. Prophylaxis against varicella zoster virus (VZV) is recommended in seropositive recipients who are not already receiving prophylaxis against CMV or HSV—however, this situation is less common and the optimal duration is uncertain due to limited data [7].

Protocols for antiviral prophylaxis vary by center, and prophylaxis is typically re-initiated even in the later post-transplant period if patients are treated for rejection, especially if T-cell depleting therapies are used. Prevention of reactivation of hepatitis B virus (HBV) is important in liver transplant recipients, who will receive immunoglobulin plus lamivudine or entecavir. Non-liver solid organ transplant recipients who are positive for HBV are monitored for HBV reactivation for 3–6 months after transplantation.

The incidence of *Pneumocystis jirovecii* pneumonia (PJP) in solid organ transplant recipients has decreased due to the use of routine prophylaxis [8]. Trimethoprim-sulfamethoxazole is the preventive drug of choice in patients without a sulfa allergy. Trimethoprim-sulfamethoxazole is also effective against nocardia, toxoplasmosis, and listeria. It has lesser protection for acute cystitis, sinusitis, and pneumococcal pneumonia. In the setting of a true sulfa allergy, dapsone, atovaquone, and pentamidine are alternatives [9]. Lung transplant recipients are at higher risk and are recommended for lifelong therapy. Other solid organ transplant recipients typically receive 6–12 months of PJP prophylaxis, although it may be modified by the presence of other risk factors such as graft dysfunction, low CD4 counts, neutropenia, concurrent CMV disease, and corticosteroid dosing [8].

Other fungal infections in the early and intermediate periods post-transplantation can be severe. Azole and other antifungal therapy may be utilized for prophylaxis against *Candida* and *Aspergillus* in higher risk patients [10]. While practice varies by transplant center, in general, lung transplant recipients are at higher risk of *Aspergillus* and often receive 3–6 months of prophylactic antifungal therapy after transplantation [11]. In other solid organ transplant recipients, the use of prophylaxis against *Aspergillus* is limited by lack of sufficient data; patients may be given prophylaxis based on risk factors for invasive disease [11]. There is also practice variation in prophylaxis against *Candida* species, with some guidelines preferring prophylaxis in gastrointestinal site transplantations (liver, pancreas, small intestine), while in other sites prophylaxis against *Aspergillus* may be more important [12]. In addition to *Candida* and *Aspergillus* species, reactivation of endemic mycosis may occur, and its incidence can be as high as 6.9% for coccidioidomycosis. Reactivation is more severe and occurs earlier (within 3 months) from donor-derived infections. Recipient reactivation usually occurs within 1 year. Symptoms can include fevers, chills, pleurisy, and cough, though severe pneumonia and multiorgan failure are possible [13]. Prophylaxis may be considered against reactivation of endemic mycoses if recipients have a history of disease prior to transplantation. In most cases, the transplant team, in consultation with a transplant infectious disease specialist, will determine the appropriate prophylaxis against invasive fungal infections. The primary care provider should be aware of possible prophylactic regimens as well as the presentation of clinical disease.

Despite usual prophylaxis, solid organ transplant recipients are susceptible to other viruses including BK virus, hepatitis C (HCV), adenovirus, and influenza. Vaccination for influenza (intramuscular inactivated vaccine), and vigilance for the other at-risk viruses is needed. In this period, solid organ transplant recipients are at risk for bacterial infections including healthcare- and hospital-acquired pneumonia as well as community-acquired pneumonia. Providers must be wary of atypical pneumonia, tuberculosis, and gastrointestinal infection with *Clostridioides difficile* (Cdiff).

Common prophylaxis regimens are shown in Table 8.2.

The late post-transplant period typically starts >6–12 months after transplant. By this time, immunosuppression is being tapered and solid organ transplant recipients are living in their home community under the care of their primary care providers in conjunction with their transplant center. Community-acquired infections are more likely and pattern similarly to the general population with pneumonia, urinary tract infections (UTI), and infectious diarrhea being common. The risk for opportunistic infections is higher if patients experience organ rejection and require intensification of immunosuppression. Unique infections affecting solid organ transplant recipients include late CMV reactivation/infection, HSV, HBV and HCV reactivation, and less commonly JC and BK virus infections. BK virus is a particular concern in renal transplant recipients in whom it can be a major cause of graft failure.

Table 8.2 Common regimens for prophylaxis against infections in solid organ transplant recipients

Infection	Prophylaxis	
Cytomegalovirus (CMV) [5]	Ganciclovir (IV), valganciclovir (PO)	
	D+/R−	Lung: 0–12 months; some centers extend >12 months Heart: 3–6 months Liver: 3–6 months Kidney: 6 months
	R+ (any donor status)	Lung: 6–12 months Heart, liver, kidney: 3 months
	D−/R−	No prophylaxis (but should have HSV/VZV prophylaxis)
HSV	If recipient is positive for HSV (1 or 2) and not receiving CMV prophylaxis, then at least 1 month is recommended. (e.g., acyclovir, but regimens vary)	
VZV	Provide if recipient is positive for VZV and negative for HSV and CMV, and not already receiving prophylaxis against CMV or HSV; optimal duration uncertain	
Fungal	Invasive (*Aspergillus*, *Candida* species): Varies by transplant center and patient risk factors; prophylaxis against *Aspergillus* often given in lung transplant recipients; against *Candida* in liver transplant recipients Endemic Varies by patient risk factors, e.g., history of prior endemic mycotic disease	
Pneumocystis jirovecii	Lung: lifelong Other organs: 6–12 months, may vary if risk factors present	

Key Considerations in Diagnosis

Solid organ transplant recipients require lifelong immunosuppression resulting in a reduction of usual signs and symptoms of inflammation that accompany infections [3]. The pragmatism and parsimonious approach we strive for in usual practice must be set aside when assessing the solid organ transplant recipient for infection. While symptoms may be muted, the actual infection may evolve rapidly and progress to a more severe infection in these immunosuppressed patients. Infections may be the result of polymicrobial infections and/or from multi-drug-resistant organisms. Comprehensive testing and more rapid escalation to invasive testing are appropriate [3].

Immunosuppression reduces the sensitivity of tests that rely on the patient's immune system such as serological tests for antibodies. Instead, direct detection of pathogens using culture, polymerase chain reaction (PCR), and similar tests of optimal specimens is preferred. This may require more invasive testing such as biopsy of infected tissue [3, 14].

Respiratory Infections

Case

A 60-year-old woman with a history of bilateral lung transplantation 2 years prior presents to the primary care clinic in the winter season with 3 days of subjective fevers, nasal congestion, rhinorrhea, dry cough, and myalgias. She is adherent to her immunosuppression regimen and has not had any episodes of rejection in the last year. On exam, her temperature is 38.0 °C, heart rate 98, blood pressure 125/70, respiratory rate 22, and oxygen saturation 97% on ambient air. Her exam reveals mild erythema of the oropharynx but no tonsillar hypertrophy and no exudate. Her lungs are clear and she has no lymphadenopathy. She received the inactivated influenza vaccine in October.

Comment:

This patient is presenting with symptoms of an upper respiratory tract infection during influenza season. She has a low-grade fever with mild tachycardia and an elevated respiratory rate. Although the patient received the influenza vaccine, not all viral subtypes are covered equally, and she is still at risk of influenza infection. Infection with other respiratory viruses including rhinovirus, coronavirus, and respiratory syncytial virus (RSV) is also possible. This patient should undergo testing with a viral respiratory PCR panel, or a rapid influenza test if the extended panel is not available. Because of the presence of cough and fever during influenza season, she should be treated empirically for influenza with oseltamivir unless contraindicated.

The absence of lymphadenopathy and sore throat make bacterial pharyngitis unlikely. Community-acquired pneumonia is also less likely without clear signs of lower respiratory tract involvement. Opportunistic infections due to mycobacterial and fungal etiologies, as well as reactivation of latent diseases, such as CMV, typically present more gradually and would not be consistent with the acuity of symptom onset in this case. Nonetheless, a chest X-ray should be obtained to evaluate for new consolidation or nodules.

Respiratory infections after solid organ transplantation are common and account for significant morbidity and mortality in this population. Bacterial pneumonia remains the most common cause of lower respiratory tract infections, with one study identifying community-acquired pneumonia (CAP) in 40.7% and healthcare-associated pneumonia (HCAP) in 38.9% of solid organ transplant recipients treated for pneumonia [15]. Solid organ transplant recipients are at higher risk of developing lower respiratory tract disease from common respiratory viruses and often develop more severe symptoms than immunocompetent hosts [16]. Solid organ transplant recipients are also more likely to develop invasive fungal pneumonia as well as bacterial and fungal co-infection in the setting of a viral respiratory illness [15]. Primary care providers must be aware of the risk factors and possible presentations of respiratory infections in solid organ transplant recipients to appropriately triage, diagnose, and treat these patients in the outpatient setting. Table 8.3 shows common respiratory infections in solid organ transplant recipients.

Table 8.3 Common respiratory infections in solid organ transplant recipients

Category of respiratory infections	Common pathogens	Common diagnostic evaluation	Treatment	Prevention
Viral*	Influenza	PCR-based nasopharyngeal swab	Neuraminidase inhibitor Oseltamivir Zanamivir	Influenza vaccination with either inactivated influenza vaccine (IIV) or recombinant influenza vaccine (RIV) Prophylaxis with oseltamivir for close contacts with influenza exposure
	Parainfluenza Human metapneumovirus Respiratory syncytial virus (RSV)	PCR-based nasopharyngeal swab	Supportive care Consider reduction in immunosuppression +/– ribavirin +/– IVIg (mixed data, only in consultation with an infectious disease specialist)	Hand hygiene No vaccination or prophylaxis available
	Adenovirus	PCR-based nasopharyngeal swab	Supportive care +/– cidofovir, only in consultation with an infectious disease specialist	Hand hygiene No vaccination or prophylaxis available
Bacterial	Streptococcus pneumoniae Haemophilus influenzae MSSA/MRSA Nocardia species Chlamydia pneumoniae Moraxella catarrhalis Legionella species Pseudomonas aeruginosa	Sputum culture Consider legionella and S. pneumoniae urine antigen tests (limited sensitivity)	Antibiotics tailored to causative agent If no pathogen identified, treat empirically with: Respiratory fluoroquinolone, or Amoxicillin-clavulanate + macrolide	Hand hygiene Vaccination for Haemophilus influenzae (Hib) and Streptococcus pneumoniae (PPSV23)

(continued)

Table 8.3 (continued)

Category of respiratory infections	Common pathogens	Common diagnostic evaluation	Treatment	Prevention
	Mycobacterium tuberculosis Non-tuberculous mycobacterium (NTM)	AFB sputum stain and culture	Antibiotics tailored to causative agent, in consultation with an infectious disease specialist	Pre-transplant testing for latent TB
Fungal	*Aspergillus* species	Sputum stain and culture Galactomannan assays on sputum and serum	Antifungal therapy, typically voriconazole, in consultation with an infectious disease specialist[a]	Prophylaxis with voriconazole early in post-transplant course (protocols vary)
	Endemic mycoses (histoplasmosis, coccidioidomycosis, blastomycosis)	Sputum or BAL culture *or* histopathologic/cytopathologic identification of organisms Serologic assays for coccidioidomycosis less sensitive in SOT recipients	Antifungal therapy, often fluconazole or itraconazole, in consultation with an infectious disease specialist[a]	None
	Pneumocystis jirovecii	Immunofluorescence stain on induced sputum or bronchoscopy sample	TMP-SMX, +/− steroids depending on degree of hypoxemia	TMP-SMX, variable duration depending on organ transplanted; lifelong after lung transplantation

[a]Also consult with transplant team due to common drug interactions between azoles and immunosuppressant medications
*The COVID-19/SARS-CoV-2 pandemic is ongoing as of this publication. Testing and treatment should follow up to date public health guidelines for high-risk populations, including solid organ transplant recipients

Diagnostic Considerations

All solid organ transplant recipients who present with a suspected respiratory viral infection should undergo evaluation with a nasopharyngeal sample tested by PCR for respiratory viral pathogens [16]. Most respiratory viral infections are restricted to the upper respiratory tract; however, solid organ transplant patients are at higher risk of developing lower respiratory tract infection and subsequent complications, including superimposed bacterial pneumonia, due to impaired cellular and humoral immunity [17]. In lung transplant recipients, development of lower respiratory tract disease may be associated with increased risk of chronic lung allograft dysfunction, though the relationship with episodes of acute rejection has not been established [18]. Identifying common viral infections, such as non-epidemic coronavirus or rhinovirus, as a cause of lower respiratory tract infection may reassure the clinician that additional evaluation is not necessary and improve antibiotic stewardship. In a solid organ transplant recipient with lower respiratory tract symptoms, the primary care provider should strongly consider obtaining chest imaging. Focal infiltrates on chest X-ray are most consistent with a bacterial pneumonia, whereas diffuse lung disease and multifocal infiltrates are more likely to represent a viral infection or non-infectious process. With a relevant exposure history and characteristic tempo of symptom onset, nodular opacities on chest X-ray may suggest a fungal etiology [19].

Chest imaging, while helpful, cannot definitively rule in or rule out bacterial, viral, or fungal etiologies of respiratory symptoms; imaging must be combined with a thorough history and the provider's best clinical judgment to determine a diagnosis. The primary care provider should have a low threshold to consult with an infectious disease specialist or a pulmonologist when interpreting the chest X-ray findings in a solid organ transplant recipient with a suspected infectious respiratory illness. Chest CT and even bronchoscopy may be indicated to differentiate infection from non-infectious causes of respiratory symptoms, including rejection in lung transplant patients, and drug fever [2]. Lung transplant recipients in particular should receive consultation with the transplant pulmonologist, both to expedite the appropriate workup and to avoid empiric treatment that may make subsequent diagnostic tests less accurate (See Chap. 7). Patients who present to clinic with signs of impending respiratory failure, hypoxemia, or any other unstable vital signs due to a suspected respiratory infection should be admitted to the hospital for inpatient evaluation and treatment. Even patients who are clinically stable may benefit from an emergency department evaluation or inpatient stay if they have higher risk for severe infection, including earlier time period since transplantation, higher level of immunosuppression, history of organ failure or chronic illness, and other risk factors, as solid organ transplant recipients can decompensate quickly.

See Chap. 9, for a broader discussion of differential diagnoses of respiratory symptoms, including non-infectious causes. Specific infectious entities are discussed below.

Respiratory Viral Illness

Influenza is an acute, febrile illness that typically manifests with respiratory symptoms or may be asymptomatic. While influenza infection is usually self-limited in immunocompetent individuals, solid organ transplant recipients may have variable presentations of influenza, ranging from atypical, non-respiratory symptoms to severe respiratory compromise [15]. Common non-respiratory symptoms of influenza infection in solid organ transplant recipients include gastrointestinal distress, sore throat, low-grade fever, or even lack of fever. Solid organ transplant recipients are also more likely to shed the influenza virus for a longer period of time than immunocompetent hosts due to inability to clear the virus, prolonging their risk of complications and possible transmission to others [15, 20, 21]. Risk of influenza infection is highest among lung transplant recipients, followed by patients with liver and kidney transplants [15]. Rates of severe influenza infection are reported between 16 and 20% in lung transplant recipients, with mortality ranging from 4 to 8% in this population [15]. Mortality is higher among solid organ transplant recipients during influenza outbreaks and was reported at 21% for lung transplant recipients in an Australian study during the 2009 H1N1 influenza epidemic [15].

If a solid organ transplant recipient presents to the primary care setting with fever and upper respiratory symptoms or cough during influenza season, the primary care provider should have a high index of suspicion for influenza infection. While it is often appropriate to treat immunocompetent hosts for influenza empirically, the Centers for Disease Control and Prevention (CDC) recommends that providers should attempt to diagnose influenza infection in solid organ transplant recipients to target therapy. While rapid influenza antigen tests are specific for influenza infection, they lack appropriate sensitivity in immunocompromised hosts [16]. More sensitive tests, including the viral respiratory PCR panels, are considered the gold standard in many institutions, and can identify the influenza subtype, which may be important in epidemic years or in cases of treatment failure. Because influenza testing varies by institution, primary care providers will need to know which tests (e.g., rapid antigen, nucleic acid amplification, PCR) are available in their location, the tests' performance characteristics, and how quickly results will be known. If a rapid influenza antigen test is negative for a solid organ transplant recipient who presents with suspected influenza and the PCR panel is not available, the patient should receive empiric influenza treatment unless contraindicated [22]. Pooled analyses of randomized controlled trials evaluating the efficacy of oseltamivir treatment in high-risk individuals have shown a decrease in the rates of hospitalization due to influenza from 3.2% to 1.6% (relative risk reduction, 50%) [23].

There are two main classes of antiviral therapy available to treat influenza infections: adamantanes (amantadine and rimantadine) and neuraminidase inhibitors (oseltamivir and zanamivir) [22, 23]. Historically, amantadanes have been active against most influenza A strains, but not influenza B. However, widespread resistance to influenza A (H3N2) and more limited resistance to influenza A (H1N1) has been reported since 2006. The neuraminidase inhibitors are active against both influenza A and B viruses, though oseltamivir resistance among certain influenza A (H1N1) strains has also been identified [23]. With these resistance patterns, the

CDC recommends oseltamivir 75 mg BID for 5 days for treatment of influenza in immunocompromised hosts; amantadanes are no longer considered first-line therapy. Providers caring for solid organ transplant patients living outside the United States should review local epidemiology and resistance patterns, and consult with local experts to guide treatment strategies. Some patients may benefit from a longer course of therapy if not significantly improved after initial treatment, particularly if levels of immunosuppression are particularly high; in this case, primary care providers should consider discussing with an infectious disease specialist. There is no data however to support doses of oseltamivir higher than 75 mg daily, though clinicians may consider increasing the duration of therapy to 75 mg daily for 10 days (or longer) in solid organ transplant patients due to prolonged viral shedding and clearance [2, 24]. Influenza changes seasonally and may have pandemic strains—it is important to follow local public health reporting and updated guidelines.

Baloxavir is a novel cap-dependent endonuclease inhibitor approved by the United States FDA in October 2018 for the treatment of acute uncomplicated influenza in patients 12 years of age and older within 2 days of symptom onset [25, 26]. Baloxavir is administered as a single-dose oral medication. In randomized controlled trials comparing baloxavir to placebo and oseltamivir, baloxavir was superior to both placebo and oseltamivir in reducing viral load 1 day after initiating treatment, with the implication that transmission rates may be reduced [27]. The role of baloxavir in treating immunosuppressed patients has not been established, although local institutions may use it in select patients, particularly if there is concern for oseltamivir resistance.

If the patient develops worsening lower respiratory symptoms including productive cough or pleuritic chest pain while on oseltamivir, one should obtain chest imaging to evaluate for bacterial co-infection or even consider treating empirically for a concomitant bacterial pneumonia. (In a lung transplant recipient, one should consult early with the transplant pulmonologist, preferably before starting antibiotics—See Chap. 7.)

Vaccination against influenza with an inactivated influenza vaccine is indicated for solid organ transplant recipients before and after transplantation [16]. However, the vaccine should be withheld in the first 2 months after transplant due to the likelihood of inadequate response [28]. Either the trivalent or quadrivalent inactivated influenza vaccine (IIV) or the recombinant influenza vaccine (RIV) may be administered intramuscularly; the live attenuated influenza nasal vaccine (LAIV) is contraindicated in solid organ transplant recipients [29]. There is no evidence indicating that solid organ transplant recipients derive additional benefit from the high-dose influenza vaccine [30, 31]. Nevertheless, some infectious disease specialists recommend the high-dose influenza vaccine in solid organ transplant recipients because of limited evidence of increased immune response, although no clinical outcome data are yet available.

In addition to influenza, infection with other viral respiratory pathogens, including respiratory syncytial virus (RSV), parainfluenza virus, human metapneumovirus, rhinovirus, and adenovirus, is common in solid organ transplant recipients [15, 17]. Similar to influenza, these respiratory viruses are spread by direct contact with aerosolized droplets [15]. The clinical syndrome is similar to infection with influenza and includes fever, cough, rhinorrhea, and myalgias, though development of lower respiratory tract symptoms with bronchiolitis and pneumonia is more common in solid organ transplant recipients than in immunocompetent individuals [17]. Nasopharyngeal swab or wash should be collected in the clinic and sent for PCR-based assays, which remain the gold standard for diagnosing respiratory viral infections in solid organ transplant recipients [2, 15]. Supportive care is the mainstay of treatment for non-influenza respiratory infections. If the patient develops hypoxia, they should be promptly admitted to the hospital. In severe cases, the transplant team should be informed; in some circumstances, the transplant team may consider whether a reduction in immunosuppression is warranted [15]. Antiviral drug therapy for certain viral pathogens in solid organ transplant recipients, including RSV and adenovirus, is under investigation [15, 17]. There are currently no accepted guidelines for the use of ribavirin in the treatment of RSV; practices vary by institution and it is typically only used in hospitalized patients with lower respiratory tract disease and a significantly depressed absolute lymphocyte count.

Infection with cytomegalovirus (CMV) can cause significant respiratory illness in solid organ transplant recipients. While infection with CMV can occur as a primary or secondary infection, the majority of cases in this patient population represent reactivation of a latent reservoir. CMV disease can manifest as either CMV syndrome, characterized by fever, malaise, and myelosuppression, or as CMV tissue-invasive disease, which can be isolated to the allograft or involve multiple organs simultaneously [32, 33]. Symptoms of CMV pneumonia are non-specific and are typically characterized by subacute onset of fevers, cough, and hypoxemia, accompanied by a range of radiographic findings including bilateral infiltrates, nodules, and areas of consolidation. Lung transplant recipients are at particularly high risk for CMV pneumonia; diagnosis requires the presence of signs or symptoms of pulmonary disease combined with the detection of CMV in bronchoalveolar lavage or lung tissue samples [34]. Because of the non-specific presentation, primary care providers should maintain a high index of suspicion for CMV pneumonia in lung transplant recipients and closely collaborate with the patient's transplant physicians to expedite evaluation and coordinate care.

Emerging respiratory infections such as COVID-19 (SARS-CoV-2) may be particularly severe in solid organ transplant recipients. At the time of this book's publication, this virus continues to be studied during the worldwide pandemic. Testing should be initiated promptly depending on local epidemiology and public health guidelines. Consultation with infectious disease specialists is indicated in a solid organ transplant recipient with suspected or confirmed COVID-19 infection.

Bacterial Pneumonia

Community-Acquired Pneumonia (CAP) is common in solid organ transplant recipients, although evidence is mixed as to whether CAP occurs more frequently in these patients compared to the general population [35, 36]. While solid organ transplant recipients are at risk for CAP from typical organisms including *Streptococcus pneumoniae, Legionella pneumophila, and Haemophilus influenza*, they are also at increased risk of infection with *Nocardia spp, Staphylococcus aureus, Pseudomonas aeruginosa,* and other gram-negative rods (GNRs) [16]. Abrupt onset of fever accompanied by cough productive of sputum should raise concern for CAP. A focal infiltrate on chest X-ray may be useful in confirming suspicion for CAP, but should not be used to rule in or rule out disease.

IDSA guidelines (2019) include recommendations for the treatment of CAP in patients with comorbidities (which include chronic heart, lung, liver, and renal disease, as well as asplenia). For solid organ transplant recipients, CAP treatment options include monotherapy with a respiratory fluoroquinolone or combination therapy with a beta-lactam (amoxicillin-clavulanate) or a cephalosporin plus either doxycycline or a macrolide [16, 37]. This treatment regimen should only be used for stable outpatients. Drug interactions are common with antibiotics and immunosuppressant medications—if starting a new antibiotic, especially a macrolide, the transplant team should be notified (See Chap. 3). The typical treatment duration is 5 days, though providers may treat longer if symptoms are not improving. However, if symptoms persist without response to antibiotic therapy, consultation with a pulmonologist should be obtained to consider additional diagnostic testing and alternate diagnoses.

Hospital admission should be expedited for any patient with CAP and unstable vital signs, and considered for certain solid organ transplant recipients who, although stable, are high risk for decompensation. Validated clinical prediction scores to stratify the need for hospitalization may be used, but only in combination with clinical judgment in this population.

As discussed above, the primary care provider who is treating a lung transplant recipient with suspected CAP should contact the patient's lung transplant specialist. Lung transplant recipients may be at risk for opportunistic infections and resistant bacteria, may already be receiving macrolides chronically for anti-inflammatory therapy, and may need an expedited evaluation for rejection.

Infection with mycobacterium, including *Mycobacterium tuberculosis, mycobacterium avian* complex (MAC), and other non-tuberculous mycobacterial (NTM) species, is an important diagnostic consideration in the solid organ transplant recipient who presents with subacute to chronic onset of respiratory symptoms. The incidence of pulmonary tuberculosis (TB) in solid organ transplant recipients depends on the incidence in the general population, epidemiologic risk factors, and new or ongoing TB exposures [38]. The frequency of active TB among solid organ transplant patients is estimated to be 20–74 times higher than the general population, with higher prevalence rates in endemic areas [39]. Rates of active TB are highest in lung transplant patients compared to other solid organ transplant recipients. Approximately two-third of active TB infections occur within the first post-transplant year, with the majority reflecting reactivation of prior disease [40]. All solid organ transplant recipients should undergo TB testing prior to transplantation to identify cases of latent tuberculosis infection (LTBI); however, not all LTBI may be identified due to anergy with end stage organ failure [41]. One-third to one-half of all cases of active TB in solid organ transplant recipients are disseminated or occur at non-pulmonary sites—thus primary care providers must maintain a high index of suspicion for pulmonary as well as disseminated disease. Active pulmonary TB in solid organ transplant recipients may manifest with non-specific symptoms such as fevers, weight loss, and fatigue, as well as productive cough, hemoptysis, and dyspnea. If the physician suspects pulmonary TB, standard TB evaluation should be pursued with a chest X-ray and sputum samples sent for acid-fast bacilli (AFB) staining and culture. Primary care providers should communicate with an infectious disease specialist and a pulmonologist to determine if more invasive diagnostic testing is warranted and to determine a treatment course if pulmonary TB is identified. Importantly, treating pulmonary TB in solid organ transplant recipients requires medication adjustment to avoid interactions between rifamycins and calcineurin inhibitors [41].

In comparison to pulmonary TB, NTM infections in solid organ transplant recipients typically occur later in the post-transplant course. However it is important to note that these infections have been described in the days to months after transplant as well [42]. NTM infections involve the lung in more than 50% of cases, with heart and lung transplant recipients being more susceptible than kidney and liver transplant recipients [2]. Manifestations of respiratory NTM infections include pulmonary infiltrates, solitary pulmonary nodules, abscesses, and cavitary lesions. Symptoms of pulmonary NTM infections are non-specific and may include chronic cough, sputum production, and less often, hemoptysis. Importantly, systemic symptoms such as fever and night sweats, may not be present [43]. In solid organ transplant recipients with suspected NTM infection, a pulmonologist should be involved early to help direct the evaluation, which may include bronchoscopy and requests for special staining, culture, and histopathology. While these pathogens are less common than other bacterial and viral causes of respiratory infection in solid organ transplant patients, they are important diagnostic considerations due to difficulty in making the diagnosis, the need for long-term, multi-drug antibiotic regimens, and potential interaction of these antibiotics with drugs used for immunosuppression [44].

Fungal Pneumonia

Invasive fungal pneumonia, particularly with *Aspergillus* species, is of concern in solid organ transplant recipients and disproportionately affects lung transplant recipients, with complicated infections affecting up to 13% of patients [45]. As opposed to the rapid symptom onset characteristic of viral or bacterial pneumonia, respiratory illness due to fungal infection usually develops over weeks or even months. Additionally, the incidence of invasive fungal infections is higher 6–12 months after transplant and mold infections, such as invasive aspergillosis, often occur >1 year after transplant [19]. Solid organ transplant recipients are also at higher risk for infection with endemic mycoses, including histoplasmosis, coccidioidomycosis, and blastomycosis, and providers should take a thorough travel history to assess risk of these infections [46]. Finally, invasive candidiasis is an important cause of infection in the solid organ transplant recipient, though it presents less commonly as pneumonia [2]. Diagnosis and treatment of invasive fungal pneumonia require the assistance of an infectious disease specialist or a pulmonologist and are often performed in the inpatient setting—thus early recognition by the primary care provider and coordinating early with specialty care are critical.

Pneumonia due to *Pneumocystis jirovecii* peaks during the first 6 months after transplantation when immunosuppression is highest. Additional risk factors include increased intensity of immunosuppression (as occurs with treatment of rejection episodes), inadequate adherence to prophylaxis, a history of CMV viremia, and lung transplantation which confers a sustained increase in risk compared to other organ transplants, leading to lifelong prophylaxis for most lung transplant recipients. *Pneumocystis jirovecii* pneumonia is typically acute or subacute in onset; however, compared to patients with HIV infection, the time course of disease presentation in solid organ transplant recipients may be more rapid. Clinicians should have a high index of suspicion for *Pneumocystis jirovecii* infection in solid organ transplant recipients who present with hypoxemia out of proportion to radiologic findings, particularly in patients who are no longer taking or who are not adherent to *Pneumocystis jirovecii* prophylaxis.

Pneumocystis jirovecii pneumonia may be diagnosed either by performing immunofluorescence on sputum samples or lower respiratory secretions. Compared to HIV-infected individuals, solid organ transplant recipients may have lower burden of organisms thus reducing the sensitivity of microscopy. PCR may be used as an alternative means to make a diagnosis of *Pneumocystis* pneumonia if the index of suspicion is high, though it does not reliably exclude airway colonization in the solid organ transplant population [47]. While evaluation for *Pneumocystis* pneumonia can be performed as an outpatient if the patient is stable and resources are readily available, often the patient will require admission for a more expedient workup, including evaluation for other causes of respiratory illness. Treatment with trimethoprim-sulfamethoxozole (TMP-SMX) is the preferred course of therapy. Low-dose daily prophylaxis with TMP-SMX, if tolerated, has the additional benefit of helping to prevent infection with *Toxoplasma* and *Nocardia* species, as well as other common causes of urinary and respiratory tract infections [19].

Gastrointestinal Infections

Case

A 54-year-old woman with a history of kidney transplantation presents with 3 weeks of diarrhea and decreased appetite. She has 3–5 loose stools daily without hematochezia, melena, or change in frequency or severity. Her immunosuppression medication dosing and adherence have not changed. She has no recent travel or change in diet or water sources. Her CMV serostatus is D+/R-. On exam, she has normal vital signs, is not orthostatic, and has a normal abdomen exam. What is the next appropriate step in her care?

Comment: This patient appears to be clinically stable, and it may be feasible to continue her evaluation as an outpatient. Initial testing should include kidney function, complete blood counts, a serum CMV PCR, and stool testing for enteric pathogens. Initial stool testing at a minimum should include common bacterial enteric pathogens and Clostridioides difficile PCR. Depending on a patient's known exposures and clinical course, testing for norovirus and parasitic infections such as cryptosporidium and giardia may be tested up front or, if deferred, then tested if initial testing results return negative and the patient continues to have symptoms. Modern stool "multiplex" panels often include bacterial, viral, and parasitic testing in a single specimen and may be sent initially, if available.

Non-infectious causes of diarrhea should also be considered. (See below as well as Chap. 9). If the above infectious testing is negative, consultation with an infectious disease or gastroenterology specialist familiar with solid organ transplant recipients should be sought, as additional tests, including endoscopy, should be considered. If she develops new or worsening symptoms, she will likely require an emergency department evaluation and consideration for expedited workup.

In solid organ transplant recipients, the most common presentation of gastrointestinal infections is diarrhea, and it affects 20–50% of patients. The Infectious Disease Society of America (IDSA) defines diarrhea as >3 soft or loose stools per day. Acute diarrhea is present for <14 days, persistent diarrhea for 14–29 days, and chronic diarrhea for >30 days. Risk factors for diarrhea in solid organ transplant recipients include being female, using tacrolimus or tacrolimus plus mycophenolate [48].

Differential Diagnosis of Infectious Causes of Diarrhea

The causes of diarrhea in solid organ transplant recipients is similar to that of the general population, including non-infectious and infectious etiologies. As in immunocompetent populations, *norovirus*, food-borne bacterial and viral illness, medications, and *Clostridioide difficile* (Cdiff) are common. However, solid organ transplant recipients are more likely to have opportunistic infections and more likely to have persistent infectious diarrhea.

Diagnostic Considerations

A good history is important when assessing diarrhea in solid organ transplant recipients. Fever more commonly indicates a viral, or invasive bacterial etiology, and rarely is caused by parasitic infections. Blood in the stool can be caused by invasive bacterial infections, *cytomegalovirus* (CMV) or Entamoeba. Watery diarrhea with or without emesis suggests viral or medication-induced diarrhea [48].

In both immunosuppressed and immunocompetent patients, fecal studies have a low overall diagnostic yield, but are often a necessary part of the evaluation. The American Society of Transplantation Infectious Diseases Community of Practice recommends a tiered approach to testing for solid organ transplant recipients presenting with diarrhea (Fig. 8.1) [48, 49]. Initial recommendations including stopping any non-immunosuppressive medications that could contribute to diarrhea and performing bacterial stool culture or, if available, stool multiplex polymerase chain reaction (PCR), Cdiff stool PCR, and serum CMV PCR or nucleotide acid

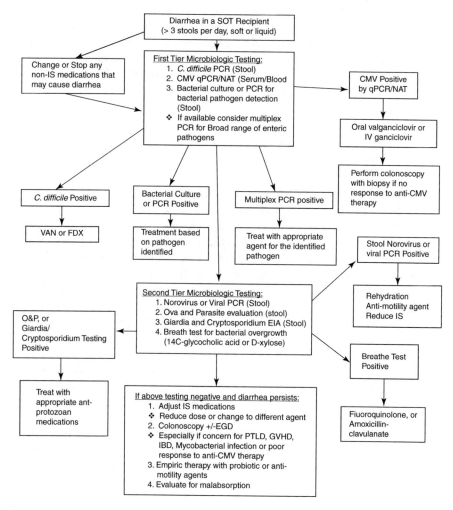

Fig. 8.1 Diagnostic approach to diarrhea in solid organ transplant [48]. (From Angarone, et al. [48] Reprinted with permission)

amplification test (NAAT). If diarrhea persists and an etiology is not identified, then additional testing should be considered for norovirus, ova and parasites, giardia stool enzyme-linked immunosorbent assay (EIA), cryptosporidium stool EIA, as well as considering a breath test for small intestine bacterial overgrowth (SIBO). If the diarrhea persists and an etiology is still not obtained, then these guidelines recommend considering discussing a potential adjustment in immunosuppressive medications that may be contributing to diarrhea, as well as colonoscopy, upper endoscopy, evaluation for malabsorption, and empiric treatment with antimotility agents or probiotics [48].

This algorithm should be adjusted for local epidemiology, the overall clinical likelihood of infectious versus non-infectious cause of diarrhea, the severity of a patient's presentation, the pattern of diarrhea (duration, relationship with intake), and the availability of a stool multiplex assay (which often tests for bacterial pathogens, norovirus, rotavirus, cryptosporidium, giardia, and Cdiff). For further discussion, see Chap. 9.

Specific Etiologies

Clostridiodes difficile (**Cdiff**) is a spore-forming anaerobic bacterium that causes infectious diarrhea in solid organ transplant recipients on the order of 1–33% depending on the type of transplant, with lowest incidence in renal transplant recipients and highest in multiorgan or heart/lung transplant recipients [50]. Cdiff infection occurs most frequently in the immediate post-transplant period; however, solid organ transplant recipients are at increased longitudinal risk. Antibiotics, notably penicillins, cephalosporins, clindamycin, and fluoroquinolones, increase risk of Cdiff infection, especially if there are multiple or prolonged courses. Specific risk factors for Cdiff in solid organ transplant recipients include age >55, repeat transplantation status, liver transplant, and treatment using anti-thymocyte globulin [48]. In solid organ transplant recipients who develop Cdiff infections, 5–16% will have a fulminant infection and the mortality rate is 2.3–8.5% [48, 50]. Cdiff is also known to increase morbidity in other infections including CMV and pneumonia, as well as cause organ dysfunction and longer hospital stays.

Diagnosis of Cdiff infections is based on both clinical and laboratory data. There is an increasing number of people who are colonized with Cdiff, and no current laboratory tests can distinguish between colonization and infection. Hence, the diagnosis of Cdiff is made when a patient experiences new onset or unexplained, clinically significant (3 loose stool/day) diarrhea in the presence of laboratory confirmation of free Cdiff toxin (toxin A or B via EIA), or toxigenic

Cdiff bacteria (Cdiff NAAT) in the stool. In the 2019 American Society of Transplantation Community of Practice guidelines for Cdiff in solid organ transplant recipients, additional recommendations include not automatically repeating negative Cdiff tests, and not "testing for cure" after an infection. Uncommonly, Cdiff may present without diarrhea, and this infection should be also considered in solid organ transplant recipients who present with fever, leukocytosis, abdominal pain, and ileus. If there is negative Cdiff standard testing and a high clinical suspicion for Cdiff infection, then further workup should be considered, including abdominal/pelvic CT imaging, colonoscopy, and repeat standard testing [50].

Treatment of Cdiff is similar in solid organ transplant recipients and immune competent patients. Treatment as of 2018 IDSA guidelines no longer uses metronidazole. First-line treatment is vancomycin 125 mg PO Q6H or fidaxomicin 200 mg BID × 10 days. Fulminant Cdiff, characterized by hypotension, ileus, or megacolon, will be managed inpatient, and is treated with vancomycin 500 mg PO Q6H plus metronidazole 500 mg IV Q8H, +/− rectal vancomycin, and possible surgery consultation. In patients with hypogammaglobulinemia (tested with quantitative immunoglobulins), treatment with IgG may reduce the risk for recurrent Cdiff infection [48]. Solid organ transplant recipients have an 8–16% risk for relapsing Cdiff infections. Treatment of recurrent Cdiff infections is well described in IDSA guidelines and includes fidaxomicin, tapering or pulsed courses of vancomycin, or vancomycin followed by rifaximin. Bezlotoxumab (10 mg/kg IV) is a human monoclonal antibody targeting Cdiff toxin B. The 2019 guidelines recommend consideration for its use in first infections and recurrences to prevent recurrent Cdiff infections [50]. Transplant infectious disease and/or gastroenterology specialists should be involved in the care of solid organ transplant recipients with recurrent Cdiff.

Fecal microbiota transplant (FMT) has been used in immunosuppressed and solid organ transplant recipients in limited studies. In immunosuppressed patients, cure rates range 78–89% but with 15% experiencing serious adverse events which included hospitalizations and 2 deaths [48]. A single-center study of 94 solid organ transplant recipients with recurrent Cdiff (78%) or severe fulminant Cdiff (22%) found an overall cure rate of 91% with FMT, and a 3-month primary cure rate of 58.7%. Adverse events were experienced in 22% consisting of mostly self-limited diarrhea, abdominal pain, FMT-related diarrhea. However, 3.2% experienced severe adverse events including 2 hospitalizations for flare of inflammatory bowel disease (IBD). The same study found that in solid organ transplant recipients with IBD, 25% experienced post FMT IBD exacerbations. In CMV-seropositive patients, 14% experienced reactivation of CMV after FMT. Notably, patients in the study also experienced severe complications of the Cdiff infection itself including death [51]. Based on this study, 2019 guidelines recommend FMT for recurrent Cdiff infections in solid organ transplant recipients [50]. Given these potential risks, it is advisable to consult a transplant infectious disease specialist when considering FMT.

Cytomegalovirus (CMV) is a double-stranded DNA virus that is part of the herpes virus family. It has varying gastrointestinal manifestations that can include esophagitis, gastritis, enteritis, colitis, and typically presents with diarrhea, abdominal pain, and fever. It can also cause hepatitis, cholangitis, and pancreatitis. Solid organ transplant recipients are at highest risk for CMV infections when the donor's serostatus is positive and recipient's serostatus is negative. Other risks include the degree of immunosuppression, acute rejection, advanced age, allograft dysfunction, and the type of transplant, with renal transplants being of highest risk [48].

As per the guidelines for work-up of diarrhea in solid organ transplant recipients, serum CMV testing with either PCR or quantitative nucleic acid amplification testing (QNAT) is a first-line test. There are some data that suggest a stool CMV PCR may be highly specific (but not sensitive), but this test is not widely available [52]. Older (2013) guidelines recommend quantitative nucleic acid amplification testing (QNAT) for both diagnosis and monitoring of CMV infections, although this test has largely been supplanted by PCR, if available. The pp65 CMV antigenemia test has historically been used for diagnosis and monitoring of CMV infections but is less standardized and more labor-intensive. Repeat serological testing is not needed after transplant, though it can help with determining susceptibility to community-acquired CMV infections in CMV-negative recipients. Viral culture of the blood and urine have poor sensitivity and specificity, respectively. Tissue invasive disease is diagnosed via CMV inclusion bodies or CMV antigens detected via immunohistochemistry on biopsy specimens obtained during colonoscopy/endoscopy. Tissue cultures and QNAT can be difficult to interpret as both infection and shedding can create positive results but may have a limited role in diagnosis [34]. Tissue diagnosis via colonoscopy should be pursued if needed to confirm the diagnosis even with a positive change in serum PCR (e.g., if there are competing diagnoses, or the patient tolerates anti-CMV therapy poorly, or if empiric therapy against CMV was attempted and the patient did not respond), or if the serum CMV PCR is negative but the clinical suspicion of CMV gastrointestinal disease is still high.

Solid organ transplant recipients with CMV gastrointestinal disease should receive consultation with an infectious disease specialist. Initial treatment is with oral valganciclovir, whereas IV ganciclovir is used for more life-threatening cases. Renal function must be monitored carefully, and doses adjusted accordingly. Treatment duration is dependent on weekly CMV viral loads. Recommendations are for 1–2 consecutive negative viral loads with a minimum treatment duration of 2 weeks. Failure to improve viral loads with therapy over the course of 6 weeks should raise the suspicion for drug resistance. Foscarnet is used if there is concern for resistance, and dose reduction or changes to immunosuppressive medications may be necessary. In some cases, genotype testing for resistance has a role [34]. After treatment, there is no evidence for benefit of secondary prophylaxis of CMV to prevent recurrent infections.

Norovirus is a single-stranded RNA virus that causes 90% of non-bacterial diarrhea, resulting in 19–21 million cases per year in the United States. Routes of infection include fecal/oral, inhalation of aerosolized emesis, or direct contact. Most immunocompetent people experience a self-limited acute diarrhea followed by up to 2 weeks of asymptomatic shedding. While some solid organ transplant recipients may present similarly, several studies suggest that chronic diarrhea is also a common presentation [53–55].

Norovirus in solid organ transplant recipients contributes to dehydration, renal insufficiency, graft dysfunction, and chronic diarrhea; it rarely causes mortality. Treatment is supportive and focuses heavily on rehydration and anti-motility agents. Reducing immunosuppressive medications has not improved the recovery for norovirus chronic diarrhea.

Other important causes of infectious diarrhea in solid organ transplant recipients include parasitic infections. Parasitic infections beside Entamoeba and giardia include cryptosporidium, cystoisospora, cyclospora, and microsporidium. Cryptosporidium is a water-borne parasite, which has been known to infect immunosuppressed and solid organ transplant recipients in epidemic outbreaks from environmental exposures. Avoidance of exposure to water sources that could be contaminated by waste products should be encouraged for all solid organ transplant recipients [56].

The COVID-19 (SARS-CoV-2) virus may present with gastrointestinal symptoms, including diarrhea. This emerging pandemic virus should be considered in the differential diagnosis of diarrhea in a solid organ transplant recipient, depending on local epidemiology and public health guidelines. The presentation, testing strategies, and treatment for solid organ transplant recipients with COVID-19 infections continues to be evaluated at the time of this book's publication. Transplant infectious disease specialists should be consulted when considering COVID-19 in a solid organ transplant recipient.

There are many non-infectious causes of diarrhea in a solid organ transplant recipient. Immunosuppressive and other medications commonly cause diarrhea—mycophenolate causes dose-dependent, direct enterocyte toxicity, while calcineurin inhibitors such as tacrolimus cause diarrhea via a macrolide promotility effect. Calcineurin inhibitors further complicate matters when diarrhea causes dehydration, leading to increased calcineurin inhibitor blood levels and renal toxicity. Sirolimus and everolimus cause diarrhea infrequently [48]. Non-immunosuppressive medications may also cause diarrhea and a thorough medication history should be gathered. Less common causes include graft versus host disease (GVHD) and post-transplant lymphoproliferative disorder. GVHD is generally rare in solid organ transplantation except for in small bowel transplants. It presents with chronic diarrhea, abdominal pain, fevers, and sometimes rash. Post-transplant lymphoproliferative disorder

(PTLD), when it involves the gastrointestinal tract, may present with chronic diarrhea, weight loss, abdominal pain, gastrointestinal bleeding, and anorexia. Risk for PTLD, from EBV activity, is thought to increase with increased immunosuppression, and is highest in multiorgan and intestinal transplants, and lowest in renal and liver transplants. Mortality rates historically for PTLD in solid organ transplantation are 50–70% [57]. (See Chaps. 9 and 10).

Urinary Tract Infections

Case
A 44-year-old woman who received a deceased donor kidney transplant 11 months ago presents with fatigue and dysuria. She was taken off of trimethoprim-sulfamethoxazole for PJP prophylaxis at 6 months post-transplant. Her post-transplant course has been complicated by a catheter-related UTI during her initial hospitalization, but none since. She had a ureteral stent post-operatively that has been removed. She has not had any episodes of rejection.

On exam she is afebrile, with otherwise normal vital signs. She has no tenderness over her transplanted kidney in the right lower quadrant, and no costovertebral angle tenderness. A urine dipstick is positive for leukocyte esterase, nitrites, and protein.

In addition to sending the urine sample for a formal urinalysis and reflexive bacterial culture, checking a complete blood count and chemistry panel, what empiric treatment should be started?

Comment:
This patient has no history of structural genitourinary tract disease, no history of resistant UTI, and no signs or symptoms concerning for a systemic infection. Her examination is reassuring without tenderness over her graft or native kidneys and she did not experience nausea or vomiting. Her diagnosis is consistent with a simple cystitis in a kidney transplant recipient.

Empiric therapy choices include fluoroquinolones, third-generation oral cephalosporins, or amoxicillin-sulbactam. Because she is past 6 months post-transplant, her duration of treatment can be 5–7 days. Longer treatment courses have not shown benefit in cases of simple cystitis. Empiric therapy with trimethoprim-sulfamethoxazole should be avoided given the risk for resistance to this antibiotic with recent use for prophylaxis. Antibiotics may be narrowed based on culture results.

If the patient develops fever, tenderness or pain over the allograft, flank pain, or vomiting, she should present to the Emergency Department as she may need volume resuscitation, IV antibiotics, and potentially urgent assessment of her allograft.

Urinary tract infections (UTIs) are common in solid organ transplant recipients, as they are in the general population. Kidney transplant recipients have higher risk for UTIs due to surgical manipulation of the genitourinary tract and the associated risk related to foreign bodies such as ureteral stents. A study of 4388 solid organ transplant recipients followed for at least 1 year found that UTI incidence varied based on the type of transplant. The overall rate of UTIs was 4.4% over the study period; the incidence of UTIs (expressed as the number of UTIs per 1000 transplant-days) was highest in kidney transplant recipients (0.45), followed by kidney-pancreas (0.22), heart (0.07), liver (0.06), and lung (0.02) [58]. The highest incidence of UTIs occur in the first 3–6 months post-transplant. Bacteremia is due to UTIs in over one-third (37%) of cases in kidney transplant recipients [59]. The wide prevalence quoted in studies of UTIs in kidney transplant recipients, 7–80%, is due to the lack of standardized diagnostic criteria, variable use of prophylactic antibiotics, and uneven follow-up duration [60].

Risk Factors

Risk factors for UTI include demographic factors, history of genitourinary diseases, and transplant-specific risks. In a study of nearly 29,000 kidney transplant recipients, 17% of men and women in the first month post-transplant developed UTIs. By 3 years after kidney transplantation, female transplant recipients experienced more UTIs than male transplant recipients, 60% versus 47%. Factors that increased risk for UTI in kidney transplant recipients were female sex, older age, indwelling catheters, diabetes, neurogenic bladder, and renal calculi [61]. Specific transplant-related risks include ureteral stents or urological structural abnormalities, vesicoureteral reflux, acute cellular rejection, and deceased-donor graft. Risks for later-onset (>6 months post-transplant) UTIs include prednisone dose >20 mg/day and serum creatinine of >2 mg/dL. However, the type of long-term immunosuppressive is not clearly associated with UTI risk [61].

UTIs in kidney transplant recipients result in serious health consequences. Blood stream infections occur in kidney transplant recipients at 40 times the annual rate of the general population. UTI caused 30–73% of blood stream infection in kidney transplant recipients and 80% of those UTIs are from gram-negative rods. In a retrospective study of 116 hospitalizations for blood stream infections in kidney transplant recipients, 83% occurred after the first year of transplant and 71% were community acquired. In this study, 57% of blood stream infectious were from a UTI source, followed by GI and surgical site infection sources. Sixty-five percent of bacteremic kidney transplant recipients developed acute kidney injury [62]. A 4-year retrospective study of kidney transplant recipients with severe UTIs requiring hospitalization found that *Klebsiella* and *E. coli* were the most common pathogens, and between a quarter and a third of those bacteria produced extended-spectrum beta-lactamase (ESBL). In these hospitalized kidney transplant recipients with UTIs, 41% experienced acute kidney injury, 3.6% experienced graft loss, and there was a 1.2% 1-year mortality [63].

Table 8.4 Classification of asymptomatic bacteriuria (AB) and urinary tract infection (UTI) in renal transplant recipients

Classification	Description	Laboratory investigations of urine
Asymptomatic bacteriuria	No urinary or systemic symptoms of infection	>10^5 CFU/mL uropathogen[a][b]
Acute simple cystitis	Dysuria, urinary urgency/frequency, or suprapubic pain; but no systemic symptoms and no ureteral stent/ nephrostomy tube/chronic urinary catheter	>10 WBC/mm^3 [c] >10^3 CFU/mL uropathogen[b]
Acute pyelonephritis/ complicated UTI	Fever, chills, malaise, hemodynamic instability, or leukocytosis (without other apparent etiology); flank/allograft pain; or bacteremia with same organism as in urine Dysuria, urgency, frequency, suprapubic pain may or may not be present	>10 WBC/mm^3 [c] >10^4 CFU/mL uropathogen[b]
Recurrent UTI	≥ 3 UTIs in prior 12-month period	As above

Reprinted from Goldman, et al., with permission [61]

WBC white blood cell, *CFU/mL* colony-forming units/milliliter

[a]While routine treatment of AB is not recommended (see Treatment section), if considering treatment of AB (e.g., in the immediate post-transplant period), a repeat urine culture is recommended (with care to minimize contamination) to assess persistence of the same uropathogen. Spontaneous resolution is common

[b]*Staphylococcus epidermidis* (except if ureteral stent), *Lactobacillus*, and *Gardnerella* sp. are unlikely to be uropathogens. Regarding CFU/mL: while most patients with UTI will have >10^5 CFU/ mL of a uropathogen in a midstream urine sample, some patients with pyelonephritis may have only 10^4–10^5 CFU/ mL of a uropathogen, and some patients with cystitis may have even fewer CFU/mL (most data on cystitis with low CFU/mL is only for *E. coli*). Not all labs report <10^4 CFU/mL

[c]While not an absolute criteria (depending on the performance characteristics of the urinalysis or presence of neutropenia), <10 WBC/mm^3 should prompt consideration of a diagnosis other than UTI

Definitions

Clinical providers must be precise in their nomenclature when describing and diagnosing urinary infections. Guidelines for classification of urinary tract infections in kidney transplant recipients are shown in Table 8.4. Other guidelines also exist for urinary tract infections in solid organ transplant recipients in general, and use similar definitions [64]. Overuse of antibiotics for asymptomatic bacteriuria can be avoided, and appropriate therapy in the setting of complicated UTIs can be selected.

Differential Diagnosis

Gram-negative rods (GNRs), with *E. coli* being most common, account for >70% of UTIs in solid organ transplant recipients. *Enterobacteriaceae, Enterococci, Pseudomonas, Staphylococcus saprophyticus, Streptococcus* species including *group B* or *viridans* can cause infections but more commonly are colonizers. Solid organ transplant recipients are at higher risk for MDR organisms. Less commonly viral and fungal urinary infection can also occur.

Specific Organisms

Carbapenem-resistant Klebsiella pneumonia (CRKP) and *extended-spectrum beta-lactamase producing Klebsiella pneumonia* (ESBL-KP) are concerning pathogens for UTIs in solid organ transplant recipients. A 2015 study of kidney transplant recipients with UTI found CRKP UTI were associated with ICU admissions, longer hospital stays, and failure of antibiotic interventions compared to susceptible klebsiella pneumonia UTIs [65].

More unusual pathogens include *Mycobacterium tuberculosis, Salmonella, CMV, and adenovirus* which mainly causes hemorrhagic cystitis. *Corynebacterium urealyticum* may be a pathogen in the setting of obstructive uropathy. Rarely *Mycoplasma hominis* and *Ureaplasma urealyticum* can cause intra-renal or perinephric abscess or graft pyelonephritis in kidney transplant recipients. *Staphylococcus epidermidis, Lactobacillus, Gardinella vaginalis* are unlikely pathogens. *Candida* species are usually asymptomatic colonizers. Rarely, they can cause upper tract infections including candidemia and ureterovesicular fungal balls [61]. A urine culture with mixed flora represents contamination.

Special consideration should be given to *BK virus* in solid organ transplant recipients. It is a polyomavirus that is ubiquitous in the environment and causes both animal and human infections. The median age of infection is 4–5 years old. Primary infection is usually a self-limited respiratory infection and rarely presents as acute cystitis. BK virus develops a lifelong latency in renal cells and transitional epithelial cells of the genitourinary tract. Immunosuppression triggers viruria that in some cases results in invasive renal infections. In kidney transplant recipients, the reactivation occurs in native kidneys and can cause a high level of renal graft failure, as high as 50–80% within 2 years of transplant. BK virus nephropathy is much rarer in non-renal solid organ transplantation, although when it does occur it tends to lead to end stage renal disease (ESRD) and significant mortality. The most common manifestations of BK virus reactivation infections are BK nephropathy and hemorrhagic cystitis. The gold standard for diagnosis of BK nephropathy is renal biopsy, although BK viral loads in the blood and urine as well as the presence of decoy cells (virally infected epithelial cells seen on cytology) assist in diagnosis and are used in screening. The key treatment of BK virus nephropathy/re-activation infections is reduction in immunosuppression [66].

Diagnostic Considerations

In solid organ transplant recipients, the presentation of UTI may lack usual lower urinary tract symptoms such as frequency, urgency, and dysuria. Instead, symptoms such as fever, malaise, and non-specific sepsis symptoms as well as leukocytosis may be the main presentation. Because of denervation of the allograft, the transplanted kidney may not be tender to palpation. Pyuria >10 WBC/mL is usually present, and lack of pyuria in the setting of UTI symptoms should spur evaluation for alternative etiologies. Notably, *E. coli* UTI in solid organ transplant recipients may only have 10^4 CFUs and still be considered a UTI by transplant infectious disease specialists [61].

Therapeutic Considerations

The Infectious Disease Community of Practice of the American Society of Transplantation guidelines (2019) recommend the following [61]: Routine urine testing in asymptomatic solid organ transplant recipients should not be performed after the first 2 months post-transplant. In the setting of asymptomatic bacteriuria, the recommendation is to observe for symptoms without treatment. However, if there is persistent asymptomatic bacteriuria with an associated creatinine rise, there is a weak recommendation for treatment with antibiotics. Simple cystitis should be treated for 5–10 days, and never for 3 days in solid organ transplant recipients. Treatment of complicated UTI/pyelonephritis should be for 14–21 days with an effort to narrow antibiotics based on urine culture data. However, the course should be extended for a longer duration if source control (such as in the setting of perinephric abscesses that require incision and drainage) is only achieved partway through the antibiotic course [61].

Specific Treatment Recommendations by Condition

Simple cystitis should be treated empirically with fluoroquinolones, amoxicillin-clavulanate, or an oral third-generation cephalosporin. Providers should be wary of the risk for trimethoprim-sulfamethoxozole resistance in patients who have received this antibiotic for prophylaxis. Empiric antibiotics should be narrowed as much as possible based on the culture results. While 7–10 days of antibiotic therapy should be utilized in the first 6 months post-transplant, 5–7 days can be considered for simple cystitis after 6 months [61].

Pyelonephritis/complicated UTIs in stable patients can be treated with ceftriaxone, ampicillin-sulbactam, or ciprofloxacin as long as prior cultures do not show antibiotic resistance. Patients with nausea and vomiting or other signs of clinical instability should be admitted to the hospital, and empiric therapy with piperacillin/tazobactam, cefepime, or a carbapenem should be initiated. Detailed inpatient management is beyond the scope of this book, but in general, consultation with a transplant infectious disease specialist is often indicated, as multi-drug-resistant organisms are increasing; the transplant team will also need to be involved, especially in severe infections (e.g., septic shock) in which reduction of immunosuppressive medications is recommended; and advanced imaging may be required to assess for upper tract disease such as renal abscess or structural abnormalities that could lead to obstruction in order to ensure source control. Treatment duration should be 14–21 days, and antibiotics should be narrowed to reflect coverage of culture results [61].

For *recurrent UTI* treatment, interventions have not been adequately tested in solid organ transplant recipients. Recommendations for solid organ transplant recipients with recurrent UTIs are identical to those for immunocompetent patients. Behavioral interventions including hydration, timed voiding, front to back wiping in females, and avoidance of serial anal and vaginal intercourse is recommended. Vaginal estrogen for post-menopausal women decreased the frequency of recurrent UTIs from 6 in the placebo group to 0.5 per year in the treatment group. Post-coital antibiotics in females, and assessment for BPH with obstruction and prostatitis in males are also recommended. Non-antimicrobial interventions such as cranberry juice and probiotics are not well supported [61]. Additionally, given the higher risk of UTIs in the solid organ transplant population, primary care providers should strongly consider consultation with an infectious disease specialist.

Early postoperative infections are usually addressed by the transplant team. For donor-derived infections trimethoprim-sulfamethoxazole used for PJP prophylaxis in the first 6–12 months will effectively serve as dual prophylaxis against many UTI organisms in kidney transplant recipients. One study showed a two-third reduction in UTIs for those receiving trimethoprim-sulfamethoxazole versus no antimicrobial prophylaxis. In patients who cannot tolerate trimethoprim-sulfamethoxazole, some authors recommend fluoroquinolones or Fosfomycin specifically for UTI prophylaxis, and guidelines are to limit such prophylaxis to the first post-transplant month [61].

Ureteral stents are utilized in kidney transplant recipients to reduce the risk of ureterovesicular anastomosis stenosis. However, ureteral stents may increase the risk for UTI, and they are typically removed within 2 weeks of transplantation to decrease the risk for UTI [61].

Infections of the Central Nervous System

Case

A 45-year-old man who underwent liver transplant 18 months prior is brought to the primary care clinic by his family who is concerned about confusion. They noticed that he has become progressively more confused and fatigued over the last 10 days. They note word-finding difficulties, trouble remembering the names of his children, and being confused about the time of day. He has been sleeping more and taking naps in the afternoon, which is unusual for him. Yesterday morning, he began complaining of a headache, and this morning he was difficult to rouse from sleep. In the office, his temperature is 38.1 °C, heart rate 92, blood pressure 104/54, respiratory rate 16, and oxygen saturation 98% on ambient air. He is sleepy but arousable and able to participate in conversation; however, he cannot recall the events of the last week and thinks the year is 1958. His strength, reflexes, and a limited cranial nerve examination of the pupils, extraocular movement, facial and oropharynx motor function is normal.

Comment:

This patient is presenting with acute to subacute onset of altered mental status accompanied by a low-grade fever. In a solid organ transplant recipient, these symptoms should prompt immediate referral to the emergency department for rapid evaluation and treatment. While the neurologic symptoms may be nonspecific, the possibility of meningoencephalitis must be considered in this population. In this case, the duration of symptoms is longer than what would be expected for bacterial meningitis; however, meningoencephalitis due to a fungal pathogen, such as cryptococcus, is of high concern.

This patient should undergo immediate testing in an emergency setting, including complete blood counts, basic chemistries, neuroimaging with contrast, and a lumbar puncture (LP). Cerebrospinal fluid should be sent for cell count with differential, glucose, protein, bacterial cultures, fungal cultures, PCR for herpes viruses (HSV, VZV, EBV, CMV), and cryptococcal antigen. Although this patient's presentation is less consistent with bacterial meningitis, empiric antibiotic therapy should be started while awaiting laboratory data. Infectious disease specialists should be consulted early to guide additional evaluation and management.

Infections of the central nervous system (CNS) are less common in solid organ transplant recipients than in prior years due to more tailored immunosuppressive regimens and routine surveillance. The current incidence of opportunistic CNS infections in this population is estimated to be 1–2%, down from 7% in previous studies [67]. However, CNS infections remain a significant cause of morbidity for solid organ transplant recipients, with some studies suggesting mortality rates as high as 44–77% [68]. Further, mortality rates with CNS fungal infections after solid organ transplantation may be as high as 90% percent. Solid organ transplant recipients may not present with typical symptoms of CNS infection, and therefore clinicians should have a high index of suspicion in a patient with fever, headache, and/ or altered mental status [68]. Like most infectious complications in solid organ transplant recipient, the risk for different CNS infections varies according to time after transplantation (See Tables 8.1 and 8.5) [69].

Diagnostic Considerations

A solid organ transplant recipient with onset of fever and altered mental status should undergo a rapid evaluation including CBC, peripheral blood cultures, and a lumbar puncture (LP) to evaluate for CNS infection. Diagnostic studies from the LP

Table 8.5 Common CNS infections in solid organ transplant recipients by time since transplantation

Time course	Infections	Special considerations
Initial 30 days post-transplant	Pre-transplant colonization Donor-derived infections Nosocomial infections (MRSA, *Candida* species, *Aspergillus* species	Viral prophylaxis in the immediate post-transplant period makes reactivation of viral infections less likely
1–6 months post-transplant	Opportunistic infections (Nocardia, Listeria, Toxoplasmosis, endemic mycoses) Reactivation of viral infections (EBV, VZV, HSV, CMV, HHV-6)	Viral prophylaxis often decreases 3–6 months after transplant, increasing risk for reactivation syndromes
>6 months post-transplant	Opportunistic infections (Nocardia, Listeria, Cryptococcus, Aspergillus) Community-acquired infections Reactivation of previous infections (Herpes viruses, JC virus)	Incidence of opportunistic fungal CNS infection is highest >12 months after transplant

Reprinted with permission from Pizzi et al. [68] with special consideration comments added

should include cell count, glucose, total protein, gram stain and bacterial culture, and measurement of the opening pressure [70]. For most solid organ transplant recipients undergoing evaluation for CNS infection, the CSF should also be sent for viral PCR including enteroviruses, HSV, VZV, EBV, and CMV. If there is concern for a fungal etiology, providers should consider sending a CSF cryptococcal antigen and India ink staining for Cryptococcus [71].

Solid organ transplant recipients are at higher risk for development of bacterial or fungal brain abscesses than immunocompetent hosts. Any solid organ transplant recipient presenting with cranial nerve deficits requires urgent brain imaging [71]. A space-occupying lesion identified on brain imaging in a solid organ transplant recipient warrants immediate neurosurgical and infectious disease consultation to direct additional evaluation and consideration of early treatment. In the case of a space-occupying lesion, the decision to pursue an LP is done in conjunction with radiology, neurosurgery, or infectious disease, depending on the resources available, due to the concern for herniation if the intracranial pressure is elevated. If analysis of the CSF is unrevealing for patients with a space-occupying lesion, brain biopsy with pathologic examination may be indicated.

Bacterial Infections of the CNS

There is a sevenfold increase in the incidence of bacterial meningitis among solid organ transplant recipients compared to the broader population [72]. Patients after solid organ transplantation who develop bacterial meningitis may not manifest typical symptoms of high fevers and meningismus due to impaired inflammatory response from immunosuppressing medications [68]. Solid organ transplant recipients are also at higher risk of CNS infection with opportunistic bacteria including *Nocardia spp*, *Mycobacterium*, and *Listeria spp*. These infections often begin as a respiratory illness and result in meningitis due to hematogenous spread of the organism [72].

If there is concern for bacterial meningitis, the solid organ transplant recipient should be evaluated in an emergency department or inpatient setting to undergo lumbar puncture and rapid administration of antibiotics until diagnostic studies return. Of note, solid organ transplant recipients with significant bacterial CNS infections may have a lower pleocytosis than immunocompetent hosts on evaluation of the cerebral spinal fluid (CSF), so providers should have a low threshold to administer antibiotics until further consultation with an infectious disease specialist is available.

Viral Infections of the CNS

Viral infections of the CNS most commonly present 1–6 months after transplantation. Herpes viruses are the most common causes of viral CNS infection in solid organ transplant recipients, including VZV, HSV, CMV, EBV, and HHV-6 [68]. Patients may present with symptoms of either a meningitis or encephalitis. A solid organ transplant recipient who presents with altered mental status, personality changes, seizures, or speech or gait disturbance should be evaluated for viral encephalitis with lumbar puncture and PCR-based assays on the CSF. As with bacterial infections, evaluation will typically require an emergency department evaluation and likely hospitalization.

EBV rarely causes encephalitis but is associated with post-transplant lymphoproliferative disorder (PTLD) in the CNS [72]. While more commonly seen in patients receiving immunomodulating drugs for rheumatologic or neurologic disease, infection with JC virus can cause progressive multifocal leukoencephalopathy (PML) in solid organ transplant recipients late in the post-transplantation course [2].

Fungal Infections of the CNS

Infection with cryptococcus is by far the most common cause of fungal meningitis and meningoencephalitis in patients after solid organ transplantation. The onset of cryptococcus infection is late in the post-transplant course, often occurring 16–21 months after transplantation [71]. Cryptococcus infection occurs after inhalation through the respiratory tract and is typically thought to represent reactivation of the infection in immunocompromised hosts, although primary infections do occur. Importantly, fever is present only 50% of the time in solid organ transplant recipients with cryptococcus meningoencephalitis. Testing for cryptococcus antigen in the CSF and the serum is the gold standard for diagnosing cryptococcus infection and is more commonly used in institutions across the United States than India ink testing. Treatment regimens vary and may involve induction therapy for 2 weeks with liposomal amphotericin B and flucytosine, followed by consolidation therapy with fluconazole for 8 weeks, and finally a lower dose maintenance regimen of fluconazole for an additional 6–12 months [71].

Aspergillus is the most common fungal etiology causing cerebral abscesses in solid organ transplant recipients [2]. Mortality for solid organ transplant recipients with aspergillus abscesses is greater than 50%, even with voriconazole or amphotericin B treatment. Providers should also be aware that *Toxoplasma gondii*, a parasitic infection, may cause brain abscesses in solid organ transplant recipients and requires prolonged antimicrobial therapy [70].

Skin and Soft Tissue Infections

Case

A 67-year-old patient with history of kidney transplantation presents to the primary care clinic with 4 days of worsening erythema, edema, and pain of the right lower extremity. The patient first noticed erythema and swelling around his great toe, which progressed to the foot and then the lower leg in the following days. Yesterday evening, he had trouble going to sleep due to pain. He does not have fever or chills. He had no trauma to the foot and does not walk barefoot. On exam, he is afebrile and vital signs are normal. His right lower extremity has erythema and edema extending from the distal foot up the knee, with increased erythema and induration medially compared to laterally. There are no areas of purulence or fluctuance. There is dryness and cracking of the skin between his toes with evidence of tinea pedis. There is no pain in the joints of the ankle or foot with range of motion.

Comment:

This patient has uncomplicated cellulitis of the lower extremity. There are no signs of systemic infection and no areas of purulence. He likely developed a bacterial superinfection of his foot due to underlying tinea pedis, which causes skin breakdown and creates a portal of entry for skin flora. A swab for bacterial culture is only indicated if purulence is present; in the absence of purulence, a skin culture is not helpful due to contamination from skin flora. In the absence of purulence or signs of an abscess, empiric treatment should be tailored to cover Streptococcus species and methicillin-sensitive S. aureus (MSSA). If there are areas of purulence, the antibiotic spectrum should be extended to cover methicillin-resistant S. aureus (MRSA); common regimens include a first-generation cephalosporin combined with antibiotic active against MRSA including doxycycline, trimethoprim-sulfamethoxazole, or clindamycin. When considering antibiotics in a solid organ transplant recipient, drug interactions should be checked, as well as dose adjustment for chronic kidney disease, a common metabolic complication. If an abscess is present, it should be treated with incision and drainage as well as an antibiotic active against MRSA. Cellulitis may be treated for a little as 5 days though the treatment course may be extended up to 14 days, depending on the individual and degree of improvement.

Signs of systemic infection from a skin and soft tissue infection should prompt immediate referral to the emergency room for laboratory evaluation, blood cultures, imaging, and possible surgical consultation. If there is concern for concomitant deep vein thrombosis, then venous duplex imaging should be obtained.

Skin and soft tissue infections (SSTIs) are extremely common in solid organ transplant recipients due to ongoing immunosuppression and may affect up to 20% of patients at some time in the post-transplant period [73]. Similar to immunocompetent hosts, SSTIs in solid organ transplant recipients may be caused by bacteria, mycobacteria, fungi, viruses, and parasites, although immunocompromised individuals are more susceptible to severe morbidity and mortality. Common skin infections may present atypically in solid organ transplant recipients because of defects in cellular and humoral immunity and may reflect either localized or disseminated disease. When assessing SSTIs in solid organ transplant recipients, providers should use a similar approach to evaluation and management of SSTIs in immunocompetent hosts, first determining if the lesion is purulent or non-purulent (see Fig. 8.2) as this directs initial diagnostic and management strategies. In immunosuppressed hosts, cutaneous lesions are commonly vesicular,

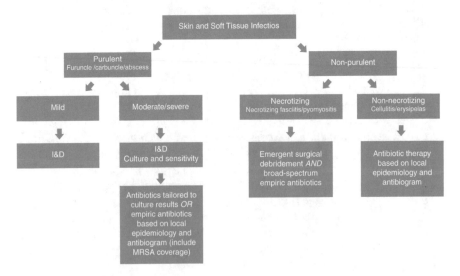

Fig. 8.2 Evaluation and management of skin and soft tissue infections

nodular, or ulcerative, and the patient's travel and exposure history becomes critically important in driving the differential diagnosis. Other, non-infectious diagnostic considerations for skin findings in a solid organ transplant recipient include drug eruptions, erythema multiforme, Sweet syndrome, and underlying malignancy [74].

Diagnostic Considerations

Appropriate diagnostic evaluation of SSTIs in solid organ transplant recipients depends on the appearance of the skin lesion, concern for disseminated disease, and the patient's exposure history. If the lesion is purulent, providers should have high suspicion for typical or atypical bacterial infection and should obtain a swab of the purulent material to send for gram stain and bacterial culture. While non-bacterial pathogens can cause purulent-appearing lesions, bacterial culture is the most appropriate first step. Blood cultures are rarely indicated in the evaluation of SSTI except when fever is present, in patients who use recreational injection drugs, and patients presenting in shock. When there is concern for disseminated infection either because of the presence of systemic symptoms or multiple similar-appearing cutaneous lesions at distant sites, providers should consider ordering both bacterial and fungal blood cultures. Vesicular lesions should be unroofed with samples sent for viral PCR to detect infection with herpes simplex virus (HSV) or varicella zoster virus (VZV) infection. Nodules or ulcerative lesions, either solitary or grouped, may be difficult to identify by visual inspection alone and referral to a surgeon or dermatologist for skin biopsy may be indicated. Tissue specimens should be sent to both the microbiology lab for culture and the pathology lab for histologic evaluation [74, 75]. Special stains and culture media may be required depending on the exposure history and differential diagnosis; primary care providers should communicate early with an infectious disease specialist and a dermatologist to ensure that appropriate testing is performed.

Cellulitis and Abscesses

Cellulitis remains the most common clinical SSTI syndrome with an incidence of 2 cases per 1000-patient years. Cellulitis is a non-necrotizing, superficial skin infection involving the epidermis and dermis. Immunosuppression is an important risk factor for SSTIs; risk increases when other conditions are present including chronic skin inflammation, poor venous or lymphatic circulation, diabetes mellitus, and obesity [75]. Furuncles, carbuncles, and cutaneous abscesses represent isolated collections of pus in the dermis and deeper tissues that require incision and drainage to fully control the source of infection. Abscesses typically present as tender, erythematous, indurated nodules, often with fluctuance and surrounding skin erythema [76]. Cellulitis and abscesses are not distinctly different entities in solid organ transplant recipients compared to immunocompetent hosts. The most important principles in diagnosis include vigilance when assessing possible cutaneous infection, understanding that the syndromes may present more subtly in solid organ transplant recipients and may progress more rapidly than in immunocompetent individuals.

Beta-hemolytic streptococci remain the most common cause of cellulitis in immunocompetent and immunocompromised hosts, followed by community-acquired *S. aureus*, including MRSA. In some studies, *S. aureus* (MSSA and MRSA) is the predominant pathogen involved in purulent cellulitis and remains the leading causes of SSTIs overall, especially in cases involving abscesses [76].

Other pathogens, including GNRs, are encountered less frequently and most often in the setting of bacteremia. Infection with atypical bacteria, such as nocardia or non-tuberculous mycobacteria, are infrequent causes of cellulitis; skin manifestations of these pathogens may also present as pustules, nodules, ulcers, and abscesses [77]. Other rare causes of SSTIs have been associated with certain exposures, such as an outbreak of nontuberculous mycobacterium after exposure to fish markets in New York City [78, 79].

The IDSA has established clear guidelines for the diagnosis and management of SSTIs; yet, rates of misdiagnosis, inappropriate antibiotic use, and hospitalization remain high [75, 80]. Of note, fever has been shown to be an unreliable indicator for the need for admission, despite traditional practice [81]. Further, other physical exam findings consistent with severe infection, such as bullae and lymphatic streaking, do not correlate with fever. Risk prediction tools for SSTI also have poor performance, lacking sensitivity in the identification of severe infections in elderly patients and populations with elevated risk, such as solid organ transplant recipients. Thus, providers must remain vigilant in their assessment of cellulitis and abscess, with low threshold for diagnostic sampling and treatment.

In typical cases of cellulitis without systemic signs of purulence, the IDSA recommends antibiotic therapy targeted at streptococci. If purulence is present or suspected, therapy should be extended to cover MRSA. Providers should choose antibiotics based on local susceptibility patterns and institutional antibiograms; typical oral regimens that cover both streptococci and MRSA include a penicillin or first-generation cephalosporin, combined with trimethoprim-sulfamethoxozole, doxycycline, or clindamycin. If a patient is already receiving trimethoprim-sulfamethoxozole for prophylaxis, an alternative agent should be selected to cover MRSA. When used for a short duration to treat purulent cellulitis, there are no particular concerns about these antibiotics interacting with immunosuppression regimens. Linezolid is another oral antibiotic active against *S. aureus*; however, its use is typically reserved for patients who cannot tolerate or have demonstrated resistance to first-line agents. Use of linezolid is also limited by cost and interactions with other common medications including selective serotonin reuptake inhibitors (SSRIs) and serotonin-norepinephrine reuptake inhibitors (SNRIs). Note that cytopenias caused by linezolid develop with long antibiotic courses and are of less concern when it is used for a short course to treat cellulitis.

Some clinicians treat both streptococci and MRSA initially, particularly in solid organ transplant recipients, although clear guidance on this approach is lacking. Recommended treatment duration for cellulitis is 5 days and may be extended if the patient is not improving as expected. While prior evidence held that abscesses could be treated with incision and drainage alone, a large randomized controlled trial demonstrated that cure rate for abscesses increased with the addition of trimethoprim-sulfamethoxozole to incision and drainage compared to incision and drainage alone, particularly in settings where MRSA is prevalent [82]. The IDSA makes a strong recommendation for clinicians to consult with an infectious disease specialist or a dermatologist in the treatment of cellulitis in solid organ transplant recipients, particularly if complicating factors are present [75].

Necrotizing Skin Infections

Necrotizing soft tissue infections (NSTIs) remain a relatively rare cause of SSTIs overall, and there is a paucity of data on NSTIs in immunocompromised patients. NSTIs are associated with high mortality rates (15–50%), and early recognition and diagnosis can be challenging. Common pathogens included GNRs, anaerobes, coagulase-negative *Staphylococcus* species, *S. aureus* species, beta-hemolytic streptococcal species, and *Enterococcus* species; however, in a single-center study on NSTIs in immunocompromised hosts, wound cultures revealed polymicrobial growth in 58.7% of cases [83]. In this study, more immunocompromised patients had positive blood cultures in the setting of NSTIs compared to immunocompetent hosts. Immunocompromised patients also had increased rates of in-hospital death associated with NSTI infection compared to immunocompetent hosts (39.1% vs. 19.4%). Additional findings included a lower WBC counts (often in the normal range) and absence of fever among immunocompromised hosts. These findings highlight the high index of suspicion needed among triaging physicians to ensure early identification and appropriate referral to an emergency care setting [84].

Vesicular Eruptions

The presence of vesicular lesions in a solid organ transplant recipient should raise suspicion for infection with a herpes virus. Reactivation of herpes simplex virus (HSV) and varicella zoster virus (VZV) are most common; however, cytomegalovirus (CMV), Epstein-Barr virus (EBV), and human herpes virus 6 (HHV-6) may cause vesicular lesions as well, though cutaneous manifestations are less common in these diseases.

HSV accounted for the vast majority of mucocutaneous infection in solid organ transplant recipients (>80%) before the introduction of antiviral prophylaxis; since then, incidence has dropped dramatically [84]. Infection with HSV produces painful, grouped vesicles on an erythematous base that coalesce into shallow ulcerations on surfaces of mucous membranes. HSV lesions in solid organ transplant recipients may take longer to heal than in immunocompetent hosts, in part due to impaired cellular immunity and prolonged viral shedding [74]. HSV-1 tends to cause oropharyngeal lesions, whereas HSV-2 has a predilection for anogenital eruptions; however, both serotypes may affect any mucocutaneous surface, particularly in solid organ transplant recipients.

Reactivation of VZV is common among solid organ transplant recipients, with shingles, or "zoster," affecting 6–7% of individuals [74]. VZV reactivation presents with grouped vesicles on an erythematous base and typically affects a single dermatome. Disseminated zoster, defined as reactivation of VZV affecting 3 or more dermatomes, is more common in immunocompromised individuals and may take longer to respond to antiviral therapy. Primary infection with VZV, also called chicken pox, is relatively uncommon in adults due to almost universal exposure during childhood. Solid organ transplant recipients should have varicella titer testing prior to transplantation, and the varicella vaccine should be considered for anyone who is seronegative for anti-varicella antibodies. It is important to note that the current VZV vaccine is a live, attenuated vaccine, and administration is contraindicated post-transplantation [85].

If HSV or VZV infection is suspected, providers should obtain a swab of vesicular lesions and send the sample for PCR testing (see above). While awaiting testing results, empiric treatment with acyclovir or valacyclovir may be initiated to reduce duration and severity of symptoms. First-line therapy for herpes labialis includes acyclovir 400 mg 5×/day for 5 days. Genital herpes may be treated with acyclovir 400 mg 5×/day for 10 days or valacyclovir 1000 mg 3×/day for 10 days. Patients with recurrent HSV could experience asymptomatic shedding for days before an outbreak occurs; thus, there may be a role for twice-daily suppressive therapy with acyclovir or valacyclovir in individuals with more than 3 outbreaks per year to reduce risk of transmission. Herpes zoster should be treated with a higher dose of acyclovir, 800 mg 5×/day for 7–10 days or valacyclovir 1000 mg 3×/day for 7 days [85]. Severe HSV or VZV infection may require hospitalization and administration of IV acyclovir. Famciclovir is also active against HSV and VZV and may be used in the treatment of these infections, though treatment duration varies.

Disseminated CMV may cause a maculopapular, vesicular, or even ulcerative eruption in solid organ transplant recipients. Cutaneous manifestations of CMV typically affect 10–20% of solid organ transplant recipients with systemic CMV disease and portend a poor prognosis [85]. Infection with HHV-6 typically causes a self-limited febrile illness with a maculopapular rash, though manifestations may be more severe in solid organ transplant recipients. Cutaneous lesions associated with EBV infection are most commonly seen in the setting of post-transplant lymphoproliferative disorder (PTLD).

Nodular and Ulcerative Lesions

Numerous bacterial and fungal pathogens can cause nodular cutaneous lesions in solid organ transplant recipients, and these lesions may or may not indicate disseminated infection. In solid organ transplant recipients, defects in cellular immunity predispose to mycobacteria, atypical bacteria, certain zoonoses (*Brucella, Bartonella*), and parasites (Leishmaniasis), all of which may present with cutaneous nodules or ulcers. As an example, up to 32% of solid organ transplant recipients with disseminated nocardia infection developed skin manifestations [78]. Some non-tuberculous mycobacteria (NTM) may produce localized nodules or ulcerated lesions (e.g., *Mycobacterium fortuitum*), while infections with *Mycobacterium abscessus* or *chelonae* are more likely to result in pustular, nodular, or papular lesions in association with disseminated infection.

The most common clinical presentation of candidiasis in solid organ transplant recipients is mucocutaneous disease, including thrush and esophageal candidiasis [86]. However, *Candida* remains the most common cause of disseminated fungal infections in solid organ transplant recipients; skin lesions occur in 10% of these patients and may be the presenting symptom in 13–36% of cases [74]. In comparison, disseminated *Aspergillus* infection is a rare cause of cutaneous lesions in solid organ transplant recipients and is unlikely to be a presenting symptom for PCPs.

Endemic fungal infections, including histoplasmosis, coccidioidomycosis, and blastomycosis, typically cause primary pulmonary infections. Primary inoculation with these pathogens causing isolated skin disease is uncommon. Solid organ transplant recipients infected with an endemic mycosis are at higher risk for disseminated disease due to impaired cellular immunity, and may develop papules, plaques, pustules, nodules, or ulcers. Skin disease is the most common extra-pulmonary manifestation of blastomycosis and may present as either verrucous or ulcerative lesions [87].

If there is concern for an endemic fungal infection, a thorough exposure history is critical. In the United States, histoplasmosis is native to the Ohio and Mississippi River Valleys and remains the most common of the endemic fungal infections overall. Coccidioidomycosis is endemic to the Southwestern United States including central California, as well as areas of Washington State and northern Mexico [88]. Blastomycosis is found predominantly in southern and southeastern states bordering the Ohio and Mississippi River Valleys, as well as upper Midwestern states in the Great Lakes region. Taking a detailed history to clarify recent travel to endemic areas, as well as exploration of concomitant pulmonary symptoms, will help clarify the diagnostic possibilities. Worldwide patterns vary—knowing local and regional patterns of endemic mycoses can aid in the diagnosis of cutaneous fungal infections.

Diagnosis of nodular and ulcerative lesions typically requires biopsy, either with a dermatologist or a surgeon, depending on the depth of the wound. These samples should be sent for microbiologic and pathologic evaluation. Empiric therapy is not recommended; rather, providers should await culture or pathology results and consider consultation or referral to an infectious disease specialist to determine treatment.

Prevention

In addition to the medications for prophylaxis against viruses and *Pneumocystis jirovecii*, solid organ transplant recipients are educated to take other measures to prevent infection, including hand hygiene, avoiding sick contacts, foods that have higher risk of bacterial contamination, and travel to locations with endemic infectious diseases. During the COVID-19/SARS-CoV-2 pandemic, solid organ transplant

Table 8.6 Vaccinations in pre- and post solid organ transplant recipients [56, 89–91]

Vaccinations	Pre-transplant	Post-transplant	Comments
Measles Mumps Rubella (MMR—live)	Yes	No	Recommended to be given prior to transplantation. This live attenuated vaccination is contraindicated after transplant
Zoster (Zostavax ®—live)	Yes	No	Live attenuated virus vaccine can be given prior to transplant
Zoster (Shingrix ®—recombinant antigen)	Yes	Yes only in low-dose immunosuppression	ACIP recommends it for patients on low-dose immunosuppression (<20 mg prednisone/day) or anticipating higher immunosuppression or recovering from higher dose immunosuppression. Subjects on moderate or high-dose immunosuppression were excluded from efficacy studies. Consult with transplant team if considering.
Varicella (live)	Yes	No	
Prevnar ® vaccine (PCV13)	Yes	Yes	At least 1 year after PPSV23
Pneumococcal vaccine (PPSV23)	Yes	Yes	At least 8 weeks after PCV13. Booster 5 years after first PPSV23 dose if <65 years of age. A last dose is given at 65 or older, again 5 years after the last PPSV23 dose
Hepatitis A vaccine			Recommended in ESLD
Hepatitis B vaccine			Recommended in ESLD, ESRD
Tetanus/diphtheria (Td)	Yes	Yes	Every 10 years
Tetanus/ diphtheria/ pertussis (Tdap)	Yes	Yes	
Influenza (inactivated)	Yes	Yes	
Influenza (live)	Yes	No	Not within 2 weeks of transplant
Meningitis (*N. meningitidis*)	Yes	Yes	
Polio (inactivated)	Yes	Yes	
Polio (live)	Yes	No	
HPV	Yes	Yes	

recipients are in the highest risk category and should limit their exposure by following public health guidelines. The primary care provider can assist by keeping vaccinations up to date (Table 8.6; see also Chap. 12). Solid organ transplant recipients should be reminded not to accept live vaccines. Additionally, the recombinant herpes zoster vaccine is currently not recommended—although it is not a live vaccine, there is a theoretical risk of precipitating acute rejection, and the use of this vaccine is still under investigation in this population. Vaccine guidelines change regularly—it is important to regularly check updated recommendations, and if in doubt, discuss with the transplant team.

Conclusion

Infection remains a significant risk in solid organ transplant recipients. A knowledge of the time course of immunosuppression and potential pathogens will assist in the evaluation and management of the solid organ transplant recipient who presents to the primary care setting with potentially infectious symptoms. Signs and symptoms of infection may present subtly in solid organ transplant recipients due to immunosuppression; hence, primary care providers must maintain a high index of suspicion when evaluating these patients in clinic. A higher level of care is often required for more severe infections because of the increased risk for complications and monitoring required due to immunosuppression, and consultation with the transplant team and an infectious disease specialist is often indicated. With timely and appropriate care, infections may be treated successfully in the solid organ transplant recipient.

References

1. Rana A, Gruessner A, Agopian V, Khalpey Z, Riaz I, Kaplan B, et al. Survival benefit of solid-organ transplantation the United States. JAMA Surg. 2015;150(3):252–9.
2. Timsit J, Sonneville R, Kalil A, Bassetti M, Ferrer R, Jaber S, et al. Diagnostic and therapeutic approach to infectious diseases in solid organ transplant recipients. Intensive Care Med. 2019;45(5):573–91. https://doi.org/10.1007/s00134-019-05597-y.
3. Fishman J. Infection in solid-organ transplant recipients. N Engl J Med. 2007;357(25): 2601–14.
4. Fishman J, Greenwald M, Grossi P. Transmission of infection with human allografts: essential considerations in donor screening. Clin Infect Dis. 2012;55(5):720–7.
5. Razonable R, Humar A, AST Infectious Disease Community of Practice. Cytomegalovirus in solid organ transplantation. Am J Transplant. 2013;13(Suppl 4):93–106.
6. Lee DH, Zuckerman RA, AST Infectious Diseases Community of Practice. Herpes simplex virus infections in solid organ transplantation: Guidelines from the American Society of Transplantation Infectious Diseases Community of Practice. Clin Transplant. 2019;33(9):e13526. https://doi.org/10.1111/ctr.13526.
7. Pergam S, Limaye AP, AST Infectious Diseases Community of Practice. Varicella zoster virus in solid organ transplantation: Guidelines from the American Society of Transplantation Infectious Diseases Community of Practice. Clin Transplant. 2019;33(9):e13622. https://doi.org/10.1111/ctr.13622.
8. Fishman JA, Gans H, AST Infectious Diseases Community of Practice. Pneumocystis jiroveci in solid organ transplantation: Guidelines from the American Society of Transplantation

Infectious Diseases Community of Practice. Clin Transplant. 2019;33(9):e13587. https://doi.org/10.1111/ctr.13587.

9. Martin S, Fishman J, the AST Infectious Diseases Community of Practice. Pneumocystis pneumonia in solid organ transplantation. Am J Transplant. 2013;13(Suppl 4):272–9.

10. Silveira F, Kusne S, the AST Infectious Diseases Community of Practice. Candida infections in solid organ transplantation. Am J Transplant. 2013;13(Suppl 4):220–7.

11. Husain S, Camargo JF. Invasive aspergillosis in solid-organ transplant recipients: guidelines from the American Society of Transplantation Infectious Diseases Community of Practice. Clin Transpl. 2019;33(9):e13544. https://doi.org/10.1111/ctr.13544.

12. Aslam S, Rotstein C, AST Infectious Disease Community of Practice Clin Transplant. Candida infections in solid organ transplantation: Guidelines from the American Society of Transplantation Infectious Diseases Community of Practice. Clin Transplant. 2019;33(9):e13623. https://doi.org/10.1111/ctr.13623.

13. Miller R, Assi M, the AST Infectious Diseases Community of Practice. Endemic fungal infections in solid organ transplantation. Clin Transplant. 2019;33(9):e13553.

14. Fishman J. Infections in immunocompromised hosts and organ transplant recipients: essentials. Liver Transpl. 2011;17(Suppl 3):S34–7.

15. Grim SA, Reid GE, Clark NM. Update in the treatment of non-influenza respiratory virus infection in solid organ transplant recipients. Expert Opin Pharmacother. 2017;18(8):767–79. https://doi.org/10.1080/14656566.2017.1322063.

16. Razonable RR, Paya CV. Infections in transplant patients. Clin Infect Dis. 2010;97:611–24. https://doi.org/10.1017/CBO9780511722240.088.

17. Abbas S, Raybould JE, Sastry S, de la Cruz O. Respiratory viruses in transplant recipients: more than just a cold. Clinical syndromes and infection prevention principles. Int J Infect Dis. 2017;62:86–93. https://doi.org/10.1016/j.ijid.2017.07.011.

18. Vu D-L, Bridevaux P-O, Aubert J-D, Soccal PM, Kaiser L. Respiratory viruses in lung transplant recipients: a critical review and pooled analysis of clinical studies. Am J Transplant. 2011;11:1071–8.

19. Fishman JA. Infection in organ transplantation. Am J Transplant. 2017;17(4):856–79. https://doi.org/10.1111/ajt.14208.

20. López-Medrano F, Aguado JM, Lizasoain M, et al. Clinical implications of respiratory virus infections in solid organ transplant recipients: a prospective study. Transplantation. 2007;84(7):851–6. https://doi.org/10.1097/01.tp.0000282788.70383.8b.

21. Paulsen GC, Danziger-Isakov L. Respiratory viral infections in solid organ and hematopoietic stem cell transplantation. Clin Chest Med. 2017;38(4):707–26. https://doi.org/10.1016/j.ccm.2017.07.012.

22. Frieden TR, Harold Jaffe DW, Stephens JW, et al. Antiviral Agents for the Treatment and Chemoprophylaxis of Influenza Recommendations of the Advisory Committee on Immunization Practices (ACIP) Morbidity and Mortality Weekly Report Hemagglutinin Neuraminidase M2 Ion Channel RNP Centers for Disease Control and Prevention MMWR Editorial and Production Staff MMWR Editorial Board Recommendations and Reports. Vol. 60; 2011. http://www.cdc.gov/flu. Accessed 20 Aug 2019.

23. Harper SA, Bradley JS, Englund JA, et al. IDSA guidelines for seasonal influenza in adults seasonal influenza in adults and children-diagnosis, treatment, chemoprophylaxis, and institutional outbreak management: clinical practice guidelines of the Infectious Diseases Society of America. https://doi.org/10.1086/598513

24. Uyeki TM, et al. Clinical practice guidelines by the Infectious Diseases Society of America: 2018 update on diagnosis, treatment, chemoprophylaxis, and institutional outbreak management of seasonal influenza. Clin Infect Dis. 2019;68(6):e1–e47.

25. FDA approves new drug to treat influenza. https://www.fda.gov/news-events/press-announcements/fda-approves-new-drug-treat-influenza. October 24, 2018. Accessed 11 Nov 2019.

26. Influenza antiviral drug baloxavir marboxil. https://www.cdc.gov/flu/treatment/baloxavir-marboxil.htm. November 18, 2019. Accessed 22 Nov 2019.

27. Hayden FG, Sugaya N, Hirotsu N, Lee N, de Jong MD, Hurt AC, Ishida T, Sekino H, Yamada K, Portsmouth S, Kawaguchi K, Shishido T, Arai M, Tsuchiya K, Uehara T, Watanabe A, Baloxavir Marboxil Investigators Group. Baloxavir marboxil for uncomplicated influenza in adults and adolescents. N Engl J Med. 2018;379(10):913–23.
28. Rubin LG, Levin MJ, Ljungman P, et al. 2013 IDSA Clinical Practice Guideline for vaccination of the immunocompromised host Clin Infect Dis. 2013. https://doi.org/10.1093/cid/cit816.
29. Frieden TR, Jaffe HW, Rasmussen SA, et al. Prevention and Control of Seasonal Influenza with Vaccines Recommendations of the Advisory Committee on Immunization Practices-United States, 2016–17 Influenza Season Morbidity and Mortality Weekly Report Recommendations and Reports Centers for Disease Control and Prevention MMWR Editorial and Production Staff (Serials) MMWR Editorial Board. Vol. 65; 2016. http://www.cdc.gov/vaccines/acip. Accessed 20 Aug 2019.
30. Natori Y, Shiotsuka M, Slomovic J, Hoschler K, Ferreira V, Ashton P, Rotstein C, Lilly L, Schiff J, Singer L, Humar A, Kumar D. A double-blind, randomized trial of high-dose vs standard-dose influenza vaccine in adult solid-organ transplant recipients. Clin Infect Dis. 2018;66(11):1698–704.
31. Mombelli M, Rettby N, Perreau M, Pascual M, Pantaleo G, Manuel O. Immunogenicity and safety of double versus standard dose of the seasonal influenza vaccine in solid-organ transplant recipients: a randomized controlled trial. Vaccine. 2018;36(41):6163–9.
32. Koval CE. Prevention and treatment of cytomegalovirus infections in solid organ transplant recipients. Infect Dis Clin. 2018;32(3):581–97.
33. Ljungman P, Griffiths P, Paya C. Definitions of cytomegalovirus infection and disease in transplant recipients. Clin Infect Dis. 2002;34(8):1094–7.
34. Kotton CN, Kumar D, Caliendo AM, Asberg A, Chou S, Danziger-Isakov L, Humar A, Transplantation Society International CMV Consensus Group. Updated international consensus guidelines on the management of cytomegalovirus in solid-organ transplantation. Transplantation. 2013;96(4):333–60.
35. Sousa D, Justo I, Dominguez A, Manzur A, Izquierdo C, Ruiz L, Nebot M, Bayas JM, Celorrio JM, Varona W, Llinares P, Miguez E, Sanchez E, Carratala J. Community-acquired pneumonia in immunocompromised older patients: incidence, causative organisms and outcome. Clin Microbiol Infect. 2013;19(2):187–92.
36. Cervera C, Agustí C, Angeles Marcos M, Pumarola T, Cofán F, Navasa M, Pérez-Villa F, Torres A, Moreno A. Microbiologic features and outcome of pneumonia in transplanted patients. Diagn Microbiol Infect Dis. 2006;55(1):47–54.
37. Metlay JP, Waterer GW, Long AC, Anzueto A, Brozek J, Crothers K, Cooley LA, Dean NC, Fine MJ, Flanders SA, Griffin MR, Metersky ML, Musher DM, Restrepo MI, Whitney CG. Diagnosis and treatment of adults with community-acquired pneumonia. An official clinical practice guideline of the American Thoracic Society and Infectious Diseases Society of America. Am J Respir Crit Care Med. 2019;200(7):e45–67. https://doi.org/10.1164/rccm.201908-1581ST.
38. Torre-Cisneros J, Doblas A, Aguado JM, Juan RS, Blanes M, Montejo M, Cervera C, Len O, Carratala J, Cisneros JM, Bou G, Muñoz P, Ramos A, Gurgui M, Borrell N, Fortún J, Moreno A, Gavalda J. Tuberculosis after solid-organ transplant: incidence, risk factors, and clinical characteristics in the RESITRA (Spanish Network of Infection in Transplantation) Cohort. Clin Infect Dis. 2009;48(12):1657–65.
39. Munoz P, Rodriguez C, Bouza C, Bouza E. *Mycobacterium tuberculosis* infection in recipients of solid organ transplants. Clin Infect Dis. 2005;40:581–7.
40. Subramanian A, Dorman S. *Mycobacterium tuberculosis* in solid organ transplant recipients. Am J Transplant. 2009;9:S57–62.
41. Aguado JM, Torre-Cisneros J, Fortún J, Benito N, Meije Y, Doblas A, Muñoz P, Snydman DR. Tuberculosis in solid-organ transplant recipients: consensus statement of the Group for the Study of Infection in Transplant Recipients (GESITRA) of the Spanish Society of Infectious Diseases and Clinical Microbiology. Clin Infect Dis. 2009;48(9):1276–84.

42. Patel R, Roberts GD, Keating MR, Paya CV. Infections due to nontuberculous mycobacteria in kidney, heart, and liver transplant recipients. Clin Infect Dis. 1994;19(2):263–73.
43. Griffith DE, Aksamit T, Brown-Elliot B, et al. An official ATS/IDSA statement: diagnosis, treatment, and prevention of nontuberculous mycobacterial diseases. Am J Respir Crit Care Med. 2007;175:367–416.
44. Keating MR, Daly JS. Nontuberculous mycobacterial infections in solid organ transplantation. Am J Transplant. 2013;13:77–82.
45. Guenette A, Husain S. Infectious complications following solid organ transplantation. Crit Care Clin. 2019;35(1):151–68. https://doi.org/10.1016/j.ccc.2018.08.004.
46. Malo J, Luraschi-Monjagatta C, Wolk DM, Thompson R, Hage CA, Knox KS. Update on the diagnosis of pulmonary coccidioidomycosis. Ann Am Thorac Soc. 2014;11(2):243–53. https://doi.org/10.1513/AnnalsATS.201308-286FR.
47. Panel on Opportunistic Infections in HIV-Infected Adults and Adolescents. Guidelines for the prevention and treatment of opportunistic infections in HIV-infected adults and adolescents: recommendations from the Centers for Disease Control and Prevention, the National Institutes of Health, and the HIV Medicine Association of the Infectious Diseases Society of America. Available at http://aidsinfo.nih.gov/contentfiles/lvguidelines/adult_oi.pdf. Accessed 11 Nov 2019, page B-2.
48. Angarone M, Snydman D, on behalf of the AST ID Community of Practice. Diagnosis and management of diarrhea in solid-organ transplant recipients: guidelines from the American Society of Transplantation Infectious Diseases Community of Practice. Clin Transplant. 2019;33(9):e13550.
49. Trinh S, Echenique I, Penugonda S, Angarone M. Optimal strategies for the diagnosis of community-onset diarrhea in solid organ transplant recipients: less is more. Transpl Infect Dis. 2017;19(2). https://doi.org/10.1111/tid.12673
50. Mullane K, Dubberke E, on behalf of the AST ID Community of Practice. Management of Clostridioides (formerly Clostridium) difficile infection (CDI) in solid organ transplant recipients: guidelines from the American Society of Transplantation Community of Practice. Clin Transplant. 2019;33(9):e13564.
51. Cheng Y, Phelps E, Ganapini V, Khan N, Ouyang F, Xu H, et al. Fecal microbiota transplantation for the treatment of recurrent and severe Clostridium difficile infection in solid organ transplant recipients: a multicenter experience. Am J Transplant. 2019 Feb;19(2):501–11.
52. Ganzenmueller T, Kluba J, Becker J, Bachmann O, Heim A. Detection of cytomegalovirus (CMV) by real-time PCR in fecal samplesfor the non-invasive diagnosis of CMV intestinal disease. J Clin Virol. 2014;61(4):517–22.
53. Angarone M, Ison M. Diarrhea in solid organ transplant recipients. Curr Opin Infect Dis. 2015;28(4):308–16.
54. Lee LY, Ladner DP, Ison MG. Norovirus infection in solid organ transplant recipients: a single-center retrospective study. Transpl Infect Dis. 2016;18(6):932–8. https://doi.org/10.1111/tid.12622.
55. van Beek J, van der Eijk AA, Fraaij PL, Caliskan K, Cransberg K, Dalinghaus M, Hoek RA, Metselaar HJ, Roodnat J, Vennema H, Koopmans MP. Chronic norovirus infection among solid organ recipients in a tertiary care hospital, the Netherlands, 2006–2014. Clin Microbiol Infect. 2017;23(4):265.e9–265.e13. https://doi.org/10.1016/j.cmi.2016.12.010.
56. Blair B. Safe living following solid organ transplantation. Infect Dis Clin N Am. 2018 Sep;32(3):507–15.
57. Bishnoi R, Bajwa R, Franke A, Skelton W IV, Wang Y, Patel N, et al. Post-transplant lymphoproliferative disorder (PTLD): single institutional experience of 141 patients. Exp Hematol Oncol. 2017;6:26.
58. Vidal E, Torre-Cisneros J, Blanes M, Montejo M, Cervera C, Aguado JM, Len O, Carratalá J, Cordero E, Bou G, Muñoz P, Ramos A, Gurguí M, Borrell N, Fortún J, Spanish Network for Research in Infectious Diseases (REIPI). Bacterial urinary tract infection after solid organ

transplantation in the RESITRA cohort. Transpl Infect Dis. 2012;14(6):595–603. https://doi.org/10.1111/j.1399-3062.2012.00744.x.

59. Silva M Jr, Marra A, Pereira C, Medina-Pestana J, Camargo L. Bloodstream infection after kidney transplantation: epidemiology, microbiology, associated risk factors, and outcome. Transplantation. 2010;90(5):581–7.
60. Goldman J, Julian K. Urinary tract infections in solid organ transplant recipients: guidelines from the American Society of Transplantation Infectious Diseases Community of Practice. Clin Transpl. 2019 Feb;21:e13507.
61. Hollier I, Ison M. The challenge of urinary tract infections in renal transplant recipients. Transpl Infect Dis. 2018 Apr;20(2):e12828.
62. Shendi A, Wallis G, Painter H, Harber M, Collier S. Epidemiology and impact of blood-stream infections among kidney transplant recipients: a retrospective single-center experience. Transpl Infect Dis. 2018;20(1). https://doi.org/10.1111/tid.12815.
63. Al Midani A, Elands S, Collier S, Harber M, Shendi A. Impact of urinary tract infections in kidney transplant recipients: a 4-year single-center experience. Transplant Proc. 2018 Dec;50(10):3351–5.
64. Vidal E, Cervera C, Cordero E, Armiñanzas C, Carratalá J, Cisneros JM, Fariñas MC, López-Medrano F, Moreno A, Muñoz P, Origüen J, Sabé N, Valerio M, Torre-Cisneros J, Study Group of Infection in Transplant Recipients (GESITRA) of the Spanish Society of Infectious Diseases, Clinical Microbiology (SEIMC); Spanish Network for Research in Infectious Diseases (REIPI). Management of urinary tract infection in solid organ transplant recipients: consensus statement of the Group for the Study of Infection in Transplant Recipients (GESITRA) of the Spanish Society of Infectious Diseases and Clinical Microbiology (SEIMC) and the Spanish Network for Research in Infectious Diseases (REIPI). Enferm Infecc Microbiol Clin. 2015;33(10):679.e1–679.e21. https://doi.org/10.1016/j.eimc.2015.03.024.
65. Brizendine K, Richter S, Cober E, van Duin D. Carbapenem-resistant Klebsiella pneumoniae urinary tract infection following solid organ transplantation. Antimicrob Agents Chemother. 2015;59(1):553–7.
66. Vigil D, Konstantinov N, Barry M, Harford A, Servilla K, Kim Y, et al. BK nephropathy in the native kidneys of patients with organ transplants: clinical spectrum of BK infection. World J Transplant. 2016;6(3):472–504.
67. Pizzi M, Ng L. Neurologic complications of solid organ transplantation. Neurol Clin. 2017;35(4):809–23. https://doi.org/10.1016/j.ncl.2017.06.013.
68. Sonneville R, Mariotte E, Brouwer MC. Cerebral complications of solid organ transplantation. Intensive Care Med. 2019;45:394–7. https://doi.org/10.1007/s00134-019-05540-1.
69. Živković SA, Abdel-Hamid H. Neurologic manifestations of transplant complications. Neurol Clin. 2010. https://doi.org/10.1016/j.ncl.2009.09.011.
70. Baddley JW, Forrest GN. Cryptococcosis in solid organ transplantation—guidelines from the American Society of Transplantation Infectious Diseases Community of Practice. Clin Transpl. 2019. https://doi.org/10.1111/ctr.13543.
71. Wright AJ, Fishman JA. Central nervous system syndromes in solid organ transplant recipients. Clin Infect Dis. 2014;59(7):1001–11. https://doi.org/10.1093/cid/ciu428.
72. van Veen KEB, Brouwer MC, van der Ende A, van de Beek D. Bacterial meningitis in solid organ transplant recipients: a population-based prospective study. Transpl Infect Dis. 2016;18(5):674–80. https://doi.org/10.1111/tid.12570.
73. Burke VE, Lopez FA. Approach to skin and soft tissue infections in non-HIV immunocompromised hosts. Curr Opin Infect Dis. 2017;30(4):354–63. https://doi.org/10.1097/QCO.0000000000000378.
74. Stevens DL, Bisno AL, Chambers HF, et al. Executive summary: practice guidelines for the diagnosis and management of skin and soft tissue infections: 2014 update by the infectious diseases society of America. Clin Infect Dis. 2014;59(2):147–59. https://doi.org/10.1093/cid/ciu444.
75. Poulakou G, Lagou S, Tsiodras S. What's new in the epidemiology of skin and soft tissue infections in 2018? Curr Opin Infect Dis. 2019;32(2):77–86. https://doi.org/10.1097/qco.0000000000000527.

76. Vermandere M, Aertgeerts B, Agoritsas T, et al. Antibiotics after incision and drainage for uncomplicated skin abscesses: A clinical practice guideline. BMJ (Online). 2018;360:1–8. https://doi.org/10.1136/bmj.k243.
77. Coussement J, Lebeaux D, van Delden C, et al. Nocardia infection in solid organ transplant recipients: a Multicenter European Case-control Study. Clin Infect Dis. 2016;63(3):338–45. https://doi.org/10.1093/cid/ciw241.
78. Sia TY, Taimur S, Blau DM, et al. Clinical and pathological evaluation of Mycobacterium marinum group skin infections associated with fish markets in New York City. Clin Infect Dis. 2016;62(5):590–5. https://doi.org/10.1093/cid/civ937.
79. Yacisin K, Hsieh JL, Weiss D, et al. Outbreak of non-tuberculous mycobacteria skin or soft tissue infections associated with handling fish – New York City, 2013-2014. Epidemiol Infect. 2017;145(11):2269–79. https://doi.org/10.1017/S0950268817001066.
80. Quirke M, Ayoub F, McCabe A, et al. Risk factors for nonpurulent leg cellulitis: a systematic review and meta-analysis. Br J Dermatol. 2017;177(2):382–94. https://doi.org/10.1111/bjd.15186.
81. Mongelluzzo J, Tu B, Grimes B, et al. Correlation of physical exam findings with fever in patients with skin and soft tissue infections. West J Emerg Med. 2017;18(3):398–402. https://doi.org/10.5811/westjem.2016.12.32838.
82. Krishnadasan A, Ph D, Abrahamian FM, et al. TMP SMX vs placebo uncomplicated skin abcess. N Engl J Med. 2016;374:82332. https://doi.org/10.1056/NEJMoa1507476.
83. Keung EZ, Liu X, Nuzhad A, Adams C, Ashley SW, Askari R. Immunocompromised status in patients with necrotizing soft-tissue infection. JAMA Surg. 2013;148(5):419–26. https://doi.org/10.1001/jamasurg.2013.173.
84. Tan H-H, Goh C-L. Viral infections affecting the skin in organ transplant recipients. Am J Clin Dermatol. 2006;7(1):13–29. https://doi.org/10.2165/00128071-200607010-00003.
85. Varicella vaccine recommendations. https://www.cdc.gov/vaccines/vpd/varicella/hcp/recommendations.html. Accessed 23 Sept 2019.
86. Grossi PA. Clinical aspects of invasive candidiasis in solid organ transplant recipients. Drugs. 2009;69(Suppl 1):15–20. https://doi.org/10.2165/11315510-000000000-00000.
87. Saccente M, Woods GL. Clinical and laboratory update on blastomycosis. Clin Microbiol Rev. 2010;23(2):367–81. https://doi.org/10.1128/CMR.00056-09.
88. Marsden-Haug N, Goldoft M, Ralston C, et al. Coccidioidomycosis acquired in Washington State. Clin Infect Dis. 2013;56(6):847–50. https://doi.org/10.1093/cid/cis1028.
89. Dooling K, Guo A, Patel M, Lee G, Moore K, Belongia E, et al. Recommendations of the advisory committee on immunization practices for use of herpes zoster vaccines. MMWR Morb Mortal Wkly Rep. 2018 Jan 26;67(3):103–8.
90. Stucchi R, Lopes M, Kumar D, Manuel O. Vaccine recommendations for solid-organ transplant recipients and donors. Transplantation. 2018;102(2S Suppl 2):S72–80.
91. Pneumococcal vaccine timing for adults. Centers for Disease Control and Prevention. 2015. https://www.cdc.gov/vaccines/vpd/pneumo/downloads/pneumo-vaccine-timing.pdf. Accessed 28 Sept 2019.

Chapter 9
Common Symptoms in the Adult Solid Organ Transplant Recipient

Kim O'Connor and Christopher J. Wong

Introduction

Solid organ transplant (SOT) recipients often return to the primary care setting after the first few months following transplantation, especially if their course has been free of serious complications. While they will still have contact with their transplant team—the frequency of which varies by transplant center as well as the patient's complications—they may present to primary care when they develop new symptoms. Patients may be unsure if the new symptoms are related to the transplanted organ, their immunosuppression, side effects of medications, or an unrelated illness. This chapter explores several common symptoms and offers an approach to the initial evaluation. As will be discussed, if the patient's presentation is concerning, close coordination with the transplant team is advised, and often transfer to an acute care setting (e.g., emergency department or admission to the hospital) may be indicated for expedited evaluation and treatment.

Respiratory Symptoms

Respiratory symptoms, including shortness of breath and cough, are common concerns of patients presenting to primary care. Cough alone is among the most common reasons for ambulatory visits: excluding visits for general follow-up, medication management, checkups, and postoperative evaluation, it is the number one reason for outpatient visits in the United States [1]. The following section focuses on addressing cough and dyspnea in solid organ transplant recipients who present to care in the outpatient setting.

K. O'Connor · C. J. Wong (✉)
Department of Medicine, Division of General Internal Medicine, University of Washington, Seattle, WA, USA
e-mail: cjwong@uw.edu

© Springer Nature Switzerland AG 2020
C. J. Wong (ed.), *Primary Care of the Solid Organ Transplant Recipient*,
https://doi.org/10.1007/978-3-030-50629-2_9

General Approach

Assess Clinical Stability

- Patients with new-onset hypoxia, severe tachypnea, signs of sepsis, or respiratory distress will need rapid evaluation and treatment in an emergency setting.
- Solid organ transplant recipients are at risk of rapid decompensation in cases of severe infection, and it is generally best to err on the side of caution when considering whether to transfer to a higher level of care.

History

History should be directed toward infectious and non-infectious causes of respiratory symptoms.

- *Core transplant history:* Important initial information to gather includes the time since transplantation and prior episodes of rejection, as the types of infections to which a solid organ transplant recipient is more susceptible may vary based on this history. (For more in-depth discussion, see Chap. 8).
- *Medications*: A thorough medication history should be taken. The degree of immunosuppression may be helpful in triaging the potential for opportunistic infections as well as the risk of decompensation.
- *Habits*: In most cases, solid organ transplant recipients have stopped smoking cigarettes prior to transplantation. However, prior smoking can still lead to complications, including lung cancer and chronic obstructive pulmonary disease. Additionally, patients may have returned to using cigarettes or vaping after transplantation. Patients should be asked about substance use, as inhaled marijuana has been associated with pulmonary aspergillosis in renal transplant recipients [2], although its precise contribution to pulmonary aspergillosis in solid organ transplant recipients overall is uncertain.
- *Exposures*: As with the general population, recent hospitalization increases the risk for multi-drug resistant organisms, and recent travel should prompt consideration for infectious illnesses not endemic to the current location.
- *Associated symptoms*:

  - Symptoms such as fever and rhinorrhea may point to an infectious source. Solid organ transplant recipients may contract community-acquired viral infections such as the common cold. However, one must be careful not to prematurely narrow the differential diagnosis if the patient is at higher risk for other opportunistic infections due to increased levels of immunosuppression. Prolonged viral infections may lead to secondary bacterial infection. Due to immunosuppression, the solid organ transplant recipient may not present with typical fevers and the absence of a fever is not reliable enough to rule out infection.
  - While a cough may be infectious (e.g., caused by an upper or lower respiratory tract infection), it is important not to assume an infectious source.

Interstitial and obstructive lung diseases, pulmonary edema, gastroesophageal reflux, and lung cancer all may feature cough as their presenting symptom. Sputum character does not reliably distinguish one cause from another. Hemoptysis should always be evaluated further—history should include asking about other symptoms of infection, including risk factors for tuberculosis, as well as symptoms of malignancy such as systemic symptoms.

- Dyspnea alone (for example, absent symptoms such as rhinorrhea, cough, angina, fever) should lead to a similar differential diagnosis as in the general population, including pulmonary embolism, congestive heart failure, pulmonary hypertension, interstitial lung disease, obstructive lung disease, and systemic illnesses such as anemia. However, one should still consider an atypical presentation of infection as well as malignancy (for example, lung cancer with a pleural effusion) (See Chap. 10).

- *Time course*: Duration and tempo of symptoms cannot solely distinguish among causes of respiratory symptoms, but may nevertheless provide clues.

  - Acute (1–2 days): Consider acute infections more highly on the differential diagnosis, especially if other infectious symptoms are present. Additionally, acute pulmonary embolism should be considered, especially if risk factors are present. However, even chronic conditions may present acutely (e.g., a lung cancer may present with an effusion that becomes symptomatic, or a decreased cardiac ejection fraction may be subclinical until it presents with decompensated heart failure).
  - Sub-acute (2 weeks): Infections, including opportunistic, may still occur. *Pneumocystis jirovecii* pneumonia may present subacutely with cough and dyspnea, although more severe and acute cases can occur in solid organ transplant recipients compared to patients with HIV. Other non-infectious causes should still be in the differential diagnosis.
  - Chronic (weeks to months): In a stable patient with chronic cough, consider traditional causes such as gastroesophageal reflux disease, postnasal drip, and reactive airways disease. Medication side effects and interstitial lung disease should also be considered. For stable outpatients with dyspnea, all causes should be considered, including anemia, heart disease, and lung disease.
  - For all of the above considerations, in the heart or lung transplant recipient, respiratory symptoms should raise concern for rejection or other transplanted organ dysfunction (see below).

- Special mention should be made for lung and heart transplant recipients.

  - Lung transplant recipients presenting with dyspnea or cough should have their workup coordinated with the lung transplant specialist, as the transplant team will often recommend an urgent workup for rejection, re-evaluate graft function, and also may perform additional tests for infection (see Chap. 7). Other diagnostic considerations include lung cancer, in which the risk is higher in lung transplant recipients compared to other solid organ transplant recipients (see Chap. 10), and airway stenosis, a unique complication of lung transplantation. Additionally, it is important to know whether the patient received a single

or double lung transplant. In single lung transplant recipients, the native lung may still be diseased—for example, in a patient with a single lung transplant for smoking-related COPD, the native lung remains at increased risk for infection, malignancy, and other complications such as pneumothorax.
–   Heart transplant recipients have a denervated donor organ, so may not present with typical angina. Dyspnea on exertion may be a sign of coronary artery disease as well as heart failure. As with lung transplant recipients, heart transplant recipients who present with dyspnea without a readily apparent non-cardiac etiology should have their care coordinated with the transplant team, as an expedited workup is likely warranted (see Chap. 6).

Examination

•   Examination should include vital signs and a thorough upper respiratory tract, pulmonary, and cardiovascular exam.
•   Abdominal exam may be useful if an intra-abdominal process leading to pulmonary symptoms is suspected.
•   In patients with dyspnea, assessment should include looking for signs of anemia or other systemic illnesses.

Differential Diagnosis

Infectious

(Infections are covered more in Chap. 8)

•   *Pneumonia*: Precise estimates on incidence of pneumonia in solid organ transplant recipients are difficult to obtain. A point-prevalence study in Europe estimated an incidence of 10 per 1000 patients per year [3]. The incidence was highest in lung transplant recipients. The majority presented late (defined as >6 months). Although this sample included outpatient care, the cases identified were primarily in hospitalized patients. Similarly, prior single-center studies showed a high mortality rate, but cases were predominantly nosocomial and early after transplantation [4].
    Several fungal infections can cause pneumonia in solid organ transplant recipients. *Pneumocystis jirovecii* is an important causative agent of opportunistic infections in the solid organ transplant population, so much so that most solid organ transplant recipients receive prophylaxis against *P. jirovecii* within the first 6–12 months after transplantation (protocols vary), with lifelong prophylaxis given to lung transplant recipients. Patients with *Pneumocystis jirovecii* pneumonia may present acutely with hypoxia and dyspnea, more commonly than in patients with HIV infection, who often present subacutely with several weeks of progressive symptoms. While prophylaxis is credited to dramatic reductions in *P. jirovecii* pneumonia, cases still occur, especially after prophylaxis has been discontinued, and have been associated with episodes of acute rejection (and

therefore increased immunosuppression), as well as cytomegalovirus (CMV) viremia; additionally, heart and lung transplant recipients are at higher risk compared to other solid organ transplant recipients [5, 6].

Infections due to *Aspergillus fumigatus* are more common than those due to *Pneumocystis jirovecii* and other fungal infections in solid organ transplant recipients [7]. Risk factors include lung and heart transplantation, CMV infection, the degree of immunosuppression, and environmental exposure [7]. Nosocomial infections may occur early after transplantation, but late infections (> 6 months post-transplant) also occur. Pulmonary infections caused by *Aspergillus* may present with cough, fever, hemoptysis, chest pain, and malaise. Patients may manifest symptoms in other organs if the infection has already spread at the time of presentation [7]. Prophylaxis is typically administered in the first few months post-transplant for lung transplant recipients and in some heart transplant recipients (protocols vary) [7].

Other fungi such as Candida species, Cryptococcus, Zygomycetes species, the endemic mycoses coccidioidomycosis and histoplasma all may cause pulmonary infections. Histoplasmosis tends to occur in the later post-transplant period with disseminated disease but can have subacute pulmonary symptoms [7]. In contrast, coccidioidomycosis tends to occur earlier post-transplant and represent reactivation [7]. Blastomycosis is considered rare even in this population [7] (see Chap. 8).

Mycobacterial infections can be divided into infections caused by *Mycobacterium tuberculosis* and those by all non-tuberculous mycobacteria. Pulmonary tuberculosis does occur, and level of suspicion is dependent on exposure and local epidemiologic risk factors. Non-tuberculous mycobacterial pulmonary infections are less common than other pathogenic infections in the solid organ transplant population, but they do occur and should be suspected in patient with chronic cough and especially if systemic symptoms are present. (See Chap. 8).

Viral infections. Most solid organ transplant recipients receive prophylaxis against CMV during the first 6–12 months after transplantation (see Chap. 8). Although considered an "early" post-transplant infection, because of effective prophylaxis in the initial post-transplant period, late cases do occur. While multiple immunosuppressive agents decrease T-cell function and increase the risk of CMV, mammalian target of rapamycin (mTOR) inhibitors do not appear to increase risk and may even lower the risk of CMV infection [8]. CMV not only may cause a viral syndrome with non-specific symptoms but also may cause end-organ damage, including pneumonia. As noted above, CMV infection increases the risk for subsequent *Aspergillus* and *P. jirovecii* infections.

A multitude of other viruses may cause respiratory infections—those that may cause lower respiratory tract symptoms include influenza and respiratory syncytial virus (RSV).

- Upper respiratory tract infections: Solid organ transplant recipients are susceptible to the common respiratory viruses that cause the common cold, similar to the general population, including rhinovirus and coronavirus. Patients with rhinorrhea and other upper respiratory tract infection (URI) symptoms, without evidence of bacterial sinusitis or lower respiratory tract disease, may be considered to have an isolated URI. However, any patient with a cough or dyspnea should have a broader differential considered in the evaluation. For lung transplant recipients, even mild respiratory viral infections may be associated with a decline in graft function and, therefore, the lung transplant team should be notified (see Chap. 7).

- COVID-19: COVID-19 (SARS-CoV-2) became a worldwide pandemic in 2020. At the time of this book's publication, the presentation, prognosis, and optimal treatment in solid organ transplant recipients is continuing to be studied. Testing should be initiated promptly depending on local epidemiology, and consultation with infectious disease specialists is warranted in this population.

Non-infectious

Immunosuppression should raise suspicion for infection in a solid organ transplant recipient who presents with respiratory symptoms. However, certain other conditions also have a higher prevalence in the solid organ transplant population.

- *Cancer*: Solid organ transplant recipients have an increased overall risk of malignancy compared to the general population, as well as higher mortality when cancers occur [9]. While studies vary, there is an increased incidence of cancers that may present with pulmonary symptoms, including lung cancer, lymphoma, melanoma, and kidney cancer, in all solid organ transplant recipients [10, 11]. Primary lung cancer, metastatic cancer to the lung, and lymphoma in the lung may present with cough or hemoptysis. Additionally, pleural effusions due directly or indirectly to malignancy may cause dyspnea and pleuritic chest pain (see Chap. 10).
- *Pulmonary embolism*: The risk of venous thromboembolism (VTE) has been shown to be increased in the postoperative period, especially in lung transplant recipients [12]. Long-term VTE risk has been reported in other solid organ transplant recipients, but the majority of studies are retrospective and the incidence rates vary widely [13, 14]. Some studies suggest an ongoing risk for renal-transplant recipients, with increased risk associated with chronic kidney disease, and not associated with immunosuppression [15, 16]. In the absence of more definitive data, one should consider that solid organ transplant recipients presenting to primary care may be at higher risk for VTE, even after the immediate post-transplantation period. As the precise degree of risk is uncertain, providers should continue to assess for traditional VTE risk factors.
- *Interstitial lung disease*: Interstitial lung disease typically presents with a variety of chronic to subacute symptoms, including dyspnea and cough. In addition to exploring traditional risk factors for ILD, in the solid organ transplant recipient, there have been case reports of ILD associated with immunosuppressive medications, including the mammalian target of rapamycin (mTOR) inhibitors sirolimus and everolimus [17–19].
- *Lung transplant recipients*: Lung transplant recipients may present with acute rejection. Acute symptomatic rejection may present with acute dyspnea and cough. Symptoms may be subtle and, therefore, lung transplant centers routinely monitor lung function. In cases of suspected rejection, consultation with the

transplant pulmonologist is critical, and other causes of dyspnea such as airway stenosis and infection will often need to be evaluated urgently (see Chap. 7). Chronic symptoms in lung transplant recipients may arise from Chronic Lung Allograft Dysfunction (CLAD), of which there are two main types – bronchiolitis obliterans syndrome (BOS), and restrictive allograft syndrome (RAS). CLAD may present with chronic dyspnea and cough (See Chap. 7).

- *Heart disease:* Cardiac causes of respiratory symptoms should be considered. Although solid organ transplant recipients are screened pre-transplantation for heart disease (see Chap. 2), they may still develop cardiovascular disease after transplantation. Solid organ transplant recipients are at increased risk of the metabolic risk factors that lead to cardiovascular disease, including diabetes, hypertension, and hyperlipidemia. Cardiovascular disease is increased in kidney transplant recipients, although data on risk in liver transplant recipients is not consistent [14, 20]. Lung transplant recipients have not been shown to have increased mortality from cardiovascular disease, possibly due to the earlier onset of graft dysfunction and lower overall mortality [20]. Heart transplant recipients are at risk for allograft vasculopathy, a form of rejection in the coronary arteries (see Chap. 6).

Causes of dyspnea or cough in solid organ transplant recipients are summarized in Table 9.1.

Table 9.1 Causes of dyspnea or cough in solid organ transplant recipients

Infectious	Non-infectious
Upper respiratory tract infection	*Pulmonary/lung disease*
Viral rhinosinusitis	COPD exacerbation
Bacterial sinusitis	Asthma exacerbation
Lower respiratory tract infection	Interstitial lung disease
Pneumonia	Pulmonary embolism
Bacterial	Pulmonary hypertension
Viral (e.g., CMV); emerging: COVID-19	Lung transplant recipients: rejection, chronic lung allograft dysfunction, airway stenosis
Fungal (e.g., *Aspergillus, P. jirovecii, Candida* species, endemic mycoses)	*Malignancy*
Mycobacterial	Primary lung cancer
Bronchitis	Lymphoma/PTLD in the lungs or mediastinum
Viral	Pleural effusion associated with malignancy
Bacterial	Metastatic disease to the lung
	Head and neck cancer/laryngeal
	Cardiac
	Heart failure
	Coronary artery disease
	Heart transplant recipients: cardiac allograft vasculopathy; rejection
	Medication side effect
	ACE inhibitors (cough)
	Gastrointestinal
	Gastroesophageal reflux disease
	Upper airway
	Postnasal drip/upper airway cough syndrome
	Metabolic
	Anemia

Additional Testing and Treatment

- Imaging: While one cannot recommend a one-size-fits-all approach, in general one should have a lower threshold to obtain imaging in solid organ transplant recipients who present with respiratory symptoms due to the increased risk of infection and malignancy, as well as their potentially blunted inflammatory response to infection. A chest X-ray is a reasonable first imaging test, but in patients with concerning symptoms, a chest CT is more sensitive.
- Specific tests for respiratory pathogens: While testing for respiratory viruses other than influenza is uncommonly performed in the general population, for solid organ transplant recipients presenting with potentially infectious respiratory symptoms, it is recommended to obtain a nasopharyngeal swab to send for PCR-based tests for viral pathogens.
- Additional testing: Solid organ transplant recipients with serious illnesses such as pneumonia frequently require additional testing such as sputum samples, bronchoscopy, and in some cases biopsy depending on the presentation, imaging findings, and response to treatment.
- If CMV is considered, consultation with an infectious disease specialist is appropriate. Imaging findings are typically bilateral, patchy, and may include ground glass opacities, air-space disease, and small nodules; however, most imaging studies of CMV pneumonitis included only a small number of SOT recipients [21]. CMV disease (in any organ) is diagnosed definitively by tissue. The CMV antigenemia assay is not sufficiently sensitive in the SOT population [22] and has been replaced by PCR [8]. Serology should be determined from reviewing the transplantation history, as CMV-negative hosts who receive organs from CMV-positive donors are at highest risk, but it is not helpful to recheck these tests in the acute setting. While in some cases if other causes are ruled out or are deemed of low likelihood, pneumonitis with CMV viremia may prompt initial treatment for presumed CMV disease, followed by invasive testing if the patient does not respond to initial treatment. However, if other causes are also likely and unable to be ruled out, then early invasive testing with bronchoalveolar lavage may be indicated both to assess for the cytopathic presence of CMV in the lung and to investigate other causes of the patient's symptoms. In lung transplant recipients in particular, bronchoscopy may be especially important to assess for rejection – consultation with the transplant pulmonologist should be obtained.
- Early consultation is generally recommended for patients with higher risk or more serious presentations. The primary care provider should have a low threshold to consult with the transplant specialist and an infectious disease specialist, and transfer to a higher level of care if necessary.
- Empiric treatment: If influenza is suspected, treatment should be initiated while waiting for confirmatory testing. For suspected community-acquired pneumonia, patients should be triaged for consideration of hospitalization for inpatient treatment. If deemed stable for outpatient treatment for community-acquired pneumonia, then empiric, guideline-concordant treatment should be started, with appropriate assessment of potential drug interactions and whether the patient is at risk for drug-resistant organisms. Empiric treatment should generally not be

started in stable patients in whom opportunistic infections are suspected, as guidance by an infectious disease specialist is usually warranted to identify appropriate testing and management. As noted above, for lung transplant recipients, the transplant team should be contacted prior to empiric treatment, as they may have recommendations to guide choice of treatment and what testing should be performed to help assess for both infection and rejection (see Chaps. 7 and 8).

- Corticosteroids: Corticosteroids for obstructive lung disease exacerbation and reactive airways should be used with caution, as it may affect evaluation of organ rejection— in lung transplant recipients in particular, corticosteroids should not be given (unless emergent) without first consulting the transplant pulmonologist.
- IV fluids: IV fluids should generally not be given to solid organ transplant recipients in the primary care setting. If the patient is sick enough to require IV fluids, then transfer to an acute care setting is indicated. In particular, IV fluids should be administered with caution and only in a well-monitored setting for lung transplant recipients, as the disruption in the lymphatic system makes these patients more susceptible to pulmonary edema. Heart transplant recipients should also generally not be given IV fluids without consultation with the transplant cardiologist, as their volume status and graft function will likely need more urgent assessment.

Follow-Up

As with any patient, if the solid organ transplant recipient being treated for a pulmonary condition does not improve, one should reconsider the initial diagnosis as well as consider co-infection with more than one organism.

Key Points
- As with all solid organ transplant recipients presenting with a new symptom, a thorough history and directed exam should be performed.
- Solid organ transplant recipients presenting with potentially infectious respiratory symptoms should generally have a nasopharyngeal swab sent for respiratory virus PCR testing.
- Solid organ transplant recipients are more likely to need advanced imaging and invasive testing for the diagnosis and treatment of serious respiratory conditions.
- Stable lung transplant recipients should not receive empiric IV fluids or corticosteroids without consulting with the transplant specialist first—they are sensitive to pulmonary edema from IV fluids, and corticosteroids can affect workup for rejection.
- A broad differential diagnosis is required for pneumonia in solid organ transplant recipients—in stable patients over 6 months since transplantation, community-acquired pneumonia is common, but other opportunistic infections can still occur.
- Solid organ transplant recipients are at increased risk for cancers that may present with respiratory symptoms.

Urinary Symptoms

Urinary symptoms are common reasons for primary care visits. Once a solid organ transplant recipient is returned to the primary care setting, it is quite likely that if the patient has urinary symptoms, the initial site of contact may be the primary care clinic rather than the specialist's office. In this section, we consider the solid organ transplant recipient who presents with dysuria and/or hematuria.

General Approach

Assess Clinical Stability

- Patients with signs of sepsis from a urinary tract source will need more rapid evaluation and treatment in an emergency setting.
- SOT recipients are at higher risk of rapid decompensation in cases of severe infection, and it is generally best to err on the side of caution.

History

- *Core transplant history:* Important initial information to gather includes the time since transplantation and prior episodes of rejection, as the types of infections to which a solid organ transplant recipient is more susceptible may vary based on this history. (For more in-depth discussion, see Chap. 8.)
- *Medications*: A thorough medication history should be taken. The degree of current immunosuppression may be helpful in triaging the potential for opportunistic infections as well as the risk of decompensation.
- *Habits*: A history of smoking increases the risk for urinary tract malignancies. Solid organ transplant recipients are generally required to stop smoking prior to transplantation. However, prior smoking continues to pose a risk for future cancers: the risk of bladder cancer is higher in former smokers compared to those who have never smoked [23].
- *Exposure*s: Recent hospitalization increases the risk for multi-drug resistant organisms, and recent travel should prompt consideration for infectious illnesses not endemic to the current location. As with the general population, certain chemical exposures increase the risk for bladder cancer.
- *Risk factors for urinary tract infections (UTIs):* Risk factors for UTIs in solid organ transplant recipients include age, female gender, and post-transplant dialysis [24]. Other risk factors identified in kidney transplant recipients include age, history of increase in immunosuppression, prior reflux kidney disease, and having a deceased donor [25]. Patients who have had urinary catheters or instrumentation are also at higher risk of UTI.

- *Prior UTIs and local resistance patterns*: Many patients have recurrent UTIs and it is helpful to review prior microbiological data to identify the prior organisms and their antimicrobial resistance.
- *Associated symptoms*:
  - Urethral discharge may be a sign of urethritis from a sexually transmitted infection. Patients should be asked about exposure history, including number of partners, type of sexual activity, and condom use, if appropriate.
  - Flank pain, fever, chills are suggestive of systemic infection such as pyelonephritis.
  - Colicky abdominal or groin pain is suggestive of nephrolithiasis.
  - Gross hematuria may be a sign of nephrolithiasis, bladder stones, coagulopathy, benign prostatic hyperplasia, or urinary tract malignancy.
- Special mention should be made for kidney transplant recipients (see Chap. 4): In the renal transplant recipient, pyelonephritis of the transplanted kidney may present with pain in the lower abdominal quadrant where the transplanted organ is typically located.

Examination

- Vital signs.
- Examination of the flank and abdomen.
- If present, vaginal symptoms should be evaluated and may require a pelvic examination.
- Prostate exam if symptoms of prostatitis.
- Kidney transplant recipients should have an examination of the abdomen that includes assessment of the transplant site (typically in the left or right lower quadrant).

Differential Diagnosis

Infectious

(Infections are covered more in Chap. 8)

- Urinary tract infections are common in all solid organ transplant recipients in the first several months after transplantation [24]. During this period, the patient will most likely remain primarily in the care of the transplant team. However, even after the first few months post-transplant, urinary tract infections continue to occur in all solid organ transplant recipients, although the incidence is highest in kidney transplant recipients [24]. UTI is a common cause of bacteremia in kidney transplant recipients [26].

- The main issues for UTIs in non-renal transplant recipients are diagnostic accuracy and choice and duration of antibiotic therapy.
- While opportunistic infections do occur in the genitourinary tract, they are less common compared to opportunistic infections at other sites. Candida UTIs do occur, with higher risk in renal transplant recipients.
- Prostatitis may occur in solid organ transplant recipients, but the exact incidence is unknown. It should be suspected if a patient has recurrent UTIs or typical symptoms. While there are case reports of unusual pathogens, including CMV and Cryptococcus, initially typical urinary pathogens should be suspected.
- Urethral discharge, vaginal discharge, and sexual contact should raise concern for sexually transmitted infections. There is little data on the solid organ transplant population as to prevalence, however.

Non-infectious

- Gross hematuria should always be evaluated. Sources can include the kidney itself (glomerulonephritis, renal cysts, renal cell carcinoma), nephrolithiasis or bladder stones, other urothelial tract malignancy, the prostate, and, for kidney transplant recipients, acute rejection.
- In renal transplant recipients, acute rejection may be asymptomatic and found only on laboratory studies, but it may also present with fever, malaise, and tenderness of the transplanted kidney. If these symptoms are present along with an increased level of creatinine, and especially if no infection is found, the transplant nephrologist should be consulted to evaluate for acute rejection.

Additional Testing and Treatment

Solid organ transplant recipients presenting with UTI symptoms (dysuria, frequency, or urgency) should have a clean-catch urinalysis performed.

- Solid organ transplant recipients are at risk for less common pathogens, drug-resistant organisms, and more severe illness. Therefore, it is recommended that solid organ transplant recipients who present with urinary tract infection symptoms should always have urine testing performed, including a culture. This practice is in contrast to low-risk patients in the general population who may be treated empirically with antibiotics based on local resistance patterns without obtaining a formal culture.
- For solid organ transplant recipients, the definition of asymptomatic bacteriuria is the same as for the general population and is defined as a urine culture with $\geq 10^5$ colony-forming units/mL in a patient with no symptoms of cystitis and no systemic symptoms [26]. Note however, that in most cases, it is not recommended to obtain a urine culture if a patient is not symptomatic.

- The definition of acute uncomplicated cystitis in a solid organ transplant recipient is the following: the presence of local symptoms (dysuria, urinary frequency or urgency, or suprapubic pain) without systemic symptoms or urinary tract instrumentation. The colony count threshold in a urine culture is a matter of some debate. Some guidelines specify a colony count of $\geq 10^5$ colony-forming units/mL, the same number as for asymptomatic bacteriuria [28]. However, many authors recommend using a lower threshold in symptomatic patients even in the general population, as some cases of true cystitis are associated with lower colony counts of between 10^2–10^5 colony-forming units/mL [27].
- In kidney transplant recipients, the definitions are similar, with formal classification as shown in Table 9.2 [26]. Some laboratories appropriately offer "reflexive" cultures to be done if pyuria is present. However, because pyuria is not an absolute criterion (although the absence should broaden the differential diagnosis), especially in patients with neutropenia, a culture should be obtained in most cases in patients with urinary tract symptoms.
- Empiric treatment:

  - For acute, uncomplicated cystitis, a fluoroquinolone, amoxicillin-clavulanate, or a third-generation cephalosporin is recommended as empiric therapy, pending culture results [26]. Guidelines vary with regard to the use of fosfomycin as first-line therapy [26, 28].
  - The choice of initial antibiotic should also be modified based on prior UTI results, if available, and local resistance patterns and whether there is a history of hospitalization or instrumentation.
  - Note that some guidelines do not recommend nitrofurantoin in solid organ transplant recipients due to risk of adverse effects [28], whereas others allow for its use if the creatinine clearance is >60 mL/min, and possibly even if >40 mL/min [26].

- Treatment duration: In contrast to simple cystitis in female patients, in which a 3-day course is appropriate, for solid organ transplant recipients (both female and male), the treatment duration is recommended for a longer period, 5–10 days [26, 28].
  Pyelonephritis: If the patient's clinical presentation is consistent with pyelonephritis, in most cases the patient should be transferred to an acute-care setting, as the patient will require IV antibiotics, additional blood tests, and blood cultures, and need close monitoring for risk of sepsis. Diagnostic criteria for pyelonephritis vary. General criteria for pyelonephritis in solid organ transplant recipients (other than kidney transplant) are the following [28]:

  - Urine culture $\geq 10^5$ colonies/mL and/or bacteremia and fever.
  - Costovertebral angle pain (or renal allograft pain in a kidney transplant recipient), chills, or cystitis criteria met (bacteriuria plus symptoms).

Table 9.2 shows the classification of simple cystitis and pyelonephritis in guidelines specifically created for kidney transplant recipients. The differences in criteria for pyelonephritis between kidney transplant and other solid organ transplants

Table 9.2 Classification of asymptomatic bacteriuria (AB) and urinary tract infection (UTI) in renal transplant recipients

Classification	Description	Laboratory investigations of urine
Asymptomatic bacteriuria	No urinary or systemic symptoms of infection	>10⁵ CFU/mL uropathogen[a][b]
Acute simple cystitis	Dysuria, urinary urgency/frequency, or suprapubic pain; but no systemic symptoms and no ureteral stent/nephrostomy tube/chronic urinary catheter	>10 WBC/mm³[c] >10³ CFU/mL uropathogen[b]
Acute pyelonephritis/ complicated UTI	Fever, chills, malaise, hemodynamic instability, or leukocytosis (without other apparent etiology); flank/ allograft pain; or bacteremia with same organism as in urine. Dysuria, urgency, frequency, suprapubic pain may or may not be present	>10 WBC/mm³[c] >10⁴ CFU/mL uropathogen[b]
Recurrent UTI	≥ 3 UTIs in prior 12-month period	As above

WBC white blood cell. *CFU/mL* colony-forming units/milliliter

Reprinted from Goldman, et al., with permission [26]

[a]While routine treatment of AB is not recommended (see Treatment section), if considering treatment of AB (e.g., in the immediate post-transplantation period), a repeat urine culture is recommended (with care to minimize contamination) to assess the persistence of the same uropathogen. Spontaneous resolution is common.

[b]*Staphylococcus epidermidis* (except if ureteral stent), *Lactobacillus*, and *Gardnerella* sp. are unlikely to be uropathogens. Regarding CFU/mL: while most patients with UTI will have >10⁵ CFU/mL of a uropathogen in a midstream urine sample, some patients with pyelonephritis may have only 10⁴–10⁵ CFU/ mL of a uropathogen and some patients with cystitis may have even fewer CFU/mL (most data on cystitis with low CFU/mL are only for *E. coli*). Not all labs report <10⁴ CFU/mL

[c]While not an absolute criterion (depending on the performance characteristics of the urinalysis or presence of neutropenia), <10 WBC/mm³ should prompt consideration of a diagnosis other than UTI

are subtle, and both guidelines require that the patient have significant systemic symptoms. In a solid organ transplant recipient, such systemic symptoms should generally prompt urgent acute care treatment and further evaluation. Blood cultures should be drawn prior to antibiotic initiation. Further treatment is beyond the scope of this chapter.

- For further discussion of urinary pathogens, risk factors, and treatment, see Chap. 8.
- The workup for gross hematuria is similar to the workup in the general population. The evaluation for infection and kidney stones is straightforward. If this evaluation is negative, then additional testing for malignancy is indicated; generally, consultation with a urologist should be undertaken to discuss cross-sectional imaging and cystoscopy. Solid organ transplant recipients are at increased risk for malignancies

that affect the urinary tract. In addition, kidney transplant recipients are at particularly increased risk for kidney cancer (see Chap. 10).
- If rejection is considered in kidney transplant recipients, urgent consultation with the renal transplant specialist is indicated.

Key Points

- As with all solid organ transplant recipients presenting with a new symptom, a thorough history and directed exam should be performed.
- If a urinary tract infection is suspected, urinalysis with culture should be obtained for all solid organ transplant recipients.
- Treatment for uncomplicated UTI in solid organ transplant recipients is typically 5–10 days.
- Consultation with the kidney transplant team is indicated for kidney transplant recipients who present with a UTI.
- For severe infections (e.g., pyelonephritis), transfer to an acute care setting should strongly be considered.

Gastrointestinal Symptoms: Diarrhea

Diarrhea is a common complaint in solid organ transplant recipients with a prevalence ranging from 20% to 50% [29]. Solid organ transplant recipients are particularly susceptible to complications from diarrheal illnesses, including volume depletion, increased toxicity of medications, organ rejection, and death. The evaluation and management of diarrhea in a solid organ transplant recipient differ compared to the general population due to a higher risk of infections, side effects due to immunosuppressive medication, and rapid clinical deterioration.

General Approach

Assess Clinical Stability

- Patients will need more rapid evaluation and treatment in an emergency setting if they have any of the following:
  - Vital sign instability
  - Signs of sepsis from a gastrointestinal (or other) source
  - Severe volume depletion requiring IV fluid resuscitation
  - Frailty and ongoing large-volume diarrhea, anticipating that volume depletion will occur imminently even if not present on initial evaluation

- – Symptoms or signs of acute gastrointestinal bleeding in addition to diarrhea
- – Acute abdomen, signs of peritonitis on exam
- – Inability to take oral medications—including immunosuppressive medications, due to ongoing nausea and vomiting

- Solid organ transplant recipients are at higher risk of rapid decompensation in cases of severe infection, and it is generally best to err on the side of caution.

History

- Core transplant history: Important initial information to gather includes the time since transplantation, prior episodes of rejection, as the types of infections a solid organ transplant recipient is more susceptible to may vary based on this history. (For more in-depth discussion, see Chap. 8.)
- Time course: Acute diarrhea (< 14 days) without obvious non-infectious source is often from an acute infectious etiology. Chronic diarrhea (> 30 days) may be infectious, but an expanded list of pathogens should be considered (see Differential Diagnosis below), as well as other non-infectious sources.
- Associated symptoms:

  - – Blood may be associated with bacterial infections (dysentery), but it is not specific—it may also be seen in inflammatory bowel disease and bowel ischemia.
  - – Nausea and emesis may indicate an ileus, obstruction, or upper gastrointestinal tract problem; however, it is nonspecific. Many infectious diarrheal illnesses do not typically cause nausea and vomiting, however.
  - – Malabsorption: Patients may give a history of an "oily sheen" in the toilet, or intolerances to certain foods.
  - – Abdominal pain: Many medication-induced causes of diarrhea may cause cramping but not typically severe pain. Severe pain should raise concern for severe bacterial infection, perforation, ischemia, and inflammatory bowel disease.

- Stool pattern: Unremitting diarrhea without association with food intake is more likely to be secretory than malabsorptive or osmotic, and more likely to be infectious. Symptom pattern in the immunosuppressed patient is not completely reliable, however.
- Medication history:

  - – Level of immunosuppression: higher doses (for example, patients with lung and heart transplants tend to have higher maintenance dosing, or patients with a history of rejection requiring recent pulse doses of corticosteroids or a higher maintenance dose) are associated with a higher risk of opportunistic infections.
  - – Mycophenolate is a component of the most commonly used regimen for many solid organ transplant recipients and frequently causes diarrhea. The medication history should be reviewed for any recent initiation or increase in dose of mycophenolate.

- Immunosuppressive medications such as tacrolimus also commonly cause magnesium wasting, requiring oral magnesium supplementation, which may in turn cause diarrhea.
- Diarrhea may affect medication levels. For chronic diarrhea, immunosuppressive medication trough levels should be reviewed and rechecked if necessary.

- Exposures:

  - Antibiotics: Patients should be asked about any recent infections that may have been treated with antibiotics, including urgent care visits or dental infections. Antibiotic exposure increases the risk of antibiotic-associated diarrhea, Clostrioides difficile infection, as well as resistant pathogens.
  - Hospitalization: Recent hospitalization increases the risk of hospital-acquired organisms.
  - Travel: Solid organ transplant recipients frequently travel and do not always have pre-travel counseling (See Chap. 12). Given the increased susceptibility to opportunistic infections, if the patient has traveled recently, they may have acquired other infectious organisms not typically seen in the patient's home region.
  - Food: Untreated sources of water may be a source of parasitic infections.

Examination

- Vitals signs
- Mucous membranes, skin turgor, and other assessment of volume depletion
- Cardiopulmonary exam
- Abdominal exam, assess for tenderness, peritoneal signs, masses
- Stool for appearance of melena, emesis (if present) for appearance of blood

Differential Diagnosis

Infectious causes of diarrhea in solid organ transplant recipients are discussed in more detail in Chap. 8. Following is a brief list (Table 9.3):

- *Clostridioides difficile* infection (CDI). *Clostridioides difficile* is the leading cause of infectious diarrhea in solid organ transplant recipients with incidence rates ranging from <1% to 23% [29, 30]. Higher rates occur in liver and lung transplant recipients and the lowest rates are in patients with kidney transplants [29, 31]. Compared to the general population, solid organ transplant recipients are at even greater risk for CDI due to immunosuppression, recent surgery, antibiotic treatments, ganciclovir prophylaxis, gastric acid suppression, and prolonged hospital stays [30]. Additional risk factors include enteral feeding, gastrointestinal surgery, obesity, cancer chemotherapy, hematopoietic stem cell transplantation, inflammatory bowel disease, and cirrhosis [32]. Although the use of multiple antibiotics, broad-spectrum antimicrobials, and longer durations

Table 9.3 Causes of diarrhea in solid organ transplant recipients

Infectious	Non-infectious
Bacterial	*Medication side effect*
Enteric pathogens (e.g., *E. coli*, *Shigella*,	Mycophenolate
Salmonella, *Campylobacter*)	Magnesium
C. difficile	Antidepressants
Viral (e.g., CMV, norovirus, rotavirus)*	Stool softeners, laxatives
Parasitic (e.g., Giardia, Cryptosporidium,	Proton pump inhibitors
Cystoisospora, Microsporidium, Cyclospora)	Metformin
	Antibiotics
	Gastrointestinal
	Irritable bowel syndrome
	Inflammatory bowel disease
	Microscopic colitis
	Small intestine bacterial overgrowth
	Malabsorption
	Malignancy
	Gastrointestinal Lymphoma/PTLD
	Colon cancer
	Neuroendocrine tumors

*The emerging coronavirus COVID-19 (SARS-CoV-2) may present with gastrointestinal symptoms including diarrhea. At the time of this publication, data on this virus' symptoms in solid organ transplant recipients continues to evolve

of antibiotic therapy clearly increase the risk for CDI, in immunosuppressed patients CDI is more likely to occur even in the absence of antibiotic use [33]. The illness spectrum of CDI ranges from asymptomatic carrier to mild or moderate diarrhea all the way to fulminant pseudomembranous colitis. In solid organ transplant recipients the development of CDI increases rates of graft dysfunction and other infections such as cytomegalovirus (CMV) or pneumonia, results in mortality rates between 2.3% and 8.5%, and is an independent predictor of death [29].

- *Cytomegalovirus.* CMV infection is defined as the presence of CMV replication in the blood (positive DNA by PCR or nucleic acid amplification testing, positive CMV antigenemia, or positive CMV culture) and can be symptomatic or asymptomatic. CMV disease is defined as CMV infection accompanied by clinical signs and symptoms. CMV disease may result in a CMV syndrome (fever, malaise, atypical lymphocytosis, leukopenia or neutropenia, thrombocytopenia, and elevated hepatic transaminases) or end-organ CMV disease, including gastrointestinal disease, pneumonitis, hepatitis, nephritis, myocarditis, pancreatitis, encephalitis, and retinitis. CMV has a predilection to infect the transplanted allograft, hence more likely causing symptoms and end-organ damage in the grafted organ [34].

    CMV infections most often occur between 30 days and 6 months after transplantation, as this is the time when immunosuppression tends to be maximal. In patients not receiving CMV prophylaxis (duration depending on the type of transplanted organ, patient and donor serostatus, and transplant center protocols), CMV infection typically occurs within 3 months of transplantation. The onset of disease may be delayed among patients receiving anti-CMV prophylaxis and also tends to occur within 3–6 months after completion of antiviral prophylaxis in CMV donor-positive/recipient-negative solid organ transplant recipients [34]. Donor and recipient CMV serostatus prior to transplantation is the most significant risk factor with the highest risk of infection occurring in CMV-seronegative recipients of a CMV-seropositive donor organ. In solid organ transplant recipients, the most common site of tissue invasive disease is the gastrointestinal tract, potentially causing esophagitis, gastritis, enteritis, and/or colitis. Typical symptoms include abdominal pain, diarrhea, and fever; however, signs may be subtle and present as mild epigastric discomfort or dyspepsia. CMV gastrointestinal disease has been associated with disorders such as inflammatory bowel disease as well as co-infection with *C. difficile*. CMV hepatitis, cholangitis, cholangiopathy, and pancreatitis also occur and may or may not have associated diarrhea [29].

In addition to causing direct symptoms and tissue-invasive disease, CMV infection can cause indirect effects such as allograft dysfunction or rejection and increased susceptibility to other opportunistic infections and death. One study demonstrated graft dysfunction in one of six patients with CMV-associated colitis [35].

- *Norovirus.* More than 90% of non-bacterial infectious diarrhea cases are due to norovirus with outbreaks occurring year-round but most commonly during the winter months. Transmission occurs via fecal-oral route, contact with contaminated surfaces, or via inhalation of aerosols from vomitus. In immunocompetent patients, norovirus tends to cause acute diarrhea lasting a few days; however, either acute or chronic diarrhea can occur in solid organ transplant recipients. Many solid organ transplant recipients with norovirus will develop weight loss and acute renal failure due to volume depletion.

- *Parasitic* causes of diarrhea in solid organ transplant recipients are less common but important to consider especially when other etiologies are not identified. Giardia and cryptosporidium are among the most common parasites to cause infection. If no diagnosis is made, then further investigation should be undertaken for more unusual pathogens such as Microsporidia, Cystoisospora, Cyclospora, and other ova and parasites [29]. As endemic parasites vary worldwide, local epidemiology should be considered.

Non-infectious Causes

- *Drug-induced diarrhea.* Drug-induced diarrhea is common in solid organ transplant recipients and may be due to the direct effects of the immunosuppressive drugs or due to other medications commonly administered including antibiotics, colchicine, or laxatives.

  - Compared to other immunosuppressive medications, mycophenolate mofetil (MMF) or mycophenolic acid (MPA) are more commonly associated with gastrointestinal side effects including nausea, vomiting, and diarrhea [35, 36].

The diarrhea associated with MMF and MPA is dose-dependent due to direct enterocyte damage. Diarrhea caused by mycophenolate may be bothersome but usually is not severe; however, in some cases, it may lead to dehydration, gastrointestinal hemorrhage, or perforations [37]. Additionally, a rarer disease similar to inflammatory bowel disease can occur.

– Calcineurin inhibitors such as tacrolimus or cyclosporine can cause diarrhea due to their macrolide effects, which can increase gut motility [29].
– Although less common, sirolimus and everolimus can also cause diarrhea.
– Non-immunosuppressive medications commonly used in solid organ transplant recipients that are frequently implicated in causing diarrhea include anti-bacterials, anti-arrhythmics, diabetic agents, laxatives, proton pump inhibitors, and magnesium supplementation. A careful review for these medications with dose adjustments or discontinuation may be appropriate with the guidance of the transplant team [29].

• *Graft-versus-host disease (GVHD).* GVHD is a multisystem disorder that occurs when the immune cells transplanted from a non-identical donor (the graft) recognize the transplant recipient (host) as foreign, thereby initiating an immune reaction that causes disease in the transplant recipient. GVHD is most commonly a complication of allogeneic hematopoietic cell transplant (HCT). It is a rare complication in solid organ transplant recipients, generally only occurring in liver and small intestine transplantation [29]. Acute GVHD usually occurs between 2 and 6 weeks after liver transplantation; however, this can be variable with late onset cases seen in other transplant settings [38]. (Small intestine transplantation is not covered in this book). The clinical presentation of solid organ transplant-associated GVHD includes skin rash, diarrhea, abdominal pain, gastrointestinal bleeding, fever, and in most cases quickly advances to become a multisystem disease affecting the bone marrow and other non-transplanted organs [29, 38]. The characteristic skin rash presents as red to violet maculopapular lesions first appearing on the hands and soles but may progress to the whole body, coalesce, and in severe cases lead to the development of vesicles or bullae. The mortality rate of SOT-associated GVHD can exceed more than 75% [38]. Diagnosis is based on clinical symptoms, pathologic changes in biopsied tissues, and systemic lymphoid chimerism.

• *Post-transplant lymphoproliferative disorder (PTLD).* Post-transplant lymphoproliferative disorder (PTLD) is an important malignancy to recognize in solid organ transplant recipients. It is a lymphoproliferative disorder with varying subtypes, often similar to B-cell lymphoma, and is associated with higher levels of immunosuppression as well as unfavorable Epstein-Barr virus serostatus (donor positive, recipient negative).

PTLD can affect virtually any organ system and has a variable presentation. Extranodal masses occur in more than half of the cases of PTLD and can involve the gastrointestinal (GI) tract, lungs, skin, liver, central nervous system, and allograft. When PTLD occurs extra-nodally, the gastrointestinal system is most commonly affected. Since PTLD can occur anywhere along the GI system, symptoms may include chronic diarrhea, weight loss, protein-losing enteropathy, abdominal pain, and anorexia [29].

- *Small intestine bacterial overgrowth (SIBO).* Small intestine bacterial over-growth may account for more than 10% of cases of chronic diarrhea in solid organ transplant recipients. SIBO occurs when bacteria colonize the upper small bowel leading to malabsorption and diarrhea. Immunosuppression, exocrine pancreatic insufficiency, achlorhydria, anatomic abnormalities (e.g., ileocecal resection and blind loop syndrome), and small bowel motility disorders predispose to SIBO. In many cases, the etiology may be multifactorial. Patients may be asymptomatic or symptoms can range from mild, mimicking irritable bowel syndrome (abdominal pain or discomfort, bloating, cramping, flatulence, chronic diarrhea), to severe, resulting in steatorrhea, malabsorption, and weight loss [39].
- *Inflammatory bowel disease (IBD).* Inflammatory bowel disease may occur de novo in solid organ transplant recipients but more commonly it presents as an exacerbation of preexisting disease. De novo development of IBD is ten times the incidence of IBD in the general population and is increased in CMV mismatch patients (seropositive donor, seronegative recipient). Recurrent IBD following transplantation appears to have a more aggressive course than de novo IBD and many patients will require escalation in medical therapy or colectomy for refractory disease. The risk of IBD recurrence post-transplantation includes active disease at the time of transplantation, short duration of IBD prior to transplantation, and the use of tacrolimus. Azathioprine and 5-aminosalicylates appear to be protective [39, 40].
- *Microscopic colitis.* Either subtype—lymphocytic colitis or collagenous colitis—can cause chronic watery diarrhea. In one study of kidney and kidney-pancreas transplant patients, the incidence of microscopic colitis was 50-fold higher in the solid organ transplant recipients compared to the general population. A definitive diagnosis requires histologic evaluation of large bowel biopsies [39].
- *Colon cancer.* Colon cancer risk may be increased in solid organ transplant recipients, and although rare, it may manifest as post-transplant diarrhea. Several studies have demonstrated a two- to threefold increased risk of colon cancer in transplant recipients. Cancers may also develop at a younger age and behave more aggressively [39].

Additional Testing and Treatment

Given the broad differential diagnosis, solid organ transplant recipients who present with diarrhea require at least basic testing. With the above history, exam, and differential diagnosis in mind, a suggested approach is shown in Fig. 9.1.

- The clinically unstable patient should be immediately transferred to an acute care setting such as the emergency department or admitted to the hospital. Signs of clinical instability include tachycardia, hypotension, orthostatic vital signs, intractable nausea or vomiting, severe abdominal pain or acute abdomen, melena, and hematemesis. Clinical judgment should be exercised in patients who are not

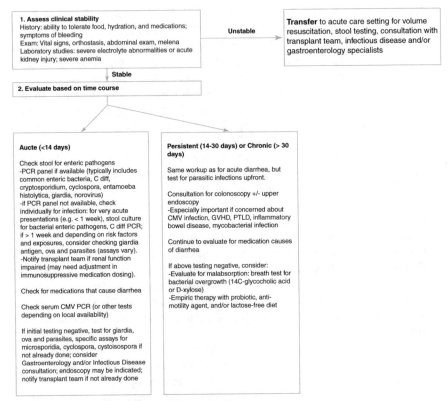

Fig. 9.1 Suggested approach to evaluation of diarrhea in solid organ transplant recipients*

immediately unstable but appear to be at risk of becoming unstable—this category includes patients who are not yet volume depleted but whose diarrhea is so profuse that they are not expected to be able to maintain hydration and patients who cannot tolerate oral intake in whom vital immunosuppressive medications may be missed. Additionally, strong consideration should be made for admitting frail or elderly solid organ transplant recipients who present with severe diarrhea, as the likelihood of volume depletion is high. The workup after admission is beyond the scope of this book, but it would typically include volume resuscitation, and an expedited workup for infectious causes of diarrhea, often with consultation from the transplant team and an infectious disease specialist; endoscopy will often be required for a tissue diagnosis and a gastroenterologist will need to be involved as well.

- In a stable patient, a workup is still recommended in almost all cases. This practice is in contrast to the general population, many of whom may be diagnosed clinically with a viral gastroenteritis and be treated with supportive care alone.
  - Medications: It is recommended to stop any medications that may be causing or worsening diarrhea. However, any potential changes in immunosuppressants should be directed by the transplant specialist. Medications are less

likely to be causal if the diarrhea is acute and severe in onset without recent medication changes; if there is associated nausea and vomiting; if there is severe abdominal pain or signs of bleeding; and if there are other signs of infection such as fever and chills.

- Acute diarrhea (<14 days):

  Compared to immunocompetent patients, the evaluation of diarrhea in solid organ transplant recipients should be worked up more expeditiously due to the risk of severe complications. For very acute cases (e.g., diarrhea of 1–3 days' duration) in solid organ transplant recipients who are >6 months since transplantation, evaluation for common bacterial pathogens and common viruses, as well as *C. difficile* is indicated. A serum CMV PCR is also a reasonable initial test as CMV colitis can occur late after transplantation, although this test by itself does not make a diagnosis of CMV colitis. For acute diarrhea in the 7–14 day period, it is additionally reasonable to consider early testing for parasitic causes, depending on the results of the initial testing (if completed) and exposure history.

  If available, a stool enteric pathogen PCR panel that includes bacterial pathogens, *C. difficile*, and common viruses is a good initial assay in addition to the serum CMV PCR. If not available, then bacterial and viral pathogens can be tested separately from the Giardia antigen and ova and parasite testing.

  If the initial testing is negative and the diarrhea persists, then consultation with a gastroenterologist is indicated, as workup for CMV colitis with endoscopy, and/or testing for SIBO, may be required.

- Persistent (14–30 days) and chronic diarrhea (>30 days):

  If the patient presents late in the course with prolonged diarrhea, then all testing for acute causes should still be performed, although bacterial enteric pathogens become less likely to be a cause. In solid organ transplant recipients, viruses such as norovirus can lead to a chronic diarrhea not typical of immunocompetent hosts. In addition, testing for parasitic causes should be performed. As mentioned above, a serum CMV PCR and a stool multi-assay for bacterial pathogens, viruses, *C. difficile*, and parasites are reasonable first steps if available.

  If the initial testing is negative, then consultation with a gastroenterologist familiar with immunosuppressed patients is appropriate for consideration of colonoscopy and possible upper endoscopy to evaluate for CMV infection, inflammatory bowel disease, microscopic colitis, and malignancy, depending on the overall clinical suspicion. Note that the definitive diagnosis of CMV infection requires biopsy for histopathology and that the CMV viral load by blood test can be negative but tissue gastrointestinal examination positive—when uncertain, a transplant infectious disease specialist should be consulted.

- Treatment is directed at the underlying etiology if found. Empiric treatment (e.g., antibiotics) is generally discouraged in a stable patient, with preference to making a correct diagnosis.
- If no clear cause is found, the primary care provider should continue to work with the transplant team and gastroenterology consultant to consider adjustments in medications, as well as further workup for malabsorption and less common causes

of diarrhea. Empiric treatment with anti-diarrheal medications is appropriate if infectious causes are ruled out; some authors also recommend a trial of probiotics.

- For a more detailed discussion of infectious causes, see Chap. 8. Note that the evaluation algorithm above differs slightly from infectious disease guidelines to reflect triage for clinical factors and time course.
- COVID-19/SARS-CoV-2: The novel coronavirus may present with gastrointestinal symptoms. Depending on local epidemiology, this virus should be considered in the differential diagnosis of solid organ transplant recipients presenting with diarrhea. However, optimal diagnostic and treatment strategies are still being determined–local public health guidelines in combination with transplant infectious disease specialists should be consulted regarding assessment for and treatment of COVID-19 in this population.

Key Points

- As with all solid organ transplant recipients presenting with a new symptom, a thorough history and directed exam should be performed.
- An early workup for infectious causes is generally indicated for solid organ transplant recipients who present with diarrhea, especially if other infectious symptoms are present and no obvious recent medication change was made.
- Infectious workup generally includes serum CMV PCR and stool tests for enteric bacterial pathogens (more likely in acute diarrhea), *C. difficile* (any duration), viruses (any duration), and parasitic causes (more likely persistent or chronic).
- Invasive testing with colonoscopy may be required if initial testing is negative, or to assess for CMV gastrointestinal disease and inflammatory bowel disease.
- Consultation with a gastroenterologist and infectious disease specialist is often indicated if the initial workup is negative, or to assist with prioritizing testing and empiric treatment.

Dermatologic Issues in Solid Organ Transplant Recipients

Skin manifestations occur commonly in solid organ transplant recipients. The most common occurrence is skin cancer. Infections, graft versus host disease, and cosmetic complications of immunosuppressive agents should also be considered.

Malignancy

The risk of malignancy increases in solid organ transplant recipients due to the long-term use of immunosuppressive therapies (see Chap. 10). The most common site to develop malignancy is the skin, accounting for up to 40% of malignancies in solid organ transplant recipients. Skin cancers in solid organ transplant recipients are more aggressive, invasive, and metastatic compared to healthy controls [41]. A variety of factors increase the development of skin cancer, including intensity and duration of immunosuppression, ethnic background, sun exposure history, and geographic location. More than 50% of skin cancers will develop in white solid organ transplant recipients with rates of approximately 6% in nonwhite solid organ transplant recipients [42, 43]. Interestingly, as opposed to white patients, in nonwhite patients two-thirds of these skin cancers develop in partial sun-exposed areas or sun-protected areas including the genitals [44]. (Note the terms "white" and "nonwhite" are listed here because these categories were used in these studies).

Regular skin exams are important in the care of the solid organ transplant recipient. The frequency of skin examination may range from once yearly if there is no history of skin cancer or actinic keratosis (AK) to every 3–6 months in the setting of nonmelanoma skin cancers, AKs, and melanomas. The recommended frequency of skin exams varies depending upon risk factors, medical history, degree of immunosuppression, and history of type and number of skin cancers. Rapidly developing tumors, aggressive tumors, or metastatic skin cancer requires more frequent exams usually every 4–6 weeks. Skin cancer exams should also include palpation of lymph nodes. Involvement of dermatologists in the care of solid organ transplant recipients is often indicated. The use of chemoprevention of skin cancer may be appropriate in some patients and should be guided by dermatologists.

Nonmelanoma Skin Cancers (NMSC)

Nonmelanoma skin cancers including squamous cell carcinomas (SCC) and basal cell carcinomas (BCC) occur the most often. However, solid organ transplant recipients are also at risk for melanoma and Kaposi sarcoma. As compared to the general population in whom BCCs are more common, solid organ transplant recipients are 65–250 times more likely to develop SCC and 6–16 times more likely to develop BCC [43, 45, 46]. As the time from transplantation increases, the risk of skin cancer also increases. Based on a large cohort of over 10,000 adult United States transplant recipients who received their primary transplant in 2003 and were followed for a median time of 6 years, the predictors of post-transplant skin cancer included the following (in order of importance): white race, history of pre-transplant skin cancer, age at transplantation ≥50 years, male sex, and thoracic organ transplant [47]. Several other large studies found similar findings and predictors for skin cancer [48, 49].

The proposed pathogenesis for higher rates of skin cancer in solid organ transplant recipients includes the effects of immunosuppressive medications in reducing immune surveillance and leading to the survival and proliferation of atypical cells; direct or contributory carcinogenic effects of the calcineurin inhibitors such as azathioprine and cyclosporine; or proliferation of oncogenic viruses [41].

In patients with very little natural skin pigment, SCC most often develops in sun-exposed areas. The development of SCC on non-sun-exposed areas is much less common overall; however, SCC in sun-protected areas more commonly occurs in patients with more pigmented skin. The development of SCC within areas of chronic inflammation and scarring is also more likely to occur in patients with more pigmented skin. In addition to examining sun-exposed areas, close inspection of the anus, genitalia, and periungual region (most often due to HPV exposure) and sites of chronic inflammation and scarring is important. SCC arising on the external ear or at mucocutaneous interfaces such as the lips, genitalia, and perianal areas tend to be more aggressive with rates of metastasis estimated to range from 10% to 30% [50].

The typical description of an SCC in immunocompetent patients includes the development of one or more red, scaly, well-demarcated superficial plaques. Lesions may also be papular, nodular, skin-colored, or pigmented or present as a cutaneous horn. The pigmented variant is more common in patients with more darkly pigmented skin. The appearance of SCC may change depending upon the location and one should maintain a high level of suspicion when evaluating persistent skin lesions.

Numerous SCC or actinic keratosis may develop in solid organ transplant recipients especially if they have light natural skin pigment and a history of extensive sun exposure. The scalp and back of the hands are common sites for multiple SCC or AKs. The incidence and mortality of SCC are increased in transplant recipients. Solid organ transplant recipients are also more likely to develop lip cancer [51]. Pain is not a typical symptom of SCC; however, in solid organ transplant recipients, this could indicate an invasive tumor which may be associated with increased overall mortality [52].

Nodular basal cell skin cancer is the most common type of BCC; however, there are other subtypes of BCC including superficial, pigmented, and infiltrating. Therefore, high clinical suspicion is needed for BCC when not presenting in the more familiar nodular manner. The typical presentation of nodular BCC in immunocompetent and solid organ transplant recipients is as a pearly papule(s) or nodule(s) with rolled borders and overlying telangiectasias in sun-exposed areas. Ulceration and focal pigmentation are often seen.

Shave, punch, or excisional biopsies may be used for the diagnosis of SCC or BCC. Ideally, biopsies should extend to at least the mid-reticular dermis in order to allow for adequate evaluation of invasive disease. Once diagnosis is confirmed, referral to dermatology surgery for additional resection is often needed.

Melanoma

Melanoma risk is increased in solid organ transplant recipients. Based on information from a large investigation conducted in the United States, it has been shown that the incidence of melanoma increases sharply in the first 4 years after transplantation before declining steadily. Risk also increases with the intensity and duration of immunosuppression. Compared to the general population, the risk of melanoma is more than twofold higher in solid organ transplant recipients with higher rates in kidney transplant recipients than in liver or lung recipients. Male sex, increasing age, and azathioprine maintenance therapy were also associated with increased rates of melanoma [53]. These risk factors along with the use of cyclosporine or sirolimus were confirmed by another large study in renal transplant recipients [54]. Transmission of melanoma from organ donors to organ recipients has also been reported. Compared to non-transplanted patients, melanoma-specific mortality is higher in transplant recipients even when stage and treatment are taken into account [55].

Although melanoma is more common in patients with less skin pigment, the risk of melanoma may still be increased in patients with more skin pigment with certain solid organ transplants. Based on a large study of renal transplant patients, it has been shown that the annual incidence of melanoma was 17 times greater in African-American transplant recipients than in the African-American general population [56].

There are four main subtypes of melanoma: superficial spreading (most common type), nodular melanoma, lentigo maligna melanoma, and acral lentiginous melanoma (the least common type). The appearance of the melanoma will vary based on the subtype but several features will be shared. Utilizing the rules of the ABCDEs when evaluating pigmented lesions is helpful. These include Asymmetry of pigmented lesions, irregularity of Borders, change or variegation of Color, large Diameter (greater than 6 mm), and Evolution. Ulceration and bleeding are generally late signs. The majority of melanomas arise de novo; however, about 30% may arise from a preexisting nevus. Although most melanomas are pigmented, some may appear to lack or contain little pigment and are referred to as amelanotic melanoma.

When suspicion for melanoma is high, punch or excisional biopsy is recommended. Sampling the entire lesion is recommended when possible. Ideally, the biopsy should reach the subcutaneous fat plane. This provides enough depth of tissue for the dermatopathologist to visualize the melanoma and provide accurate staging parameters that guide treatment decisions and prognosis.

Kaposi Sarcoma

Immunosuppression increases the risk of the herpes human virus-8 (HHV-8)-associated Kaposi sarcoma (KS). Rates of KS are highest in males, patients with less skin pigment, and lung transplant recipients. KS develops rapidly after organ transplantation with a mean interval of 13 months [42].

KS lesions may be faint, red-purple macules, papules, plaques, tumors, or nodules. They are often oval and may form along the lines of skin cleavage. In people with more skin pigment, lesions may be more subtle and easy to miss. Assessing for KS should including looking for hues of red and purple on a darker background, and assessment of associated local lymphadenopathy. Koebnerization (lesions occurring in areas of trauma) can occur. Cutaneous and/or mucosal lesions occur approximately 90% of the time. Most common areas of involvement are the trunk and central face, especially the nose. Visceral involvement develops in 25–30% of renal transplant recipients and 50% of heart or liver transplant recipients. The most frequently involved organs include the GI tract, lungs, and lymph nodes [42].

Punch or excisional skin biopsy is recommended for diagnosis and allows for the evaluation of the dermis and subcutis.

Infection

Immunosuppression in the setting of solid organ transplantation predisposes patients to the development of dermatologic infections. Etiology may be bacterial, mycobacterial, viral, or fungal. Often patients will experience co-infections. Human papilloma virus–associated warts are also common. The characteristic appearances of these infections may be altered in the setting of a transplant. Consequently, microbiologic and histologic tests should not be delayed. Within the first 3 months after transplantation, common bacterial and viral infections predominate. In the later period after transplantation, more rare bacterial infections and opportunistic infections such as those caused by fungi may be seen. (See Chap. 8).

Graft-Versus-Host Disease (GVHD)

GVHD is a multisystem disorder which is most commonly a complication of allogeneic hematopoietic cell transplant (HCT) and occurs when the immune cells transplanted from a non-identical donor (the graft) recognize the transplant recipient (host) as foreign, thereby initiating an immune reaction that causes disease in the transplant recipient. The development of GVHD is very rare in solid organ transplant patients but it is potentially lethal. Solid organ transplant–associated GVHD most commonly occurs in liver and small bowel transplants recipients usually between 2 and 6 weeks after transplantation. Late onset cases, however, have been seen in other transplant settings [38].

The clinical presentation of solid organ transplant–associated GVHD is variable. The organs most frequently involved are the skin, liver, and intestinal mucosa. In most cases, GVHD quickly advances to a multisystem disease that affects the bone marrow and other non-transplanted organs [38].

There is both an acute and a chronic form of cutaneous GVHD. Acute disease usually develops within 2–4 weeks of stem cell infusion around the time of engraftment. Chronic cutaneous GVHD usually develops within a mean of 4 months after transplantation [57]. Acute disease typically presents as red to violet maculopapular lesions first appearing on the hands and sole but may progress to the whole body, coalesce, and in severe cases lead to the development of vesicles or bullae or a toxic epidermal necrolysis-like picture. Chronic cutaneous GVHD manifests with mucocutaneous lesions and sclerotic (resembling scleroderma) and non-sclerotic (lichen planus-like) skin lesions. In rare cases, hyperacute cutaneous GVHD can occur with the onset prior to day 14 following transplant. Hyperacute GVHD manifests with high fevers and more severe skin disease [58].

The mortality rate of solid organ transplant–associated GVHD can exceed more than 75% [38]. Skin biopsy may support clinical impression; however, skin biopsies are not always reliable in differentiating GVHD from drug eruptions, viral exanthems, eruption of lymphocyte recovery, and toxic erythema or chemotherapy.

Dermatology involvement is encouraged to aid in diagnosis and treatment. Systemic therapy is generally required for management of patients with acute GVHD. High-potency topical steroids may be helpful in patients with limited skin disease and no systemic involvement.

Cosmesis

Immunosuppressive medications have been associated with a variety of cosmetic skin changes, including but not limited to acne, alopecia, hypertrichosis, sebaceous hyperplasia, stomatitis, gingival hyperplasia, and Cushingoid features. When new dermatologic conditions develop, a review of potential medication side effects is necessary. Common immunosuppressives that may cause cosmetic skin changes include azathioprine, cyclosporine, glucocorticoids, mycophenolate mofetil, rapamycin, and tacrolimus.

> **Key Points**
> - Routine skin exams are recommended for solid organ transplant recipients because of the high incidence of skin cancers.
> - A complete skin exam is indicated, as skin cancers may arise in partial sun-exposed areas or sun-protected areas, especially in patients with more skin pigment.
> - The incidence of both basal cell carcinoma and squamous cell carcinoma is increased in solid organ transplant recipients, but in contrast to the general population, squamous cell carcinoma is relatively more common than basal cell carcinoma.

Conclusion

Care of the solid organ transplant recipient will require the primary care provider to be familiar with common symptoms that may be first encountered in the outpatient clinic, including respiratory symptoms, urinary symptoms, diarrhea, and skin problems. The initial approach to evaluating these symptoms requires recognizing key differences between solid organ transplant recipients and the general population, including having an expanded differential diagnosis, being aware of medication side effects, considering an increased risk of infection and malignancy, and knowing when a workup needs to be performed more quickly or with more testing. In many cases, earlier consultation or triage to a higher level of care is necessary. With attentive care, the primary care provider can appropriately evaluate, triage, and manage the solid organ transplant recipient who presents to the outpatient clinic with these symptoms.

References

1. Rui P, Okeyode T. National Ambulatory Medical Care Survey: 2016 National Summary Tables. Available from: https://www.cdc.gov/nchs/data/ahcd/namcs_summary/2016_namcs_web_tables.pdf accessed 6/3/2019.
2. Marks WH, Florence L, Lieberman J, Chapman P, Howard D, Roberts P, Perkinson D. Successfully treated invasive pulmonary aspergillosis associated with smoking marijuana in a renal transplant recipient. Transplantation. 1996;61(12):1771–4.
3. Giannella M, Muñoz P, Alarcón JM, Mularoni A, Grossi P. Bouza E; PISOT study group. Pneumonia in solid organ transplant recipients: a prospective multicenter study. Transpl Infect Dis. 2014;16(2):232–41. https://doi.org/10.1111/tid.12193.
4. Bonatti H, Pruett TL, Brandacher G, Hagspiel KD, Housseini AM, Sifri CD, Sawyer RG. Pneumonia in solid organ recipients: spectrum of pathogens in 217 episodes. Transplant Proc. 2009;41(1):371–4. https://doi.org/10.1016/j.transproceed.2008.10.045.
5. Wang EZ, Partovi N, Levy RD, Shapiro RJ, Yoshida EM, Greanya ED. Pneumocystis pneumonia in solid organ transplant recipients: not yet an infection of the past. Transpl Infect Dis. 2012;14(5):519–25. https://doi.org/10.1111/j.1399-3062.2012.00740.x.
6. Iriart X, Challan Belval T, Fillaux J, Esposito L, Lavergne RA, Cardeau-Desangles I, Roques O, Del Bello A, Cointault O, Lavayssière L, Chauvin P, Menard S, Magnaval JF, Cassaing S, Rostaing L, Kamar N, Berry A. Risk factors of Pneumocystis pneumonia in solid organ recipients in the era of the common use of posttransplantation prophylaxis. Am J Transplant. 2015;15(1):190–9. https://doi.org/10.1111/ajt.12947.
7. De La Cruz O, Silveira FP. Respiratory fungal infections in solid organ and hematopoietic stem cell transplantation. Clin Chest Med. 2017;38(4):727–39. https://doi.org/10.1016/j.ccm.2017.07.013.
8. Koval CE. Prevention and treatment of Cytomegalovirus infections in solid organ transplant recipients. Infect Dis Clin N Am. 2018;32(3):581–97. https://doi.org/10.1016/j.idc.2018.04.008.
9. Acuna SA, Fernandes KA, Daly C, Hicks LK, Sutradhar R, Kim SJ, Baxter NN. Cancer mortality among recipients of solid-organ transplantation in Ontario. Canada JAMA Oncol. 2016 Apr;2(4):463–9. https://doi.org/10.1001/jamaoncol.2015.5137.
10. Lengwiler E, Stampf S, Zippelius A, Salati E, Zaman K, Schäfer N, Schardt J, Siano M, Hofbauer G, The Swiss Transplant Cohort Study. Solid cancer development in solid organ transplant recipients within the Swiss transplant cohort study. Swiss Med Wkly. 2019;149:w20078. https://doi.org/10.4414/smw.2019.20078.
11. Engels EA, Pfeiffer RM, Fraumeni JF Jr, Kasiske BL, Israni AK, Snyder JJ, Wolfe RA, Goodrich NP, Bayakly AR, Clarke CA, Copeland G, Finch JL, Fleissner ML, Goodman MT, Kahn A, Koch L, Lynch CF, Madeleine MM, Pawlish K, Rao C, Williams MA, Castenson D, Curry M, Parsons R, Fant G, Lin M. Spectrum of cancer risk among US solid organ transplant recipients. JAMA. 2011;306(17):1891–901. https://doi.org/10.1001/jama.2011.1592.
12. Aboagye JK, Hayanga JWA, Lau BD, Bush EL, Shaffer DL, Hobson DB, Kraus PS, Streiff MB, Haut ER, D'Cunha J. Venous thromboembolism in patients hospitalized for lung transplantation. Ann Thorac Surg. 2018;105(4):1071–6. https://doi.org/10.1016/j.athoracsur.2017.10.041.
13. Sáez-Giménez B, Berastegui C, Loor K, López-Meseguer M, Monforte V, Bravo C, Santamaría A, Roman A. Deep vein thrombosis and pulmonary embolism after solid organ transplantation: an unresolved problem. Transplant Rev (Orlando). 2015;29(2):85–92. https://doi.org/10.1016/j.trre.2014.12.005.
14. Tsai HI, Liu F, Lee CW, Kuo CF, See LC, Chung TT, Yu HP. Cardiovascular disease risk in patients receiving organ transplantation: a national cohort study. Transpl Int. 2017;30(11):1161–71. https://doi.org/10.1111/tri.13010.
15. Abbott KC, Cruess DF, Agodoa LY, Sawyers ES, Tveit DP. Early renal insufficiency and late venous thromboembolism after renal transplantation in the United States. Am J Kidney Dis. 2004;43(1):120–30.

16. Tveit DP, Hypolite I, Bucci J, Hshieh P, Cruess D, Agodoa LY, Welch PG, Abbott KC. Risk factors for hospitalizations resulting from pulmonary embolism after renal transplantation in the United States. J Nephrol. 2001;14(5):361–8.
17. Siddiqui AS, Zimmerman JL. Everolimus associated interstitial pneumonitis in a liver transplant patient. Respir Med Case Rep. 2016;19:15–7. https://doi.org/10.1016/j.rmcr.2016.06.004.
18. Baas MC, Struijk GH, Moes DJ, van den Berk IA, Jonkers RE, de Fijter JW, van der Heide JJ, van Dijk M, ten Berge IJ, Bemelman FJ. Interstitial pneumonitis caused by everolimus: a case-cohort study in renal transplant recipients. Transpl Int. 2014;27(5):428–36. https://doi.org/10.1111/tri.12275.
19. Champion L, Stern M, Israël-Biet D, Mamzer-Bruneel MF, Peraldi MN, Kreis H, Porcher R, Morelon E. Brief communication: sirolimus-associated pneumonitis: 24 cases in renal transplant recipients. Ann Intern Med. 2006;144(7):505–9.
20. Gillis KA, Patel RK, Jardine AG. Cardiovascular complications after transplantation: treatment options in solid organ recipients. Transplant Rev (Orlando). 2014;28(2):47–55. https://doi.org/10.1016/j.trre.2013.12.001.
21. Franquet T, Lee KS, Müller NL. Thin-section CT findings in 32 immunocompromised patients with cytomegalovirus pneumonia who do not have AIDS. AJR Am J Roentgenol. 2003;181(4):1059–63.
22. Moon SM, Sung H, Kim MN, Lee SO, Choi SH, Kim YS, Woo JH, Kim SH. Diagnostic yield of the cytomegalovirus (CMV) antigenemia assay and clinical features in solid organ transplant recipients and hematopoietic stem cell transplant recipients with CMV pneumonia. Transpl Infect Dis. 2012;14(2):192–7. https://doi.org/10.1111/j.1399-3062.2011.00703.x.
23. Freedman ND, Silverman DT, Hollenbeck AR, Schatzkin A, Abnet CC. Association between smoking and risk of bladder cancer among men and women. JAMA. 2011 Aug 17;306(7):737–45. https://doi.org/10.1001/jama.2011.1142.
24. Vidal E, Torre-Cisneros J, Blanes M, Montejo M, Cervera C, Aguado JM, Len O, Carratalá J, Cordero E, Bou G, Muñoz P, Ramos A, Gurguí M, Borrell N, Fortún J, Spanish Network for Research in Infectious Diseases (REIPI). Bacterial urinary tract infection after solid organ transplantation in the RESITRA cohort. Transpl Infect Dis. 2012;14(6):595–603. https://doi.org/10.1111/j.1399-3062.2012.00744.x.
25. Parasuraman R, Julian K, AST Infectious Diseases Community of Practice. Urinary tract infections in solid organ transplantation. Am J Transplant. 2013;13(Suppl 4):327–36. https://doi.org/10.1111/ajt.12124.
26. Goldman JD, Julian K. Urinary tract infections in solid organ transplant recipients: guidelines from the American Society of Transplantation infectious diseases Community of Practice. Clin Transpl. 2019;21:e13507. https://doi.org/10.1111/ctr.13507.
27. Meyrier A. Sampling and evaluation of voided urine in the diagnosis of urinary tract infection in adults. In: UpToDate, Post, TW (editor). UpToDate, Waltham, MA. Accessed online 1/27/2020.
28. Vidal E, Cervera C, Cordero E, Armiñanzas C, Carratalá J, Cisneros JM, Fariñas MC, López-Medrano F, Moreno A, Muñoz P, Origüen J, Sabé N, Valerio M, Torre-Cisneros J, Study Group of Infection in Transplant Recipients (GESITRA) of the Spanish Society of Infectious Diseases, Clinical Microbiology (SEIMC), Spanish Network for Research in Infectious Diseases (REIPI). Management of urinary tract infection in solid organ transplant recipients: consensus statement of the Group for the Study of infection in transplant recipients (GESITRA) of the Spanish Society of Infectious Diseases and Clinical Microbiology (SEIMC) and the Spanish network for research in infectious diseases (REIPI). Enferm Infecc Microbiol Clin. 2015;33(10):679.e1–679.e21. https://doi.org/10.1016/j.eimc.2015.03.024.
29. Angarone M, Snydman DR. Diagnosis and management of diarrhea in solid-organ transplant recipients: guidelines from the American Society of Transplantation infectious diseases Community of Practice. Clin Transpl. 2019;33:e13550.
30. Cusini A, Béguelin C, Stampf S, Boggian K, Garzoni C, Koller M, Manuel O, Meylan P, Mueller NJ, Hirsch HH, Weisser M, Berger C, van Delden C, Swiss Transplant Cohort Study.

Clostridium difficile infection is associated with graft loss in solid organ transplant recipients. Am J Transplant. 2018;18(7):1745–54. https://doi.org/10.1111/ajt.14640.

31. Boutros M, Al-Shaibi M, Chan G, Cantarovich M, Rahme E, Paraskevas S, Deschenes M, Ghali P, Wong P, Fernandez M, Giannetti N, Cecere R, Hassanain M, Chaudhury P, Metrakos P, Tchervenkov J, Barkun JS. Clostridium difficile colitis: increasing incidence, risk factors, and outcomes in solid organ transplant recipients. Transplantation. 2012;93(10):1051–7. https://doi.org/10.1097/TP.0b013e31824d34de.

32. Loo VG, Bourgault AM, Poirier L, Lamothe F, Michaud S, Turgeon N, Toye B, Beaudoin A, Frost EH, Gilca R, Brassard P, Dendukuri N, Béliveau C, Oughton M, Brukner I, Dascal A. Host and pathogen factors for Clostridium difficile infection and colonization. N Engl J Med. 2011;365(18):1693–703.

33. Ponticelli C, Passerini P. Gastrointestinal complications in renal transplant recipients. Transpl Int. 2005;18(6):643–50.

34. Razonable RR, Humar A. Cytomegalovirus in solid organ transplant recipients-guidelines of the American Society of Transplantation infectious diseases Community of Practice. Clin Transpl. 2019;33(9):e13512. https://doi.org/10.1111/ctr.13512.

35. Arslan H, Inci EK, Azap OK, Karakayali H, Torgay A, Haberal M. Etiologic agents of diarrhea in solid organ recipients. Transpl Infect Dis. 2007;9:270–5.

36. Al-Absi AI, Cooke CR, Wall BM, Sylvestre P, Ismail MK, Mya M. Patterns of injury in mycophenolate mofetil-related colitis. Transplant Proc. 2010;42(9):3591–3. https://doi.org/10.1016/j.transproceed.2010.08.066.

37. Behrend M. Adverse gastrointestinal effects of mycophenolate mofetil: aetiology, incidence and management. Drug Saf. 2001;24(9):645–63.

38. Zhang Y, Ruiz P. Solid organ transplant-associated acute graft-versus-host disease. Arch Pathol Lab Med. 2010;134(8):1220–4.

39. Pant C, Deshpande A, Larson A, O'Connor J, Rolston DD, Sferra TJ. Diarrhea in solid-organ transplant recipients: a review of the evidence. Curr Med Res Opin. 2013;29(10):1315–28. https://doi.org/10.1185/03007995.2013.816278.

40. Hampton DD, Poleski MH, Onken JE. Inflammatory bowel disease following solid organ transplantation. Clin Immunol. 2008;128(3):287–93. https://doi.org/10.1016/j.clim.2008.06.011.

41. Athar M, Walsh SB, Kopelovich L, Elmets CA. Pathogenesis of nonmelanoma skin cancers in organ transplant recipients. Arch Biochem Biophys. 2011;508(2):159–63. https://doi.org/10.1016/j.abb.2011.01.004.

42. Euvrard S, Kanitakis J, Claudy A. Skin cancers after organ transplantation. N Engl J Med. 2003;348(17):1681.

43. Greenberg JN, Zwald FO. Management of skin cancer in solid-organ transplant recipients: a multidisciplinary approach. Dermatol Clin. 2011;29(2):231.

44. Chung CL, Nadhan KS, Shaver CM, Ogrich LM, Abdelmalek M, Cusack CA, Malat GE, Pritchett EN, Doyle A. Comparison of posttransplant dermatologic diseases by race. JAMA Dermatol. 2017;153(6):552–8. https://doi.org/10.1001/jamadermatol.2017.0045.

45. Moloney FJ, Comber H, O'Lorcain P, O'Kelly P, Conlon PJ, Murphy GM. A population-based study of skin cancer incidence and prevalence in renal transplant recipients. Br J Dermatol. 2006;154(3):498.

46. Krynitz B, Olsson H, Lundh Rozell B, Lindelöf B, Edgren G, Smedby KE. Risk of basal cell carcinoma in Swedish organ transplant recipients: a population-based study. Br J Dermatol. 2016;174(1):95–103. Epub 2015 Dec 21.

47. Garrett GL, Blanc PD, Boscardin J, Lloyd AA, Ahmed RL, Anthony T, Bibee K, Breithaupt A, Cannon J, Chen A, Cheng JY, Chiesa-Fuxench Z, Colegio OR, Curiel-Lewandrowski C, Del Guzzo CA, Disse M, Dowd M, Eilers R Jr, Ortiz AE, Morris C, Golden SK, Graves MS, Griffin JR, Hopkins RS, Huang CC, Bae GH, Jambusaria A, Jennings TA, Jiang SI, Karia PS, Khetarpal S, Kim C, Klintmalm G, Konicke K, Koyfman SA, Lam C, Lee P, Leitenberger JJ, Loh T, Lowenstein S, Madankumar R, Moreau JF, Nijhawan RI, Ochoa S, Olasz EB, Otchere E, Otley C, Oulton J, Patel PH, Patel VA, Prabhu AV, Pugliano-Mauro M, Schmults CD,

Schram S, Shih AF, Shin T, Soon S, Soriano T, Srivastava D, Stein JA, Sternhell-Blackwell K, Taylor S, Vidimos A, Wu P, Zajdel N, Zelac D, Arron ST. Incidence of and risk factors for skin cancer in organ transplant recipients in the United States. JAMA Dermatol. 2017;153(3):296.
48. Park CK, Fung K, Austin PC, Kim SJ, Singer LG, Baxter NN, Rochon PA, Chan AW. Incidence and risk factors of keratinocyte carcinoma after first solid organ transplant in Ontario, Canada JAMA Dermatol. 2019. https://doi.org/10.1001/jamadermatol.2019.0692. [Epub ahead of print].
49. Kang W, Sampaio MS, Huang E, Bunnapradist S. Association of Pretransplant skin cancer with posttransplant malignancy, graft failure and death in kidney transplant recipients. Transplantation. 2017;101(6):1303.
50. Veness MJ. Defining patients with high-risk cutaneous squamous cell carcinoma. Australas J Dermatol. 2006;47(1):28.
51. Laprise C, Cahoon EK, Lynch CF, Kahn AR, Copeland G, Gonsalves L, Madeleine MM, Pfeiffer RM, Engels EA. Risk of lip cancer after solid organ transplantation in the United States. Am J Transplant. 2019;19(1):227. Epub 2018 Sep 5.
52. Kwatra SG, Mills KC, Zeitany A, Pearce DJ, Williford PM, D'Agostino RB Jr, Yosipovitch G. Pain and nonmelanoma skin cancer in transplant patients. J Am Acad Dermatol. 2012;67(6):1387.
53. Robbins HA, Clarke CA, Arron ST, Tatalovich Z, Kahn AR, Hernandez BY, Paddock L, Yanik EL, Lynch CF, Kasiske BL, Snyder J, Engels EA. Melanoma risk and survival among organ transplant recipients. J Invest Dermatol. 2015;135(11):2657.
54. Ascha M, Ascha MS, Tanenbaum J, Bordeaux JS. Risk factors for melanoma in renal transplant recipients. JAMA Dermatol. 2017;153(11):1130.
55. D'Arcy ME, Coghill AE, Lynch CF, Koch LA, Li J, Pawlish KS, Morris CR, Rao C, Engels EA. Survival after a cancer diagnosis among solid organ transplant recipients in the United States. Cancer. 2019;125(6):933.
56. Hollenbeak CS, Todd MM, Billingsley EM, Harper G, Dyer AM, Lengerich EJ. Increased incidence of melanoma in renal transplantation recipients. Cancer. 2005;104(9):1962.
57. Vargas-Díez E, García-Díez A, Marín A, Fernández-Herrera J. Life-threatening graft-vs-host disease. Clin Dermatol. 2005;23(3):285.
58. Hymes SR, Alousi AM, Cowen EW. Graft-versus-host disease: part I. pathogenesis and clinical manifestations of graft-versus-host disease. J Am Acad Dermatol. 2012;66(4):515.e1–18; quiz 533-4.

Chapter 10
Cancer Risk in the Adult Solid Organ Transplant Recipient

Deborah Greenberg

Introduction

Cancer is a leading cause of morbidity and death in solid organ transplant (SOT) recipients [1–3]. The overall malignancy risk is higher in this population for a variety of reasons, including factors related to the recipient's underlying medical conditions, oncogenic viruses, and therapeutic immunosuppression. This increased risk is often expressed as excess absolute risk (EAR) of developing cancer compared to the general age-matched population, the standardized incidence ratio (SIR)—the number of observed cancers in solid organ transplant recipients divided by the expected number of cases in the general population, or the standardized mortality ratio (SMR)—the observed cancer deaths in solid organ transplant recipients compared to the expected in the general population. The cancers with the greatest increased incidence are skin cancer, post-transplant lymphoproliferative disorders (PTLD), and solid tumors of the lung, liver, and kidney [4]. Malignancy in solid organ transplant recipients is often more aggressive, more difficult to treat, and portends a poorer prognosis compared to the non-transplant population [2]. Solid organ transplant recipients have an increased risk of cancer-related death that is greater than twice the general population [2, 5]. Screening for precancerous and cancerous lesions as well as risk factors for post-transplant malignancy such as viral infections and smoking is paramount prior to transplantation. Following solid organ transplantation, increased surveillance is essential for early diagnosis and treatment of this potentially devastating complication. The primary care provider can play a vital role in the prevention and diagnosis of cancer in solid organ transplant recipients.

D. Greenberg (✉)
Division of General Internal Medicine, Department of Medicine, University of Washington, Seattle, WA, USA
e-mail: debbiegr@uw.edu

© Springer Nature Switzerland AG 2020
C. J. Wong (ed.), *Primary Care of the Solid Organ Transplant Recipient*,
https://doi.org/10.1007/978-3-030-50629-2_10

Overview

In the United States, a solid organ transplant recipient's risk for post-transplant cancer is estimated to be 1000–1500 per 100,000 person-years. This is over 2 times that of the general population and an EAR of 0.7% per year [4]. The cumulative 5-year, 10-year, and 20-year incidence of non-cutaneous cancer following transplantation is roughly 4–7% [6], 10–15% [7, 8], and 20–30% [8], respectively. In general, the risk increases with age and has been found to be higher in men [4], although a Catalonian study of kidney transplant recipients found a significant increased risk in women only (SIR 1.18) [8]. Patients transplanted at a younger age have the greatest overall increased risk of cancer (15–30 times the risk of peers) compared to patients transplanted later in life (risk 2 times greater if transplanted at age > 65 years) [9]. The mean time to develop post-transplant solid tumors is 4–6 years [3, 10]. Lung transplant recipients have the highest cumulative incidence of non-cutaneous malignancy followed by heart, liver, and then kidney recipients [6]. Cancer mortality following solid organ transplantation is also significantly elevated compared to the general population (SMR 2.84) [3]. Using mortality data from over 11, 000 solid organ transplant recipients with cancer in the Transplant Cancer Match Study, D'Arcy and colleagues found that death from certain cancers was higher in this population compared to patients with the same cancer but no prior transplantation. This increase in cancer-specific mortality was particularly true for melanoma, bladder cancer, and breast cancer [11].

Immunosuppression magnifies known risk factors for cancer including host behaviors (smoking, alcohol intake, sun exposure) and oncogenic infectious agents, primarily viral. Proposed mechanisms of malignant pathogenesis in solid organ transplant recipients beyond immunosuppression and oncogenic infections include chronic inflammation, immune activation, and loss of immune surveillance from underlying medical conditions. Similarities have been drawn between the increased risk of cancer in patients with human immunodeficiency virus (HIV) and patients who have received solid organ transplantation. While the increased risk of several types of cancers is similar between these immunosuppressed patient populations, transplant recipients have increased susceptibility to some malignancies, including colorectal and thyroid cancers, which are not increased in the patients with HIV.

Overall survival following the diagnosis of malignancy in the post-transplantation setting is poor. In a study of post-liver transplantation recipients, 10-year overall survival was 49.4% in patients who developed a solid organ cancer compared to 88.3% without cancer [7]. Treatment of malignancy following solid organ transplantation is not straightforward. Consideration must be given to the overall prognosis of the patient, the need for maintenance immune suppression to prevent graft rejection, and the increased risk for infection, organ dysfunction, and drug interactions.

Predisposing Factors

Underlying Medical Conditions and Behaviors

Certain underlying chronic medical conditions for which the patient may undergo solid organ transplantation such as end-stage renal disease (ESRD), cirrhosis, and chronic obstructive pulmonary disease (COPD) are themselves associated with an increased risk of malignancy. Patients treated with dialysis for end-stage renal disease (ESRD) are at significantly increased risk for cancers of the kidney, bladder, thyroid, liver, skin, lungs, and multiple myeloma even without kidney transplantation [12, 13]. Patients with COPD are at higher risk for lung cancer and colorectal cancer (CRC) than the general population. In a Swedish study, patients with COPD were at significantly increased risk of post-lung transplantation skin cancer (SIR 27), lung cancer (SIR 19.8), CRC (SIR 11.4), and non-Hodgkin lymphoma (NHL) (SIR 39) compared to those without COPD [14].

Smoking and alcohol are risk factors for malignancy in the general population, especially for cancers of the head and neck, esophagus, lungs, kidney, and urinary tract. Solid organ transplant recipients who used tobacco or alcohol in excess prior to transplantation or who resume use following transplantation are at increased risk for de novo malignancy. As an example, patients who received a liver transplant for alcoholic liver disease and those with a prior history of alcohol abuse have a two- to threefold increased risk of de novo solid tumors following transplant [15–17]. A history of prior smoking or active smoking are also independent risk factors (RR 8.5, 4.4, respectively) for post-liver transplant de novo smoking-related (lung, oral, esophageal, urinary tract) cancers [15–17].

Obesity has been identified as an independent risk factor for de novo malignancy following liver transplantation, especially in non-smoking-related malignancies [15].

Oncogenic Infections

Epstein-Barr virus (EBV), human herpes virus 8 (HHV-8), human papilloma virus (HPV), hepatitis B, hepatitis C, cytomegalovirus (CMV), and the Merkel cell polyomavirus have been implicated as causative agents in malignancies that develop after solid organ transplantation.

Human papillomavirus (HPV), a sexually transmitted, double-stranded DNA virus that infects mucosal and cutaneous epithelial cells, is typically held in check by T-cell-mediated immunity. Certain high-risk strains (hrHPV), especially 16 and 18, are felt to be a causative agent and promote growth of certain types of oral, cervical, vaginal, vulvar, penile, and anal cancers. Loss of cell-mediated immunity due to post-transplant immunosuppressive medications leads to viral reactivation in latently infected cells, reduces a patient's ability to spontaneously clear new HPV infections, and subsequently leads to malignant transformation and promotion in mucosal and cutaneous epithelial cells [18]. As a consequence, HPV-related precancerous and cancerous lesions are seen more frequently in solid organ transplant recipients [4, 19]. The role of HPV in squamous cell carcinoma of the skin in post-transplant patient is less clear but may be a contributing factor [18].

Epstein-Barr virus (EBV) is a major contributor in most cases of post-transplant lymphoproliferative disorder (PTLD) [20]. Iatrogenic immunosuppression leads to poor immune control of EBV, B-cell transformation, and proliferation through a variety of mechanisms.

Immunosuppressive Medications

Immunosuppression likely plays the largest role in the increased cancer incidence seen in solid organ transplant recipients. The interactions between immunity and cancer development are unique to this patient population due to the need for therapeutic immunosuppression to prevent graft rejection following solid organ transplantation. Immunosuppressant medications promote malignant tendencies of oncogenic viruses, but some are also likely carcinogenic themselves. A variety of mechanisms that create an imbalance in the immune response, as well as direct DNA damage, have been proposed. The type, intensity, and duration of immunosuppressive agents all seem to contribute to the malignancy risk.

Immunosuppressants in general, but calcineurin inhibitors (CNIs) in particular, contribute to malignancy development following solid organ transplantation largely through their impact on T cells. With CNIs, specifically cyclosporine and tacrolimus, this appears to be a dose-dependent and cumulative dose effect [15]. As the name suggests, CNIs inhibit calcineurin, a phosphatase important in T-cell proliferation. A higher mean blood concentration of calcineurin inhibitor or a greater cumulative dose is associated with a greater risk of post-transplant malignancy. In a study of 247 liver transplant recipients, patients with the highest tacrolimus blood mean concentrations were twice as likely to develop solid organ tumors [7].

The anti-proliferation agent azathioprine has also been implicated in the promotion of malignancy in solid organ transplant recipients. Azathioprine, which impacts DNA repair mechanisms and boosts photosensitivity, is associated with elevated risk of nonmelanoma skin cancers and PTLD. In a meta-analysis incorporating data from 27 studies, azathioprine increased the incidence of squamous cell carcinoma of the skin in a variety of transplant recipients (HR 1.56) compared to other immunosuppression regimens [21].

Immunosuppressive medications which may be associated with a lower risk of post-transplant malignancy include sirolimus, a mammalian target of rapamycin (mTOR) inhibitor, and mycophenolate mofetil (MMF) and its active metabolite, mycophenolic acid (MPA). mTOR inhibitors may have an antineoplastic effect in some settings and look promising in reducing the impact of squamous cell skin cancer in post-transplantation populations, although this finding has not been consistently seen [22–26].

Donor-Transmitted Cancer

Rare reports of cancers thought to be transmitted by the donor organ have occurred. Living donors are screened based on age and gender appropriate guidelines. Despite adequate screening, donor-derived cancers may occur as frequently as once per 5000 living donations [1].

Skin and Lip Cancer

Nonmelanoma skin cancer (NMSC) is the most common cancer seen in solid organ transplant recipients [27, 28]. In contrast to the general population, squamous cell carcinoma (SCC) is more commonly seen than basal cell carcinoma (BCC) by a ratio of 4:1 [1]. Solid organ transplant recipients are at much greater risk (30- to 50-fold) of nonmelanoma skin cancers including SCC (50- to 100-fold), BCC (tenfold), Merkel cell carcinoma (MCC), and Kaposi's sarcoma (50-fold) compared to the general population [1, 27]. They also have poorer outcomes from these malignancies, including death (SMR 29.82) [3, 22].

In a large study of US solid organ transplant recipients, the overall incidence rate of skin cancer was 1437 per 100,000 person-years with the vast majority (94%) being SCC (1355 per 100,00 person-years). Melanoma is much less common to (125 per 100,000 person-years) [27]. The incidence of squamous cell skin cancer following solid organ transplantation may be declining with changes in the intensity and types of therapeutic immunosuppression regimens [29]. Medications including calcineurin inhibitors and azathioprine appear to confer a greater risk of SCC compared to mTOR inhibitors.

Risks for post-transplant SCC include pre-transplant skin cancer, age > 50 years at time of transplant, male gender, white race, time period during which the transplant was performed (reflecting immunosuppression regimen used in that era), and type of organ received [27, 29]. Heart transplant recipients have the highest risk, followed by lung transplant recipients. The SIRs in a Norwegian study were 51.9 for SCC, 2.4 for melanoma, and 54.9 for Kaposi's sarcoma. Additional risk factors in this study included sun exposure and time since transplant. Not surprisingly, human herpesvirus 8 (HHV-8) infection was a risk factor for Kaposi's sarcoma [29].

Patients should be screened regularly for skin changes and receive education regarding the use of sunscreen, sun exposure avoidance, and the need to report any skin changes to their primary care provider. Potentially precancerous lesions such as actinic keratoses should be treated aggressively as they have a greater chance of malignant transformation (30%) compared to the general population (1–10%). Following an initial diagnosis of skin cancer, solid organ transplant recipients are at high risk for recurrent skin cancer [22].

Solid organ transplant recipients also have a higher incidence of in situ (SIR 26.2) and invasive lip cancer (SIR 15.3) [30]. Risk factors for cancer of the lip in this population include male gender, white race, prior NMSC, and treatment with azathioprine or cyclosporine. In addition to a thorough skin exam, primary care providers should examine the lips for any changes as part of their regular examination in this population.

PTLD (Post-Transplant Lymphoproliferative Disorder)

Epidemiology

In the United States, post-transplant lymphoproliferative disorder (PTLD) represents 20% of post-SOT malignancy and is the second most common cancer following solid organ transplantation [4]. In the adult solid organ transplant population, non-Hodgkin lymphoma (NHL), particularly diffuse B-cell lymphoma, is a feared complication. The risk of non-Hodgkin lymphoma is sevenfold greater than the general population with an incidence of 194 per 100,000 person-years and an excess risk of 168.3 per 100,000 person-years [4]. Non-Hodgkin lymphoma was the most common cancer-related death (SMR 16.6) in a cohort of liver and cardiothoracic transplant recipients [5]. Both nodal and extra-nodal lymphomas occur more frequently in solid organ transplant recipients. The risk is lower if the transplant occurs between the ages of 35 and 50 years as opposed to <35 or > 50 years. The risk for non-Hodgkin lymphoma varies by the type of organ transplanted (lung > heart, liver > kidney). The risk of death from NHL is significantly higher in this patient population compared to non-transplant patients (SMR 9.76) [3]. Heart and lung transplant recipients are at the greatest increased risk of death from NHL [3]. PTLD causes significant risk to the patient due to the need to reduce immunosuppression, the potential for the cancer directly involving the allograft, and the impact of treatment (e.g. chemotherapy, surgery, radiation, antiviral therapy), which can further cause infection, organ dysfunction, and mortality.

Pathophysiology and Classification

PTLD is a heterogeneous, typically multisystem, group of lymphoid disorders. PTLD is due largely to the EBV-fueled proliferation of the recipient's lymphoid cells, primarily B cells, and has a wide range of clinical presentations. EBV plays a role in many cases of PTLD, especially those occurring in the early (<1 year) post-transplant period. Primary EBV infection from the donor organ or the community can be causal in adults, but more commonly occurs in children who were EBV

Table 10.1 2017 World Health Organization histopathological classification of PTLD [20]

Non-destructive PTLDs
Plasmacytic hyperplasia
Infectious mononucleosis
Florid follicular hyperplasia
Polymorphic PTLD
Monomorphic PTLDs
B-cell neoplasms
Diffuse large B-cell lymphoma
Burkitt lymphoma
Plasma cell myeloma
Plasmacytoma
Other
T-cell neoplasms
Peripheral T-cell lymphoma, NOS
Hepatosplenic T-cell lymphoma
Other
Classical Hodgkin lymphoma PTLD

Reprinted with permission

seronegative at the time of transplant. In the vast majority of cases, previously latent EBV-infected recipient B lymphocytes multiply in the setting of impaired T-cell immunity from therapeutic immunosuppression. PTLD originating from the donor organ is generally limited to the allograft in EBV seropositive recipients but can be more widespread in EBV naïve patients who receive an EBV-positive organ. Cases of EBV-negative PTLD are less common although may be increasing and associated with a later onset and poorer outcomes [20, 31].

There are six main subtypes of PTLD (Table 10.1). Monomorphic PTLD, the most common form of PTLD in adult solid organ transplant recipients, encompasses B- and less frequently T-cell lymphomas. Plasmacytic hyperplasia typically manifests as early involvement of lymph tissue, is seen in EBV seronegative recipients, and can regress spontaneously. Polymorphic PTLD is the most common subtype seen in children.

Risk Factors

Overall, the lifetime risk of PTLD is approximately 1–4% in adults and 8% in children [32, 33]. Incidence ranges vary based on organ transplanted and period of time studied (range 3 years to 20 years): 1–3% with kidney and liver transplant, 1–12% in heart and lung recipients, and 20–30% with small bowel transplant [20, 31]. Risk factors for PTLD include not only the type of transplant, but also age and EBV status of the patient at the time of transplantation and the type and intensity of immunosuppression (Table 10.2). Younger patients (age 0–35 years), particularly those who are EBV seronegative at time of transplantation, have the highest risk [32, 33]. Lung and heart recipients over age 50 years also have higher risk, perhaps due to the immunosuppressive regimens used for these transplants [6, 20]. Because

Table 10.2 Risk factors for PTLD[a]

Type of transplant
Small intestine > heart, lung > liver, kidney
Age
Younger age
Heart and lung transplant recipients over age 50
EBV serostatus
Donor positive/recipient negative (D+/R−) highest risk
Type of immunosuppression
T-cell depleting induction therapies (e.g., OKT3 ®, ATG)

[a]Precise estimates vary by study; general risk factors and trends are shown in this table

latent EBV-infected B lymphocytes are held in check by cytotoxic T-lymphocytes (CTLs), immunosuppression regimens that impair or deplete these T cells, such as the induction agents muromonab-CD3 (OKT3 ®) and anti-thymocyte globulin (ATG), increase risk for B-cell proliferation and PTLD [34].

Presentation

Patients may be asymptomatic, but common symptoms are non-specific including sore throat, fever, night sweats, abdominal pain, weight loss, and fatigue [20]. Patients may also present because of site-specific symptoms, such as a new-onset cough with lung involvement, bleeding in gastrointestinal tract PTLD, or altered mental status or headache with central nervous system disease. Patients should be monitored closely if they develop new symptoms and PTLD considered if symptoms do not improve or resolve as expected.

PTLD tends to occur early (within 1 year of transplant), late (4–7 years or more after transplant), or very late (>7–10 years after transplant) [4, 20, 33]. In a group of US kidney transplant recipients with PTLD, 58% occurred in the first year after transplantation [32]. EBV-negative PTLD tends to occur later. PTLD can involve nodal and extra-nodal sites. Extra-nodal sites may include the allograft (10–15% of cases), and can lead to organ dysfunction, or may involve the central nervous system (CNS) (5–20% of cases), skin, GI tract (20–30% of cases), lungs, or liver [35]. PTLD primarily involved the allograft in years 0–2 post-transplant, CNS in years 2–7, and GI tract in late disease (>7 years).

Evaluation of patients with suspected PTLD is the same as the work-up of suspected lymphoproliferative disorder in a non-transplant patient. Physical exam should be comprehensive, especially if the patient only has constitutional symptoms; a thorough lymph node exam should be performed. Directed additional exam may be indicated based on risks and symptoms, such as a neurologic exam if CNS involvement is suspected.

Laboratory testing can be used to bolster suspicion of potential PTLD and includes complete blood count, liver and kidney function, electrolytes, uric acid, lactate dehydrogenase, serum, and urine protein electrophoresis. EBV viral load testing can be used to monitor treatment, but its role in the diagnosis of PTLD is not as clear [20, 31, 35].

Advanced imaging studies (e.g., cross-sectional imaging such as CT and MRI) are frequently needed to make a diagnosis of PTLD. Additionally, imaging studies are used to identify a biopsy site and for staging. Excisional biopsy is the key to diagnosis whenever possible. If the optimal approach to obtaining a tissue sample is uncertain, early consultation with a hematologist-oncologist and the transplant team is recommended. There is no separate staging or scoring system for PTLD.

Because of late presentations, and symptoms potentially far from the allograft, patients are likely to present to primary care, not recognizing that they may have a transplant-related condition—therefore a high index of suspicion is critical to making this diagnosis.

Treatment

Prognosis after a diagnosis of PTLD is poor. Overall survival in kidney transplant recipients with PTLD ranges from 53% to 64% at 5 years [32, 36] and 45% at 10 years [36]. These survival outcomes are markedly decreased compared to a 5-year overall survival post-kidney transplant without PTLD of 80% [32]. In a French study of adult kidney transplant recipients, predictors of poor prognosis included widespread PTLD, late-onset PTLD, age > 55 years at PTLD diagnosis, T-cell lymphoma, elevated creatinine and LDH levels, and monomorphic histology [36]. Risk factors for a poor prognosis include EBV-negative lesions, allograft involvement, and tumor monoclonality.

Treatment of PTLD often is a multi-pronged approach. Initially, immunosuppression intensity is reduced, if possible, to allow the host's own CTLs to suppress the EBV-associated proliferation. Reductions are patient dependent and can range between 25 and 100%. Plasmacytic hyperplasia PTLD may resolve with this approach. Other forms of PTLD often need additional therapies. Surgical therapy can be used for localized disease. Rituximab monotherapy is used in some patients with CD-20-positive PTLD. Chemotherapy can be added or used without rituximab for more aggressive tumors, patients who fail rituximab, and those with CD-20 negative disease. Although response rates to chemotherapy regimens is reasonable, there is significant treatment-related mortality. In a trial of 152 patients with CD-20 positive PTLD treated initially with rituximab and then chemotherapy, if complete remission was not achieved, the overall complete response rate was 70% with a median survival of 6.6 years and a treatment-related mortality of 8% [37]. Additional therapies include antiviral agents and immunotherapy. Recent adoptive immunotherapy uses autologous or HLA-matched EBV-specific cytologic T cells to target EBV without the widespread risks of cytotoxic chemotherapy and shows promise in early trials [20, 38].

Prevention

Ideally, prevention or early detection or PTLD could help improve outcomes [39]. In some centers, high-risk patients are followed with periodic EBV PCR (polymerase chain reaction). The frequency of such monitoring varies (every 1–2 weeks) during the initial year post-transplantation. If the EBV viral load is rising, several measures may be considered depending on the individual patient. The immunosuppression can be reduced if possible. Rituximab and antiviral agents have also been used in this setting [33].

Lung Cancer

Solid organ transplant recipients have a two-fold increased risk of developing lung cancer compared to the non-transplant population with an incidence of 173.4 per 100,000 person-years and an excess risk of 85.3 per 100,000 person-years [4]. Transplanted patients are more likely to develop squamous cell carcinoma of the lung than non-transplanted patients and less likely to be diagnosed with adenocarcinoma [40]. The risk for post-transplant lung cancer is higher in lung transplant recipients (>six-fold increase compared to general population) than in recipients of other organs [4]. The incidence is also significantly elevated in heart transplant recipients over age 60 years [6]. The 5-year cumulative incidence of lung cancer following any organ transplant was 0 in patients <35 years of age at transplant but was highest in female heart recipients aged >60 years (3.77%) and lung recipients aged >60 years (females, 3.87%; males, 3.76%) [6].

In single-lung transplant recipients, there is an increased risk of lung cancer in the native lung that is high in the first 6 months and then persists at a lower level thereafter [4]. This increase in risk may be due to the same risk factors, such as smoking, which ultimately lead to transplantation. Some of these early cancers may have been present at the time of transplant and may represent a previously subclinical foci now free from immune surveillance.

In a retrospective review of 633 lung transplantations in Spain, smoking was a risk factor in 74% of patients diagnosed with lung cancer post-lung transplantation [41]. However, the risk is also higher in non-smokers, suggesting another mechanism such as chronic inflammation or recurrent infection.

In a population-based study of solid organ transplant recipients over age 65 subsequently diagnosed with lung cancer, the average time to cancer diagnosis was 3 years post-transplant. The study compared three groups with non-small cell lung cancer (NSCLC): those who had not undergone transplant, those who had undergone lung transplant, and those who underwent transplant of kidney, liver, or heart. Lung cancer was more likely diagnosed at an early stage in transplant recipients, and patients with prior lung transplant were more likely to undergo surgical intervention. With advanced disease due to NSCLC, transplant recipients were more likely to receive no treatment [40]. Lung cancer-specific survival did not differ in the non-transplanted, non-lung transplanted, and lung transplant patients.

In general, solid organ transplant recipients who develop lung cancer are treated with stage-specific appropriate therapies similar to those given to non-transplant patients, although changes in immunosuppression regimens often accompany traditional therapy.

Kidney and Urothelial Cancers

Solid organ transplant recipients have a four- to five-fold increased risk of renal cell carcinoma. The incidence in one large study was 97 per 100,000 person-years, with an excess incidence of 76.1 per 100,000 person-years [4]. Kidney cancer risk is highest among kidney transplant recipients but also elevated in liver and heart transplant recipients. Renal cell carcinoma is seen in roughly 0.005% of the general population but in as many as 0.3% of patients with end-stage renal disease [42]. This risk increases further following renal transplantation with an estimated risk of 0.7% over the ensuing 3–4 years. The risk is particularly high in patients with acquired polycystic kidney disease. The risk of kidney cancer is highest in the native kidneys but can also be seen in the renal allograft [43]. The risk of renal carcinoma is highest in the first year and again in years 4–15 following transplant. These later cancers may be due in part to carcinogenic effects of immunosuppressive medications as there is not a similar increased risk of kidney cancer in patients with HIV. The estimated mortality in patients with RCC post renal transplant is 15% at a mean follow-up of 4.2 years [43].

Urothelial (bladder, ureter, and renal pelvis) cancers are also more common in patients with ESRD with an estimated incidence of 0.5% [42]. In the United States, solid organ transplant recipients are also at increased risk for urothelial cancer post-transplantation but not to the same degree as renal cell carcinoma, with an SIR of 1.52 and 2.05 for cancers of the bladder and renal pelvis, respectively [4]. In a study of kidney transplant recipients in Catalonia, bladder cancer incidence in men was greatly increased (SIR 16.35) [8].

Presentation of kidney and urothelial cancers in solid organ transplant recipients is similar to non-transplant patients. The patient may present with hematuria, or, less commonly, pain. However, compared to non-transplant patients, patients who have undergone transplant are more likely to present incidentally [44], as tumors may be found when abdominal imaging is performed for other reasons. New onset of symptoms, especially gross hematuria, requires evaluation, typically with cross-sectional imaging and/or cystoscopy.

HPV-Associated Cancer

Cervical, vulvar, vaginal, penile, anal, and oral squamous cell carcinoma are associated with certain high-risk strains of HPV (hrHPV). Although there is an increase incidence of HPV-related oropharyngeal and anogenital (anal, vulvar, vaginal, and penile) cancers in solid organ transplant recipients, there is conflicting evidence regarding a possible increase in the risk of cervical cancer [4, 45–49]. The discrepancy among studies regarding cervical cancer risk is likely due to vigorous pre- and post-transplant cervical cancer screening and treatment of precancerous lesions in some populations [49]. Ideally, patients would receive the HPV vaccine prior to transplantation, although it is unclear whether the immune protection offered by the vaccine persists in the setting of immunosuppression [50]. The proposed mechanism for the increased incidence of these cancers is reactivation of hrHPV strains, viral replication, and subsequent tumor promotion in the setting of immunosuppressive medication to prevent graft rejection [18].

Solid organ transplant recipients have at a two- to sixfold increased risk of anal intraepithelial neoplasia (AIN) and anal squamous cell cancer (ASCC) [4, 19, 51, 52]. The risk is slightly higher in women. Other risk factors include age, cigarette smoking, HPV-related anogenital disease (abnormal Pap smear or anogenital warts), receptive anal intercourse, prior sexually transmitted infections (STIs), duration of immunosuppression, and HIV infection [53] [51]. These lesions may be diagnosed using anal Pap testing and subsequent high-resolution anoscopy for abnormal cytology. Ongoing studies seek to determine the role of anal HPV screening and cytology in high-risk groups post-transplantation to reduce progression to invasive ASCC [54].

The rate of HPV-associated gynecological cancers—cervical, vulvar, and vaginal cancers or their precursors—is also increased in women following solid organ transplantation. Studies consistently show at least a two- to threefold increase in the incidence of low- and high-grade cervical intraepithelial neoplasia (CIN) or invasive cervical cancer [19, 45–48]. In a large cohort study of cancer in solid organ transplant recipients in the United States, the risk for cervical cancer (SIR 1.03, EAR 0.2) and vaginal cancer (SIR 2.35, EAR 0.5) were not significantly elevated, but vulvar cancer (SIR 7.6, EAR 6.5) was increased [4]. In another large study of US solid organ transplant recipients, cervical carcinoma in situ (CIN3) was more common in the transplant population (SIR 3.3) as was vaginal carcinoma in situ (SIR 10.6) and vulvar carcinoma in situ (SIR 20.3) [47]. Differences in data likely reflect differences in statistical analysis, case numbers, and definitions in each study. Additional risk factors beyond hrHPV include smoking, multiple sexual partners, and other STIs [49].

Head and Neck Cancer

Solid organ transplant recipients have a roughly threefold higher risk of non-cutaneous head and neck squamous cell carcinoma (HNSCC) [4, 19]. While HNSCC is not a common cancer in the general population (roughly 4% of total malignancies), it is estimated to represent about 15% of cancers in solid organ transplant recipients [55]. Risk factors for the development of HNSCC include smoking and alcohol use. Most of these cancers are found in the oral cavity or oropharynx. In a retrospective, single institution study, the median time to diagnosis was 5.9 years and 75% of the post-transplant HNSCCs were HPV-positive. Five-year overall survival was much better in patients with HPV-positive tumors compared to those without (67% versus 32%) [56]. Solid organ transplant recipients with malignancy of the oral cavity or oropharynx are more than twice as likely to die from their cancer than the general population (SMR 2.44) [3].

Thyroid Cancer

Solid organ transplant recipients have 2–3 times the risk of thyroid cancer as the general population (EAR 20.3 per 100,000 person-years) [4, 57]. The large majority of thyroid cancers diagnosed in solid organ transplant recipients are papillary thyroid cancer, mimicking the distribution seen in the population at large. The period of greatest increased risk occurs in the first year following transplantation (SIR 4.2) and rises again after more than 5 years after transplantation (SIR 2.29) [58]. This early increase may be due in part to subclinical thyroid cancers at the time of transplantation or overdiagnosis in patients who undergo more intensive medical surveillance than the general population. There does not appear to be an increased risk of thyroid cancer recurrence or mortality in solid organ transplant recipients who are treated for thyroid cancer [3]. Identified risk factors in the transplant population include long duration (>5 years) since transplantation, dialysis, younger age at time of transplantation (age < 20), type of organ transplanted (kidney highest), older current age, and female gender [58].

Hepatobiliary Cancer

The risk of liver cancer in solid organ transplant recipients is increased 11- to 12-fold with an incidence of 120 per 100,000 person-years and excess risk of 109.6 per 100,000 person-years [4]. The vast majority of cases (89.4%) occurs in liver transplant recipients with a risk >40-fold greater than the general population. Over 95% of these cancers are reported in the first 6 months following transplant and because of methods used to report time of diagnosis, many of these cancers may represent cancers found in the explanted liver. However, in a large cohort study of solid organ transplant recipients in the United States that excluded these early cancers, there was still an increased risk of hepatocellular carcinoma in liver transplant recipients (SIR 1.5) and cholangiocarcinoma in liver (SIR 2.9) and non-liver (SIR 1.8) transplant recipients [58]. Increased risk for HCC was seen in patients with

HBV (RR 3.2), HCV (RR10), non-insulin-dependent diabetes (RR 2.5) [59]. The incidence of cholangiocarcinoma was highest in patients with a history of azathioprine use and primary sclerosing cholangitis.

Colorectal Cancer

Solid organ transplant recipients have a one- to threefold increased risk of colorectal cancer (CRC) [4, 45, 59]. Diagnosis of CRC typically is made during the sixth decade, and lung transplant recipients are at greatest risk (SIR 2.34) [60]. In a large population-based study, solid organ transplant recipients had a slightly increased risk of colon cancer compared to the general population (SIR 1.12) after a median follow-up of 3.7 years. Most of the cancers were located in the proximal colon (52%), and proximal CRC had the highest risk compared to the general population (SIR 1.69). This excess risk of proximal CRC increased over time since transplantation with a risk 2–3 times higher than age-matched controls 12 or more years after transplant (SIR 2.68). In contrast, CRC in the distal colon and rectum were not seen more frequently [60]. CRC in solid organ transplant recipients age < 50 years was increased in proximal colon (SIR 2.52) and distal colon (SIR 1.77) but not the rectum, whereas older patients had increased risk only in the proximal location (SIR 1.64) [60]. The propensity for proximal location and increased risk in patients under the age of 50 years for post-transplant CRC may have implications when screening this population. When considering CRC screening options, one should consider screening earlier than age 50, and using colonoscopy rather than fecal immunochemical testing, as colonoscopy is better able to detect proximal lesions [61].

Underlying medical conditions contribute to the increased risk of CRC. Patients with lung or liver transplantation performed for a condition known to confer increased CRC risk have an even greater risk of CRC after transplant. Patients with cystic fibrosis have an elevated risk of colon cancer at baseline [62], and this is further increased after lung transplantation (SIR 27.0) [60]. Similarly, patients who received liver transplantation for primary sclerosing cholangitis (PSC) had a significantly increased risk (SIR 4.49) of CRC. This additional risk was seen even in the absence of known inflammatory bowel disease.

Oncogenic risk from immunosuppressive medications is also seen with CRC. Maintenance immunosuppression regimens with cyclosporine and azathioprine are associated with greater risk of proximal CRC when compared to regimens using tacrolimus and MMF (incidence rate ratio, IRR 1.53) [60].

Limited information is available regarding survival following a diagnosis of CRC in solid organ transplant recipients. In a retrospective review from the Mayo Clinic, median overall survival after diagnosis was 30.8 months. Stage-specific survival at 5 years for stage 1, stage 2, stage 3, and stage 4 disease was 77%, 50%, 42.3%, and 0%, respectively. Compared to patients with CRC but no history of transplantation, solid organ transplant recipients with CRC had increased cancer-specific mortality (adjusted HR 1.77) [11].

Kaposi's Sarcoma

Kaposi's sarcoma, a cutaneous malignancy associated most frequently with HIV infection, is caused by human herpes virus 8 (HHV8). Solid organ transplant recipients, as with patients with HIV, also have a significantly increased risk of Kaposi's sarcoma (SIR 61.45, EAR 15.2) [4]. HHV8 is endemic in certain regions and thus Kaposi's is more likely to occur in Mediterranean than other Western populations. In a large population-based cohort of solid organ transplant recipients in the United States, the highest risk for Kaposi's sarcoma was associated with male gender, non-white race, non-US citizenship, lung transplantation, and a prior diagnosis of cutaneous squamous cell carcinoma. The highest incidence occurred in the first year following transplantation [63].

Cancers Without an Apparent De Novo Increased Risk Following Solid Organ Transplantation

Non-HPV-Associated Gynecologic Cancers

Endometrial and ovarian cancer incidence were not increased in either a large cohort study in the United States [4] or in a meta-analysis of studies in worldwide [19].

Breast Cancer

Breast cancer is the most common cancer among women in the United States. The overall risk of breast cancer in solid organ transplant recipients varies across studies but is likely similar to age- and gender-matched controls [4, 64]. In some studies, the incidence of breast is actually lower than the general population [4]. Unfortunately, the risk may be higher in some populations including younger women (aged <35 years) and men [65], and outcomes for those who develop breast cancer are less favorable. Once a solid organ transplant recipient is diagnosed with breast cancer, the risk of dying from breast cancer may be twice that in the general population, especially in kidney transplant recipients [11, 65]. In part, poorer outcomes reflect the more aggressive and advanced nature of these cancers at the time of diagnosis, but also uncertainties in treatment options for solid organ transplant recipients with breast cancer. Interactions between cancer therapies and immunosuppression, concerns for rejection and graft loss, and other patient-specific factors must be considered when developing a treatment regimen for these patients and may limit use of more novel biologic and immunologic agents [65].

Breast cancer screening recommendations in solid organ transplant recipients are the same as the general population. Women of average risk should be screened every other year beginning at age 50 and continuing through age 74 [65], although guidelines vary. It is not known whether women who have had solid organ transplantation would benefit from earlier or more frequent screening. When considering the use of screening tests, factors such as life expectancy should be taken into consideration. Some patients with relatively short life expectancy due to other complications of transplantation may not benefit from screening.

Cancer Screening and Prevention Pre-Transplantation

It is important that transplant recipients are free of cancer prior to transplantation. On the other hand, it is not clear that pre-transplant cancer screening reduces the risk of post-transplantation malignancy. Screening guidelines generally mimic guidelines for the general population with the addition of screening based on individual risk factors [57, 66]. A thorough physical examination (including skin and oral cavity) as well as age- and gender- appropriate breast, cervical, colon, lung, and prostate cancer screening are typically recommended. Risk reduction strategies include vaccinations, smoking cessation, and alcohol reduction.

Pre-renal transplant screening for malignancies that are more common in the population with ESRD and dialysis, such as renal cell carcinoma, thyroid cancer, and multiple myeloma may be appropriate. Patients with ESRD are at increased risk of renal and other urothelial cancers, partially due to acquired cystic disease of the kidneys and analgesic overuse, and some have advocated for screening prior to transplantation in patients who have been on dialysis for >3 years [67]. Potential screening tests proposed by the American Society of Transplantation include urinalysis, urine cytology, and imaging of the native kidneys in high-risk patients [68].

Pre-Transplant Evaluation of Patients with Prior Cancer

Patients with a history of pre-transplant malignancy (PTM) unrelated to the transplant indication currently make up 7% of solid organ transplant recipients in population-based studies [12], have roughly a 5% risk of cancer recurrence [12], and may be at greater risk of cancer-related death than solid organ transplant recipients without a prior history of cancer [69–73]. In a Swedish study of 10,448 solid organ transplant recipients, 4% had a history of PTM. These patients were 3 times more likely to die from cancer than patients without a history of pre-transplant malignancy (HR 3.6) [72]. Cancers most likely to recur include breast, kidney, urothelial, hematologic, and gastrointestinal malignancies [72, 74]. As another example, among 21,415 patients receiving a kidney transplant in Australia and New Zealand, 3% had a history of PTM; 3.5% of these patients had post-transplant cancer recurrence and 8.7% developed a second primary cancer compared to 13.2% of cancer-free patients who developed a first cancer after transplantation. Cancer recurrence was seen most frequently with urinary tract cancers, breast cancer, and melanoma. Cancer-related death was not more common in the patients with a prior history of cancer in this study [75].

A history of malignancy is not an absolute contraindication for transplant in all patients [71]. The waiting period prior to solid organ transplant listing varies based on the type, stage, and aggressiveness of the cancer as well as the urgency and indication for transplant. Some guidelines recommend disease-free intervals for specific cancers. Wait times prior to renal transplantation are typically 2–5 years based on data from the Cincinnati Transplant Tumor Registry in which >50% of recurrent malignancies occurred in the first 2 years following transplantation and only 13% occurred >5 years after transplant surgery [75]. Waiting periods prior to transplantation have come under increased scrutiny [76]. In Norway, where the waiting period is 1 year, there was no difference in overall survival in kidney transplant recipients with or without a prior cancer history [70]. Further studies are needed to clarify cancer-specific risk of recurrence, cancer-specific death, and the continued need for wait times. Consultation with the patient's oncologist is always appropriate.

Screening and Prevention Post-Transplantation

Given the increased risk of cancer following solid organ transplantation compared to the general population, strategies to reduce cancer risk and identify malignancy in early stages are important. Education regarding the role of diet, exercise, weight control, sun protection, sexually transmitted disease prevention, smoking abstinence, and limiting alcohol intake are essential. Routine cancer screening recommendations have been developed for identification of precancerous lesions and early stage diagnosis when possible. Cancer screening in solid organ transplant recipients must be individualized, taking into account the patient's overall health, life expectancy, and goals to avoid excess testing, over-diagnosis, and unnecessary treatment.

Clinical practice guidelines are frequently transplant-organ specific, often parallel protocols for the general population and are largely based on expert opinion as trials on the performance of cancer screening tests in SOT recipients are lacking. Guidelines for renal transplant are the most comprehensive. In general, the range of recommendations include the following [77]:

Skin and Lip Cancer Screening SOT recipients should undergo a thorough clinical skin examination (CSE) at least annually by a provider. High-risk patients may need more frequent examinations. Patients should be encouraged to avoid the sun or adequately cover with clothing and sunscreen [57].

Gynecologic Cancer Screening Papanicolaou (Pap) cytology and pelvic examination every 1–5 years [57, 78]. Screening intervals similar to those for HIV-infected individuals is recommended by many organizations [18]. The American Society of Transplantation recommends Pap screening at 6 -month intervals for the first year following transplant and then annually. HPV testing in these guidelines is used to reduce the screening interval to yearly if negative, and to continue screening every 6 months if hrHPV positive. Other groups recommend screening based on guidelines for the general population or using a modified strategy of reducing screening frequency if Pap and HPV testing is consistently negative [57, 79]. (See Chap. 12, for further description of these recommendations). Vulvar, vaginal, and anal inspection is also prudent given the increased risk of the cancers. The upper age of Pap screening and pelvic examination in solid organ transplant recipients has not been determined. HPV vaccination in the unvaccinated should be considered, although the age for which this is efficacious has not been determined. Currently, the FDA has approved the use of the HPV vaccine in men and women up to age 45 years. Waiting 1 year following transplant to initiate the series has been recommended to prevent any theoretical impact on the allograft [18].

Breast Cancer Screening Mammogram recommendations largely follow those for the general population with mammography every 1–2 years based on individual risk and shared decision-making. Whether a subset of patients should be considered higher risk warranting earlier or more frequent screening is not yet clear [57].

Colorectal Cancer Screening Guidelines typically follow recommendation for the general population with type of study and frequency based on individual risk and shared decision-making [57]. Given the propensity for proximal lesions and younger age at onset, screening guidelines in this population warrant further study.

Prostate Cancer Screening Some organizations recommend annual prostate-specific antigen (PSA) and digital rectal examinations if life expectancy is at least 10 years; however, many recommend no screening [57].

Lung Cancer Screening There are no recommendations for or against lung cancer screening in SOT recipients except a recommendation against screening in kidney transplant recipients by the American Society of Transplantation [57, 80]. Current smokers are often excluded from transplant consideration and solid organ transplant recipients are strongly encouraged to abstain from smoking. These guidelines were published prior to the generally accepted use of low-dose CT screening for lung cancer in high-risk individuals (5-year risk >3.6%) in the general population. Given the more aggressive nature of lung cancer in solid organ transplant recipients, particularly lung and heart recipients, it is unclear whether they would also benefit from annual screening. This had not been addressed screening guidelines.

Liver Cancer Screening Every 6–12 month alpha-fetoprotein (AFP) and screening ultrasound are recommended in patients with hepatitis B or C or those with cirrhosis [57].

Kidney and Urothelial Cancer Screening Screening with urinalysis, cytology, or ultrasound is not recommended in renal transplant recipients [80]. There are no specific recommendations in other organ recipients [57].

PTLD Screening Every 3-month review of symptoms and physical examination for PTLD is recommended during the first 12 months post-transplant and then annually in kidney transplant recipients [80]. No specific recommendations exist for other transplant populations [57].

Anogenital Cancer Screening No current, specific recommendations. Ongoing studies to determine if periodic HPV and cytology screening may reduce invasive ASCC [54].

Thyroid Cancer Screening No guideline recommendations supporting screening for thyroid cancer either with physical examination or ultrasound.

Conclusion

Cancer is currently the second leading cause of death in solid organ transplant recipients [3]. With improvement in surgical techniques, immunosuppression regimens, and treatment of complications such as infection and cardiovascular disease, the incidence of and death from cancer in this population becomes a bigger contributor to overall survival. Studies are beginning to clarify the incidence of and risk factors for a variety of cancers more commonly seen in this population and the particular subgroups at highest risk. It is hoped that this information can be used to test needed prevention and screening strategies to reduce the impact of cancer in a population that has already endured enough pain and suffering.

References

1. Chapman JR, Webster AC, Wong G. Cancer in the transplant recipient. Cold Spring Harb Perspect Med. 2013;3(7):a015677.
2. Miao Y, Everly JJ, et al. De novo cancers arising in organ transplant recipients are associated with adverse outcomes compared with the general population. Transplantation. 2009;87(9):1347–59.
3. Acuna SA, Fernandes KA, et al. Cancer mortality among solid-organ transplantation in Ontario, Canada. JAMA Oncol. 2016;2(4):463–9.
4. Engels EA, Pfieffer RM, et al. Spectrum of cancer risk among US solid organ transplant recipients. JAMA. 2011;306(17):1891–901.
5. Na R, Grulich AE, et al. De novo cancer-related death in Australian liver and cardiothoracic transplant recipients. Am J Transplant. 2013;13(5):1296–304.
6. Hall EC, Pfeiffer RM, et al. Cumulative incidence of cancer after solid organ transplantation. Cancer. 2013;119(12):2300–8.
7. Carenco C, Assenat E, et al. Tacrolimus and the risk of solid cancers after liver transplant: a dose effect relationship. Am J Transplant. 2015;15:678–86.
8. Buxeda A, Redondo-Pachón D, et al. Gender differences in cancer risk after kidney transplantation. Oncotarget. 2019;10(33):3114–28.

9. Webster AC, Craig JC, Simpson JM, Jones MP, Chapman JR. Identifying high risk groups and quantifying absolute risk of cancer after kidney transplantation: a cohort study of 15,183 recipients. Am J Transplant. 2007;7(9):2140–51.
10. Carenco C, Faure S, et al. Solid, non-skin, post-liver transplant tumors: key role of lifestyle and immunosuppression management. World J Gatroenterol. 2016;22(1):427–34.
11. D'Arcy ME, Coghill AE. Survival after a cancer diagnosis among solid organ transplant recipients in the United States. Cancer. 2019;125:933–42.
12. Acuna SA, Huang JW, et al. Cancer recurrence after solid organ transplantation: a systematic review and meta-analysis. Transplant Rev. 2017c;31:240–8.
13. Maisonneuve P, Agodoa L, et al. Cancer in patients on dialysis for end-stage renal disease: an international collaborative study. Lancet. 1999;354:93–9.
14. Eckstrom M, Riise GC, Tanash HA. Risk of cancer after lung transplantation for COPD. Int J COPD. 2017;12:2841–7.
15. Carenco C, Faure S, et al. Incidence of solid organ cancers after liver transplantation: comparison with regional cancer incidence rates and risk factors. Liver Int. 2015;35:1748–55.
16. Watt KD, Pedersen RA, et al. Long-term probability of and mortality from de novo malignancy after liver transplantation. Gastroenterology. 2009;137(6):2010–7.
17. Herrero JI, Lorenzo M, et al. De novo neoplasia after liver transplantation: an analysis of risk factors and influence on survival. Liver Transpl. 2005;11(1):89–97.
18. Chin-Hong PV, Reid GE, AST Infectious Disease Community of Practice. Human papillomavirus infections in solid organ transplant recipients: guidelines from the American Society of Transplantation Infectious Diseases Community of Practice. Clin Transpl. 2019;00:e13590.
19. Grulich AE, Van Leeuwen MT, et al. Incidence of cancers in people with HIV/AIDS compared to immunosuppressed transplant recipients: a meta-analysis. Lancet. 2007;370:59–67.
20. Allen UD, Preiksaitis JK, AST Infectious Diseases Community of Practice. Post-transplant lymphoproliferative disorders, EBV infection and disease in solid organ transplantation: guidelines from the American Society of Transplantation Infectious Diseases Community of Practice. Clin Transpl. 2019;23:e13652.
21. Jiyad Z, Olsen CM, et al. Azathioprine and risk of skin cancer in organ transplant recipients: systematic review and meta-analysis. Am J Transplant. 2016;16:3490–503.
22. Brin L, Zubair AS, Brewer JD. Optimal management of skin cancer in immunosuppressed patients. Am J Clin Dermatol. 2014;15(4):339–56.
23. Chockalingam R, Downing C, Tyring SK. Cutaneous squamous cell carcinomas in organ transplant recipients. J Clin Med. 2015;4(6):1229–39. https://doi.org/10.3390/jcm4061229.
24. Asgari MM, Arron ST, et al. Sirolimus use and risk of cutaneous squamous cell carcinoma (SCC) in solid organ transplant recipients (SOTRs). J Am Acad Dermatol. 2015;73(3):222–50.
25. Karia PS, Azzi JR, et al. Association of sirolimus use with the risk for skin cancer in a mixed-organ cohort of solid-organ transplant recipients with a history of cancer. JAMA Dermatol. 2016;152(5):533–40.
26. De Fijter JW. Cancer and mTOR inhibitors in transplant recipients. Transplantation. 2017;101(1):45–55.
27. Garrett GL, Blanc PD, et al. Incidence of and risk factors for skin cancer in organ transplant recipients in the United States. JAMA Dermatol. 2017;153(3):296–303.
28. Mithoefer AB, Supran S, Freeman RB. Risk factors associated with the development of skin cancer after liver transplantation. Liver Transpl. 2002;8(10):939–44.
29. Rizvi SMH, Aagnes B, et al. Long-term change in the risk of skin cancer after organ transplantation. A population-based nationwide cohort study. JAMA Dermatol. 2017;153(12):1270–7.
30. Laprise C, Cahoon EK. Risk of lip cancer after solid organ transplantation in the United States. Am J Transplant. 2019;19(1):227–37.
31. Nagle SJ, Reshef R, Tsai DE. Posttransplant lymphoproliferative disorder in solid organ and hematopoietic stem cell transplantation. Clin Chest Med. 2017;38:771–38.
32. Caillard S, Dharnidharka V, et al. Posttransplant lymphoproliferative disorders after renal transplantation in the United States in era of modern immunosuppression. Transplantation. 2005;80(9):1233–43.

33. Peters AC, Akinwumi MS, et al. The changing epidemiology of posttransplant lymphoprolif-erative disorder in adult solid organ transplant recipients over 30 years: a single-center experi-ence. Transplantation. 2018;102(9):1553–62.
34. Bakker NA, van Imhoff GW, Verschuuren EA, van Son WJ. Presentation and early detection of post-transplantation lymphoproliferative disorder after solid organ transplantation. Transpl Int. 2007;20:207–18.
35. Dierickx D, Habermann TM. Post-transplantation lymphoproliferative disorders in adults. NEJM. 2018;378(6):549–62.
36. Caillard S, Porcher R, et al. Post-transplantation lymphoproliferative disorder after kidney transplantation: report of a nationwide French registry and the development of a new prognos-tic score. J Clin Oncol. 2013;31(10):1302–9.
37. Trappe RU, Dierickx D, et al. Response to rituximab induction is a predictive marker in B-cell post-transplant lymphoproliferative disorder and allows successful stratification into rituximab or R-CHOP consolidation in an international, prospective, multicenter phase II trial. J Clin Oncol. 2017;35(5):536–43.
38. Chiou FK, Beath SV, et al. Cytotoxic T-lymphocyte therapy for post-transplant lymphoprolif-erative disorder after solid organ transplantation in children. Pediatr Transplant. 2018;22:e13133.
39. Aidabbagh MA, Gilman MR. The role of antiviral prophylaxis for the prevention of Epstein-Barr virus-associated posttransplant lymphoproliferative disease in solid organ transplant recipients: a systematic review. Am J Transplantation. 2017;17:770–81.
40. Sigel K, Veluswamy R, et al. Lung cancer prognosis in elderly solid organ transplant recipi-ents. Transplantation. 2015;99(10):2181–9.
41. Pérez-Callejo D, Torrente M, et al. Lung cancer in lung transplantation: incidence and out-come. Postgrad Med J. 2018;94:15–9.
42. Kompotiatis P, Thongprayoon C, et al. Association between urologic malignancies and end-stage renal disease: a meta-analysis. Nephrology. 2019;24(1):65–73.
43. Chewcharat A, Thongprayoon C, et al. Incidence and mortality of renal cell carcinoma after kidney transplant: a meta-analysis. J Clin Med. 2019;8:530–45.
44. Tsivian M, Caso JR, Kimura M, Polascik TJ. Renal tumors in solid organ recipients: clini-cal and pathologic features. Urol Oncol. 2013;31(2):255–8. https://doi.org/10.1016/j.urolonc.2010.11.006.
45. Adami J, Gabel H, et al. Cancer risk following organ transplantation: a nationwide cohort study in Sweden. Br J Cancer. 2003;89(7):1221–7.
46. Collett D, Mumford L, et al. Comparison of malignancy in recipients of different types of organ: a UK registry audit. Am J Transplant. 2010;10(8):1889–96.
47. Madeleine MM, Finch JL, et al. HPV-related cancers after solid organ transplantation in the United States. Am J Transplant. 2013;13(12):3202–9.
48. Hortlund M, Arroyo Muhr LS, et al. Cancer risks after solid organ transplantation and after long-term dialysis. Int J Cancer. 2017;140(5):1091–101.
49. Liao JB, Fisher CE, Madeleine MM. Gynecologic cancers and solid organ transplantation. Am J Transplant. 2019;19:1266–77.
50. Kumar D, Unger ER, et al. Immunogenicity of the quadrivalent human papillomavirus vaccine in organ transplant recipients. Am J Transplant. 2013;13:2411–7.
51. Patel HS, Silver AR, et al. Human papillomavirus infection and anal dysplasia in renal trans-plant recipients. Br J Surg. 2010;97(11):1716–21.
52. Meeuwis K, Melchers W, et al. Anogenital malignancies in women after renal transplantation over 40 years in a single center. Transplantation. 2012;93(9):914–22.
53. Grulich AE, Poynten IM, et al. The epidemiology of anal cancer. Sex Health. 2012;9:504–8.
54. Rosales BM, Langton-Lockton J, et al. Transplant recipients and anal neoplasia study: design, methods and participant characteristics of a prevalence study. Transplant Direct. 2019;5:e434.
55. Harris JP, Penn I. Immunosupression and the development of malignancies of the upper airway and related structures. Laryngoscope. 1981;91(4):520–8.
56. Alsidawi S, Price KA, et al. Characteristics and long-term outcomes of head and neck squa-mous cell carcinoma after solid organ transplantation. Oral Oncol. 2017;17:104–9.

57. Kitahara CM, Yanik EL, et al. Risk of thyroid cancer among solid organ transplant recipients. Am J Transplantation. 2017;17:2911–21.
58. Koshiol J, Pawlish K, et al. Risk of hepatobiliary cancer after solid organ transplant in the United States. Clin Gastroenterol Hepatol. 2014;12(9):1541–9.e3.
59. Safaeian M, Robbins HA, et al. Risk of colorectal cancer after solid organ transplantation in the United States. Am J Transplantation. 2016;16:960–7.
60. Merchea A, Shahjehan F, et al. Colorectal cancer characteristics and outcomes after solid organ transplantation. J Oncol. 2019;2019:1–8.
61. Zorzi M, Hassan C, et al. Divergent long-term detection rates of proximal and distal advanced neoplasia in fecal immunochemical test screening programs: a retrospective cohort study. Ann Int Med. 2018;169(9):602–7.
62. Maisonneuve P, Marshall BC, Knapp EA, Lowenfels AB. Cancer risk in cystic fibrosis: a 20-year nationwide study from the United States. J Natl Cancer Inst. 2013;105:122–9.
63. Cahoon EK, Linet MS, et al. Risk of Kaposi sarcoma after solid organ transplantation in the United States. Int J Cancer. 2018;143:27141–2748.
64. Wong G, Au E, Badve SV, Lim WH. Breast cancer and transplantation. Am J Transplantation. 2017;17:2243–53.
65. US Preventive Services Task Force, Siu AL. Screening for breast cancer: US preventive services task force recommendation statement. Ann Intern Med. 2016;164(4):279–96.
66. Martin P, DiMartini A, et al. Evaluation for liver transplantation in adults: 2013 practice guideline by the American association for the study of liver diseases and the American Society of Transplantation. Hepatology. 2014;59:1144–65.
67. Holley JL. Screening, diagnosis, and treatment of cancer in long-term dialysis patients. Clin J Am Soc Nephrol. 2007;2:604–10.
68. Kasiske BL, Cangro CB, et al. The evaluation of renal transplant candidates: clinical practice guidelines. Am J Transplant. 2001;1:3–95.
69. Dahle DO, Grotmol T, et al. Association between pretransplant cancer and survival in kidney transplant recipients. Transplantation. 2017;101(10):2599–605.
70. Acuna SA, Sutradhar R, Kim SJ, Baxter N. Solid organ transplantation in patients with pre-existing malignancies in remission: a propensity score matched cohort study. Transplantation. 2018;102(7):1156–64.
71. Acuna SA, Lam W, et al. Cancer evaluation in the assessment of solid organ transplant candidates: a systematic review of clinical practice guidelines. Transplant Rev. 2018;32(1):29–35.
72. Brattström C, Granath F, Edgren G, Smedby KE, Wilczek HE. Overall and cause-specific mortality in transplant recipients with a pretransplantation cancer history. Transplantation. 2013;96(3):297–305. https://doi.org/10.1097/TP.0b013e31829854b7.
73. Acuna SA, Huang JW. Outcomes of solid organ transplant recipients with preexisting malignancies in remission: a systematic review and meta-analysis. Transplantation. 2017b;101:101471–81.
74. Penn I. Evaluation of transplant candidates with pre-existing malignancies. Ann Transplant. 1997;2(4):14–7.
75. Viecelli AK, Lim WH, et al. Cancer-specific and all-cause mortality in kidney transplant recipients with and without previous cancer. Transplantation. 2015;99(12):2586–92.
76. Watschinger B, Budde K, et al. Pre-existing malignancies in renal transplant candidates- time to reconsider waiting times. Nephrol Dial Transplant. 2019;34:1–9.
77. Acuna SA, Huang JW, et al. Cancer screening recommendations for solid organ transplant recipients: a systematic review of clinical practice guidelines. Am J Transplantation. 2017;17:103–14.
78. US Preventive Services Task Force, Curry SJ, Krist AH, et al. Screening for cervical cancer: US preventive services task force recommendation statement. JAMA. 2018;320(7):674–86.
79. Moscicki AB, et al. Guidelines for cervical cancer screening in immunosuppressed women without HIV infection. J Low Genit Tract Dis. 2019;23(2):87–101.
80. Kasiske BL, Vazquez MA, et al. Recommendations for the outpatient surveillance of renal transplant recipients. J Am Soc Nephrol. 2000;11(Supple 15):S1–86.

Chapter 11
Metabolic Complications in the Adult Solid Organ Transplant Recipient

Anna Golob and Jennifer Wright

Introduction

Solid organ transplantation is increasing in incidence, its recipients are benefiting from improved long-term survival, and the age of transplant survivors is increasing. These factors will lead to both an increase in the metabolic complications faced by solid organ transplant recipients, as well as the increased likelihood that these patients will be cared for in the primary care setting. Primary care providers regularly manage metabolic conditions such as hypertension and diabetes. For the solid organ transplant recipient, addressing these conditions is often a price of success—with longevity comes the need for the chronic work to maintain health. Primary care providers can, and should, play a vital role in the screening, prevention, diagnosis, and treatment of metabolic complications in solid organ transplant recipients.

A. Golob (✉)
Department of Medicine, Division of General Internal Medicine, University of Washington, Seattle, WA, USA

VA Puget Sound Healthcare System, Seattle, WA, USA
e-mail: zilanna@uw.edu

J. Wright
Department of Medicine, Division of General Internal Medicine, University of Washington, Seattle, WA, USA
e-mail: sonic@uw.edu

© Springer Nature Switzerland AG 2020
C. J. Wong (ed.), *Primary Care of the Solid Organ Transplant Recipient*,
https://doi.org/10.1007/978-3-030-50629-2_11

Cardiovascular Disease

Epidemiology

Cardiovascular disease (CVD), including atherosclerotic-related heart disease and structural heart disease, is common after solid organ transplantation, despite screening for heart disease prior to transplantation (see Chap. 2 for discussion of pre-transplant testing). In patients who have undergone kidney transplantation, CVD risk is higher than in the general population and is the most common cause of death [1]. The rates of myocardial infarction at 12 and 36 months after kidney transplantation is 5% and 11%—while this rate is lower than in patients with end-stage renal disease awaiting transplant, it is still 10–30 times higher than in the general population [2]. Long-term rates of CVD are also high in patients who have received a liver transplant, with an average rate of 12% for cardiovascular events that occur after 6 months, although studies vary widely in cardiovascular outcomes measured and duration of follow-up [3]. With nonalcoholic steatohepatitis (NASH) becoming a leading cause of liver transplantation (see Chap. 5), it is predicted that cardiovascular disease will become more common, as transplantation for NASH is associated with higher rates of cardiovascular complications compared to other indications [4]. Heart transplant recipients are not only at risk for conventional cardiovascular disease but also have the unique risks of cardiac allograft vasculopathy (CAV) of the coronary vessels as well as graft rejection. Cardiac allograft vasculopathy occurs in 30% of heart transplant recipients by 5 years, and in 50% at 10 years [5] (See Chap. 6). Lung transplant recipients frequently have metabolic risk factors [6], but long-term survival is most impacted by graft dysfunction, malignancy, and infectious complications, with cardiovascular disease representing a comparatively smaller proportion of causes of death [7].

Pathophysiology

Risk factors for cardiovascular disease in solid organ transplant recipients include traditional risk factors, organ-related risk factors, and post-transplant factors secondary to medications.

Traditional cardiac risk factors such as hypertension (HTN) and diabetes are common, particularly in kidney transplant recipients and liver transplant recipients who had end-stage liver disease due to NASH. In most cases, solid organ transplant recipients are required to quit smoking prior to transplantation, but tobacco use can recur after transplantation.

Organ-specific risk factors are less commonly encountered and not necessarily modifiable. These include uremic cardiomyopathy, the term used to describe the pathologic cardiac hypertrophy that can occur in patients with advanced kidney disease [8], and hepatopulmonary syndrome and cirrhotic cardiomyopathy in advanced liver disease [4]. Heart transplant recipients have a unique set of factors that contribute to an elevated CVD risk. In the short term, transplant graft failure is the most common cause of cardiovascular death in heart transplant recipients. In the years following transplant, cardiac allograft vasculopathy (CAV), a unique form of immunologically mediated coronary artery disease, becomes increasingly common and problematic, with an incidence of approximately 50% at 10 years post-transplant [5], contributing to >10% of annual deaths after the first-year post-transplant [9] (See Chap. 6).

Many of the immunosuppressive medications used after solid organ transplantation contribute to the development of CVD risk factors (see Table 11.1, and Chap. 3).

Observational data not specific to solid organ transplant recipients has found an increased risk of cardiovascular events in patients treated with high-dose corticosteroids, defined as >7.5 mg of prednisolone or equivalent daily [11]. There are several mechanisms by which this association likely occurs: Corticosteroids often cause fluid retention and associated hypertension; glucose intolerance; secondary diabetes; weight gain; and worsened lipid profiles.

Calcineurin inhibitors (CNIs) similarly can lead to the development of several established cardiovascular risk factors. Hypertension is a common side effect of CNIs, which cause renal vasoconstriction and direct nephrotoxicity [10]. New-onset diabetes after transplant (NODAT) is also associated with the use of CNI (see section on "Diabetes" below for details).

Sirolimus and everolimus, mammalian target of rapamycin (mTOR), inhibitors, can lead to increased cholesterol levels. In kidney transplant recipients, sirolimus has been associated with a higher risk of all-cause mortality despite the lower risk of malignancy compared to other maintenance immunosuppression regimens [12]; therefore, it has been inferred that sirolimus may have worse cardiovascular outcomes than other immunosuppressive agents, although this potential association requires further study (See Chap. 3 for further discussion of medication side effects).

Table 11.1 Immunosuppressive medications and cardiovascular risk factors

	Corticosteroids	Calcineurin inhibitors: tacrolimus	Calcineurin inhibitors: cyclosporine	mTOR inhibitors: sirolimus/ everolimus
HTN	++	+	++	
Diabetes (NODAT)[a]	++	++	+	+
Dyslipidemia	++	+	++	+++
Renal impairment		+	+	Proteinuria
Weight gain	++			

[a]NODAT new-onset diabetes after transplant
Adapted from Munagala [10] reprinted with permission

Table 11.2 KDIGO screening recommendations for CVD risk factors in kidney transplant recipients [13]

Cardiovascular risk factor	Interval	Test/target
Diabetes (NODAT)[a]	Weekly for first 4 weeks Every 3 months for first year Annually thereafter	Fasting glucose, oral glucose tolerance test, or hemoglobin A1c
Hypertension	Measure blood pressure at every visit	Maintain a blood pressure of <130/<80 mmHg
Dyslipidemia	2–3 months after transplant Annually thereafter	Lipid panel LDL goal <100 mg/dL

[a]*NODAT* new-onset diabetes after transplant

Screening

Due to the increased risk of developing hypertension, diabetes, and dyslipidemia following solid organ transplantation, more intensive screening is performed than what is generally recommended for the general population. See Table 11.2 for the screening recommendations recommended by the Kidney Disease: Improving Global Outcomes (KDIGO) Transplant Work Group for CVD risk factors in kidney transplant recipients [13]. These are evidence-based guidelines that are likely applicable to other solid organ transplant recipients.

In addition to the above screening, heart transplant recipients are typically screened aggressively for the development of CAV with coronary angiography, often starting the first-year post-transplant [9]. This approach is favored rather than using symptoms to guide surveillance because the transplanted heart is denervated, resulting in a lack of classic angina symptoms (see Chap. 6).

Prevention and Treatment

- Hypertension: Blood pressure management is overall similar to the approach in the general population.

  - Target blood pressure: In general, blood pressure should be maintained at <130 mm Hg systolic and <80 mm Hg diastolic, although this goal should be individualized based on a patient's risk factors and tolerance to medications.
  - Lifestyle: Dietary modification such as the DASH diet, exercise, and maintaining a normal body weight are all important.
  - Medications: Studies are lacking to guide a single best approach to pharmacotherapy in solid organ transplant recipients.

Calcium channel blockers: Because calcineurin inhibitors are a common cause of blood pressure elevation, though to be at least partly mediated by renal vasoconstriction, many providers preferentially use dihydropyridine calcium channel blockers (CCBs) such as amlodipine as the first-line agent in treatment. A review of kidney transplant recipients found that CCBs resulted in less graft loss compared to placebo and fewer side effects such as hyperkalemia and anemia compared to angiotensin-converting enzyme inhibitor (ACE-i) therapy [14] (See Chap. 4). Nondihydropyridine CCBs should be avoided or discussed with the transplant team before using, as they may increase the levels of both CNIs and mTOR inhibitors (see Chap. 3).

Beta-blockers: While no longer first-line therapy for hypertension in the general population, beta-blockers are still often used in the solid organ transplant population because of concerns for adverse effects of other anti-hypertensive medications. As with non-transplant patients, they should be used with caution in patients with reactive airways, hypoglycemia unawareness, or baseline bradycardia. In heart transplant recipients, beta-blockers should be used with caution as the donor heart is denervated and may be more dependent on a higher heart rate as well as more sensitive to the effect of beta blockers (see Chap. 6).

Angiotensin-converting enzyme inhibitors (ACE-i) and angiotensin receptor blockers (ARBs): These medications are often avoided early after transplantation because of the risk of renal insufficiency during treatment with the higher doses of calcineurin inhibitors used early post-transplant, as well as the risk of hyperkalemia with the concomitant use of trimethoprim-sulfamethoxazole for *Pneumocystis jirovecii* pneumonia prophylaxis. However, there is also data to support the long-term benefits of ACE-i therapy in kidney transplant recipients, with a small randomized controlled trial finding long-term cardiovascular benefit in patients treated with ACE-i compared to placebo, in addition to other anti-hypertensive medications if needed [15]. Furthermore, these medications should be considered in patients with proteinuria. Although ACE inhibitors and ARBs can often be well tolerated 3–6 months after transplantation in a stable patient, because of the risk of worsening renal function, it is still advisable to discuss with the transplant team before starting ACE-i or ARB therapy. They should be avoided in kidney transplant recipients who have known renal artery stenosis.

Diuretics: Although thiazide diuretics are first-line anti-hypertensive therapy for the general population, they should be used with caution in solid organ transplant recipients. Thiazide diuretics can worsen the already increased risk of hyperuricemia, dyslipidemia, and hyperglycemia in solid organ transplant recipients. Acute kidney injury can occur if the patient is at risk for volume depletion. There may be an increased risk of squamous cell skin cancer although studies are not conclusive; solid organ transplant recipients are already at increased risk of these malignancies (see Chap. 10). As with ACE-i and ARB use, it is best to discuss with the transplant team prior to initiating treatment with thiazide diuretics.

- Dyslipidemia: Management of dyslipidemia is the same as in the general population with the exceptions that drug interactions are more common, and treatment is routine for kidney and heart transplant recipients.
  - Patients already on statin therapy prior to transplantation: In general, it is recommended to reduce statin therapy by 50% prior to initiation of calcineurin inhibitor therapy, unless the patient is already on pravastatin, rosuvastatin, or fluvastatin, which have fewer drug interactions. The other option is to switch to pravastatin, rosuvastatin, or fluvastatin prior to starting a calcineurin inhibitor.
  - Indications: All heart transplant recipients should receive statin therapy unless contraindicated, as early use may decrease the incidence of CAV [16] (see Chap. 6). Most kidney transplant recipients should be treated with statin therapy (see Chap. 4). Liver and lung transplant recipients should be treated if they meet other indications for statin therapy.
  - Initiation: If lower-intensity therapy is indicated, then pravastatin is the preferred statin because of fewer drug interactions with calcineurin inhibitors. If higher-intensity statin therapy is indicated, rosuvastatin is a suitable option, again because of fewer drug interactions with calcineurin inhibitors. Fluvastatin is an acceptable choice with regard to drug interactions, but is low potency and less commonly used. While there is some data for supporting the use of other statins in reducing CAV in heart transplant recipients, because of drug interactions other statins are generally avoided. If statins other than pravastatin or rosuvastatin are considered, it is best to discuss with the transplant team or a transplant pharmacist first.
- Aspirin: Aspirin use for primary prevention of cardiovascular disease in the general population is no longer routinely recommended by the American College of Cardiology/American Heart Association [17], but guidelines vary and its use may be considered on a case-by-case basis. Primary prevention studies generally excluded immunosuppressed patients however. In the solid organ transplant population, aspirin is recommended for all heart transplant recipients. Currently, there is minimal data regarding aspirin for primary prevention in other solid organ transplant recipients. In a post hoc analysis of a trial of folate therapy in kidney transplant recipients, aspirin use was not associated with reduction in cardiovascular outcomes or all-cause mortality, and had no effect on kidney function [18]. However, whether this result can be generalized is uncertain, and aspirin is still used variably in the kidney transplant population [19]. For liver and lung transplant recipients, the use of aspirin for primary prevention should be individualized. In patients who have known cardiovascular disease, aspirin should be prescribed for secondary prevention, similar to non-transplant patients, as long as there are no contraindications.

Modification of the immunosuppressive medication regimen by the transplant team may be considered for the management of hypertension, dyslipidemia, and diabetes, especially if these metabolic conditions are severe or life-threatening. However, any reduction in dosing must be balanced against the risk for allograft rejection. Corticosteroid doses are routinely lowered as much as possible post-transplant, but switching a patient from tacrolimus to another agent is less commonly done despite the increased risk of diabetes and hypertension, because tacrolimus otherwise has better immunosuppression performance characteristics [20]. CNIs also generally have more favorable outcomes in comparison to mTOR inhibitors [12].

Diabetes Mellitus

Epidemiology

New-onset diabetes after transplant (NODAT) is a common complication among solid organ transplant recipients and contributes to the increasing prevalence of cardiovascular disease (CVD) in this population [21, 22]. NODAT is diagnosed in concordance with the World Health Organization (WHO) or American Diabetes Association (ADA) criteria for diagnosing diabetes in the general population (Table 11.3), with the exception that hemoglobin A1c is not recommended as a diagnostic test until at least 3 months post-transplant to allow for new hemoglobin to be synthesized and glycated for an adequate period.

The reported prevalence of NODAT has ranged from 2.5 to 53% of solid organ transplant recipients, with variation based on type of organ transplant and criteria used to define diabetes (e.g., use of fasting plasma glucose vs oral glucose tolerance test) [22].

Table 11.3 Diagnostic criteria for new-onset diabetes after transplant (NODAT) [22]

Symptoms of diabetes (polyuria, polydipsia, and/or unexplained weight loss) with random plasma glucose >200 mg/dL
Fasting plasma glucose >126 mg/dL. Abnormal fasting plasma glucose should be confirmed on two separate days. (Prediabetes: FPG between 100 and 126 mg/dL)
Two-hour plasma glucose >200 mg/dL during an oral glucose tolerance test (OGTT) done using a glucose load of 75 grams, as per WHO guidelines. (Prediabetes: 2 hours OGTT PG 140–199 mg/dL)
Hemoglobin A1c >6.5% (Note that HbA1c should NOT be used until at least 3 months post-transplant to allow for new hemoglobin to be synthesized and glycated) (Prediabetes: HbA1c 5.7–6.4%)[a]

[a]Note that hemoglobin A1c is not among the 2003 consensus guideline diagnostic criteria, but nevertheless used by many experts based on more recent diabetes guidelines in the general population

Pathophysiology

Both traditional and transplant-specific risk factors contribute to the development of NODAT. As with the general population, traditional risk factors include age >40, obesity (BMI >30), family history of diabetes, and being a member of certain racial and ethnic groups [23]. Transplant-specific risk factors are primarily related to immunosuppressive medication side effects. Corticosteroids decrease insulin secretion, increase insulin resistance, increase hepatic gluconeogenesis, and increase plasma glucose and hence diabetes incidence in a dose-dependent fashion [22]. Multiple studies have demonstrated a higher risk of NODAT in solid organ transplant recipients treated with steroid-containing regimens compared to steroid-free regimens. For example, a study of over 25,000 kidney transplant recipients followed for 3 years found a 42% increased risk for NODAT in those who received glucocorticoids compared to those who did not [24]. Of note, even in solid organ transplant recipients who do not receive steroids, the risk of NODAT is still elevated compared to the general population due to side effects from the other commonly used immunosuppressants.

Calcineurin inhibitors (CNIs) are suspected to increase risk for NODAT by decreasing insulin synthesis and secretion [25]. Notably, tacrolimus carries a higher risk of NODAT than cyclosporine [10] but because it is associated with more favorable outcomes it remains the more commonly used CNI.

For mammalian target of rapamycin (mTOR) inhibitors including sirolimus, the mechanism for NODAT is increased insulin resistance. This effect seems to be amplified when these medications are paired with calcineurin inhibitors. Of note, azathioprine and mycophenolate mofetil do not appear to increase diabetes risk [22].

(See also Chap. 3 for discussion of side effects of immunosuppressive medications).

Screening

Patient care guidelines for solid organ transplant recipients recommend frequent screening for NODAT [13, 21]. This includes weekly fasting serum glucose levels for the first 4 weeks, followed by fasting glucose levels, oral glucose tolerance test (OGTT), or HbA1c at 3, 6, and 12 months post-transplant, and annually thereafter (Table 11.4). Abnormal fasting glucose levels should be verified either by repeating the test on another day or by obtaining an HbA1c or OGTT.

Table 11.4 Recommended screening for NODAT among solid organ transplant recipients

Condition	Interval	Test
New-onset diabetes after transplant	Weekly for first 4 weeks then At 3, 6, and 12 months then Annually thereafter	Fasting serum glucose or Oral glucose tolerance test (OGTT) or hemoglobin A1c[a]

[a]Do not use HbA1c until after 3 months post-transplant

Prevention and Treatment

As with the general population, solid organ transplant recipients with identified risk factors for diabetes including prediabetes, obesity, metabolic syndrome, or a family history of diabetes should be counseled on lifestyle changes including weight loss (if overweight or obese), a healthy diet, and exercise to reduce their risk of developing NODAT.

Management of NODAT may vary based on its timing and etiology. In the immediate post-transplant period, NODAT may be related to high doses of corticosteroids in which case it is best managed with insulin therapy and is anticipated to improve as corticosteroid doses are reduced. However, when diabetes persists after corticosteroids are decreased or stopped, or develops as a later complication after SOT, management principles are similar to those for the general population as per current ADA guidelines. These typically begin with lifestyle modification, then oral or injectable non-insulin agents, followed by insulin, unless glucose derangements are profound, in which case insulin may be preferred as initial therapy. Caution should be taken to avoid specific diabetes medication side effects/contraindications to which transplant patients may be particularly vulnerable. For example, solid organ transplant recipients with NODAT and post-graft estimated glomerular filtration rate (eGFR) <30 ml/min/1.73 m^2 should not be treated with metformin, and caution should be used with sulfonylureas due to risk of hypoglycemia. Thiazolidinediones (TZDs) are usually avoided due to risk of fluid retention, decreased bone density, and liver injury. Some providers have reported successful use of dipeptidyl peptidase 4 (DPP4) inhibitors and glucagon like peptide (GLP) 1 receptor agonists in solid organ transplant recipients. However, there is minimal published data on their use in this population. Similarly, there is little experience for the use of sodium-glucose cotransporter (SGLT) 2 inhibitors, and their use would need to weigh improved cardiovascular outcomes against the increased risk of genitourinary infections in patients who are already immune suppressed.

If a patient's diabetes is difficult to control, the primary care provider may discuss with the transplant team whether a change in the immunosuppressive regimen is feasible. The transplant specialist may consider such strategies as reducing or stopping corticosteroids or reducing the calcineurin inhibitor dose. However, most experts do not recommend switching from tacrolimus to cyclosporine unless there are additional tacrolimus-related adverse events. Additionally, worsening of diabetes is not generally an indication to switch from a calcineurin inhibitor to a mTOR inhibitor [22].

There is not a consensus on the optimal target HbA1c for solid organ transplant recipients with NODAT; many experts recommend aiming for a HbA1c <7.0 mg/dL, but this should be individualized to balance the benefit of improved glycemic control against the risks of hypoglycemia and adverse effects of medications. Of note, the HbA1c may not be reliable in the setting of anemia or use of erythropoietin stimulating agents, in which case home glucose measurements should be used to adjust therapy. In difficult-to-control cases, referral to an endocrinologist is appropriate.

Chronic Kidney Disease

Epidemiology

The development of chronic kidney disease (CKD) following solid organ transplantation is both common and ominous. In a study of non-renal solid organ transplant recipients, using a definition of GFR <30 ml/min/1.73 m^2, the prevalence of CKD at 5 years was 18.1% in liver transplant recipients, 15.8% in lung transplant recipients, and 10.9% in heart transplant recipients [26]. In a study of liver transplant recipients, 65% had stage 3 or greater CKD (GFR of <60 mL/min/1.73 m^2) at 10 years [27]. Kidney transplant recipients are at risk for chronic kidney disease both from graft dysfunction and etiologies common to all solid organ transplant recipients (See Chap. 4). It is important to be aware of solid organ transplant recipients' kidney function as it has significant implications for their health and life expectancy. In a large observational study of patients who underwent non-renal transplants, renal failure (defined as ESRD or GFR of <30 mL/min/1.73 m^2) was associated with an increased risk of death, with a relative risk of 4.55 compared to transplant recipients who did not develop renal failure [26].

Pathophysiology

Risk factors for the development of CKD after SOT can be divided into four groups: pre-transplant risk factors, peri-operative complications, immunosuppressive medications used post-transplant, and risks unique to kidney transplant recipients (Table 11.5).

Table 11.5 Causes of chronic kidney disease in solid organ transplant recipients

Pre-transplant risk factors
Hypertension
Diabetes
Conditions related to organ failure, e.g., cardiorenal syndrome, hepatorenal syndrome
Peri-operative complications
Acute kidney injury (various causes)
Immunosuppressive medications
Calcineurin inhibitors (tacrolimus, cyclosporine)
Factors unique to kidney transplant recipients[a]
BK virus nephropathy (BKVN)
Allograft rejection
Anatomic
Transplanted renal artery stenosis
Ureteral obstruction

[a]See Chap. 4

Pre-transplant risk factors include risk factors seen in the general population such as hypertension and diabetes, in addition to issues specific to end-stage organ dysfunction. For example, patients with liver cirrhosis and heart failure often have low effective circulating volume, which can affect kidney function. Creatinine alone is a poor indicator of pre-transplant kidney function, as many patients awaiting transplant have low muscle mass due to their underlying disease. A combination of GFR calculation and measurement of urine protein and creatinine offers a better understanding of a patient's kidney function prior to transplantation.

Organ transplant operations themselves carry significant risk that can impact the kidney. Intra- or postoperative hypotension and hypoperfusion can lead to acute kidney injury, and in turn, may lead to chronic kidney disease. In addition, there are organ-specific operative issues that may contribute such as use of cardiopulmonary bypass in heart transplantation [1].

Immunosuppressant medications are a large contributor to development of CKD in solid organ transplant recipients. Calcineurin inhibitors, including cyclosporine and tacrolimus, are known to cause renal impairment. Despite this, tacrolimus is a first-line immunosuppressive medication due to lower rates of graft loss and rejection, and improved patient survival [28]. Calcineurin inhibitors cause renal vasoconstriction that can lead to acute kidney injury, and chronic use can lead to interstitial fibrosis and renal impairment. mTOR inhibitors, such as sirolimus, are used much less frequently that CNIs, but also carry notable risk of kidney dysfunction. This class of medications is associated with proteinuria, and patients need to be monitored for development of this complication [28] (see Chap. 3).

Patients who have received a kidney transplant may experience a unique set of renal complications. The underlying disease that initially led to kidney failure may recur in the transplanted organ (e.g., IgA nephropathy). Rejection may lead to graft failure and recurrent kidney failure. In addition, BK virus nephropathy is a common cause of nephropathy in kidney transplant recipients. BK viremia develops in approximately 20% of adult kidney transplant recipients, and approximately 1–10% develop nephropathy related to secondary tubulointerstitial nephritis and/or ureteral stenosis [28–30] (see Chap. 4).

Screening

Post-transplant kidney function is monitored regularly. The intensity of monitoring will be greatest during the peri-operative period and then decrease in frequency as the patient transitions to general outpatient care. In general, quarterly monitoring of serum creatinine and annual urine protein is performed in most solid organ transplant recipients after the acute postoperative period.

For example, the Kidney Disease: Improving Global Outcomes (KDIGO) Transplant Work Group recommends the following for patients beginning 3 months after their kidney transplant [13]:

1. Creatinine and an estimated GFR should be monitored every 2 weeks months 4–6, monthly for months 7–12, and then at least every 3 months indefinitely.
2. Urine protein measurement is recommended every 3 months for the first year and then annually.

In the case of kidney transplant recipients, plasma BK virus PCR testing is also recommended. Guidelines and practice vary by transplant center regarding the recommended frequency of BK virus monitoring, but in general it is more frequently, e.g., every 3 months, for the first 1–2 years and then may decrease in frequency to annually, or only as part of the evaluation for a concerning change in kidney function.

Prevention and Treatment

Prevention and treatment of CKD in solid organ transplant recipients largely mimics strategies in the general population including avoidance of nephrotoxic medications, avoidance of hypovolemia/hypoperfusion, and management of hypertension and diabetes. The benefits and risks when using ACE-inhibitors is similar to the discussion above regarding hypertension management. On the one hand, ACE-inhibitors and ARBs are the medications of choice in patients with chronic kidney disease, especially if proteinuria is present. On the other hand, they should be used with caution as they may decrease GFR and worsen hyperkalemia. There is no consensus yet as to the routine use of ACE-inhibitors and ARBs in solid organ transplant recipients, but it is common practice to avoid their use in the early period after solid organ transplantation (e.g., 0–6 months). They should be avoided in kidney transplant recipients with known renal artery stenosis.

An issue that is unique to the solid organ transplant recipient is the management of chronic kidney disease due to calcineurin inhibitors. As noted previously, despite its many potential adverse effects, tacrolimus remains a first-line immunosuppressive medication. As time since a patient's transplant extends and the risk of acute rejection decreases, the goal tacrolimus level can be decreased, in turn decreasing some of the nephrotoxic effects of the medication. If the primary care provider identifies worsening chronic kidney disease, in addition to assessing for other causes, the transplant team should be contacted to discuss potential reduction in immunosuppressive medication and/or consultation with a nephrologist.

Due to immunosuppressive medications that block T-cell activity, solid organ transplant recipients have significant difficulty with clearing viral infections. As noted previously, BK virus and related nephropathy is commonly seen in renal transplant recipients. There is no targeted anti-viral therapy for BK virus; management is largely through reduction in the level of immunosuppression if possible.

Gout

Epidemiology

Hyperuricemia is common in solid organ transplant recipients, experienced in up to 84% and leading to clinical gout in as many as 28% [31]. Kidney and heart transplant recipients have a higher risk of developing gout than liver transplant recipients [31]. The reasoning behind this is unclear; factors could include variation in rates of post-transplant diuretic use and presence of other common comorbid conditions.

Pathophysiology

The calcineurin inhibitors (CNIs) cyclosporine and tacrolimus are known to cause hyperuricemia, which can lead to gout. The mechanism is hypothesized to be a combination of both decreased excretion and increased accumulation of uric acid due to the medication's effects on the kidney. Based on limited data, it appears that the risk of hyperuricemia is independent of drug trough levels [32], and cyclosporine may have an increased risk of new-onset gout after transplant compared to tacrolimus [33]. For example, in a study of patients followed after renal transplant, the 3-year cumulative incidence of a new diagnosis of clinical gout was 7.6%, with a higher risk on cyclosporine than tacrolimus (adjusted hazard ratio 1.24) [34].

In addition, other risk factors for gout are common in solid organ transplant recipients including chronic kidney disease and hypertension, again often related to calcineurin inhibitor therapy. In addition to CNIs, diuretics that are commonly used to treat hypertension further increase serum uric acid.

Screening/Surveillance

The American Society of Transplantation guidelines recommend checking serum uric acid levels once, 2–3 months post-transplant [34]. Additional routine surveillance may vary between transplant centers. Asymptomatic hyperuricemia is generally not treated pharmacologically but could result in dietary modifications and inform assessment of new symptoms such as joint pain in the future.

Treatment

The typical therapies used to treat acute gout flares in the general population include high-dose non-steroidal anti-inflammatory drugs (NSAIDs), colchicine, or prednisone, but there are special considerations for the treatment of acute gout flares in solid organ transplant recipients.

Oral prednisone or intra-articular corticosteroids are the treatment of choice for the treatment of acute gout flares in solid organ transplant recipients. Systemic prednisone should be used with caution if the patient has hypervolemia, poorly controlled diabetes, or a history of serious infectious complications. Furthermore, if the patient has had episodes of rejection treated with corticosteroids, or there is concern for ongoing rejection, then corticosteroids could make assessment of rejection more difficult. It is advised to contact the transplant team before giving systemic corticosteroids to a solid organ transplant recipient.

NSAIDs generally should be avoided in this population. Both NSAIDs and CNIs can cause renal impairment, in part secondary to afferent arteriole vasoconstriction. When they are taken in combination, the risk of kidney injury and complications of this such as hyperkalemia are heightened [33].

Colchicine use is also limited in most solid organ transplant recipients due to potentially dangerous drug interactions. Colchicine levels are increased, potentially to toxic levels, when used with strong CYP3A4 inhibitors or P-glycoprotein inhibitors, including CNIs and sirolimus. As a result, a significantly decreased dose is recommended if colchicine is used at all for patients on these immunosuppressive medications.

New additions to the acute gout treatment armamentarium are the urate oxidase medication rasburicase and the IL-1 inhibitor anakinra. Rasburicase is given by injection, with weight-based dosing. It acts by decreasing uric acid levels rather than by an anti-inflammatory effect like other medications used to treat acute gout. However, this class of medications has considerable cost and side effects, which include bronchospasm, urticaria, and with repeated use patients can develop neutralizing antibodies. Interleukin 1 inhibitors such as anakinra have also been used off-label for treatment of gout in solid organ transplant recipients [33], but these medications are not readily available, are expensive, and many providers have not had experience using them.

Prevention

Allopurinol and febuxostat are xanthine oxidase inhibitors that reduce uric acid production and in turn, reduce a patient's uric acid level and risk of gout. Allopurinol is the first-line therapy for prevention of symptomatic gout in most solid organ transplant recipients due to its efficacy and low cost. However, prescribers should be aware of a potentially dangerous interaction between allopurinol and azathioprine. Azathioprine, a purine synthesis inhibitor, is prescribed to some solid organ transplant recipients, typically in combination with a CNI and prednisone. Because it is also metabolized by xanthine oxidase, levels can become dangerously high and result in devastating side effects if prescribed in combination with allopurinol [33].

Febuxostat is the other currently available xanthine oxidase inhibitor. Similarly to allopurinol, it should not be used in combination with azathioprine. In addition, due to recent data indicating that febuxostat is associated with higher risk of both cardiovascular and all-cause mortality compared to allopurinol [35], it is considered a second-line medication.

Probenecid, which increases excretion of uric acid in the urine, is not recommended in solid organ transplant recipients with significant CKD and may have interactions with mycophenolate and cyclosporine. For these reasons, it is typically avoided [33].

Lifestyle and dietary modifications, including weight loss, reducing consumption of foods sweetened with high-fructose corn syrup, and reducing intake of alcohol and other high purine foods should also be recommended. In addition, it is important to review medications used to treat the patient's comorbid conditions. For example, thiazides and loop diuretics typically increase serum uric acid. When possible, patients with gout should have these medications substituted with losartan (see caution above regarding ARBs), which is uricosuric, or a calcium channel blocker, such as amlodipine, which can also result in a reduction in serum uric acid levels and reduced risk of gout [36].

For complex cases such as being unable to use standard medications, a rheumatologist familiar with transplant recipients should be consulted. Patients with urate nephropathy should have a nephrologist involved in their care.

Osteoporosis

Epidemiology

Osteoporosis is a frequent metabolic complication in solid organ transplant recipients, who have a fivefold increased risk compared to patients without a solid organ transplant [37]. The prevalence of osteoporotic fractures in solid organ transplant recipients has been reported to be as high as 65 percent [38], although it appears to be decreasing in recent years, perhaps due to greater awareness, prevention, and treatment. Lung transplant recipients appear to have a higher risk for osteoporosis than other solid organ transplant recipients, likely related to extensive exposure to glucocorticoids both pre- and post-transplant [37].

Pathophysiology

Solid organ transplant recipients often have both pre- and post-transplant risk factors for decreased bone mineral density. Pre-transplant risk factors include complications of the specific disease states leading to organ failure, e.g., altered bone mineral metabolism in patients with chronic kidney and liver disease and reduced calcium and vitamin D absorption in patients with cystic fibrosis, as well as general factors such as malnutrition, malabsorption, secondary hypogonadism, decreased weight-bearing exercise, low body weight, and exposure to alcohol or tobacco that are frequent in this population. Additionally, many transplant candidates have had extensive exposure to glucocorticoids prior to transplant [39].

The rate of bone loss appears to be greatest in the first 6–12 months after solid organ transplantation [40] and is related to both nonpharmacologic and pharmacologic insults. These include complications of surgery itself, such as acute and chronic kidney injury, as well as decreased mobility and nutrition in the event of extensive post-surgical hospitalization and lengthy rehabilitation courses. However, the most dominant post-transplant risk factor for osteoporosis is the medication used for immunosuppression. Glucocorticoids, which rapidly decrease bone density in doses as low as prednisone 2.5 mg per day [41] by directly inhibiting osteoblast bone building activity and stimulating osteoclast bone resorptive activity, are often used in high doses during the first 6 months after transplant. Calcineurin inhibitors (CNIs) including cyclosporine and tacrolimus have also been shown to decrease bone density in animal models by stimulating osteoclast bone resorptive activity [42], although clarifying this risk has been more challenging to study in solid organ transplant recipients who often receive glucocorticoids in combination with CNIs. Additionally, CNIs often cause kidney injury that further adversely impacts bone metabolism.

The rate of bone density loss appears to slow after the first post-transplant year, likely due to decreased immunosuppressive medication dosing as well as improved mobility and nutritional status.

Screening

Most professional transplant society guidelines and transplant experts do recommend screening for osteoporosis, prevalent fractures, and low serum 25-hydroxy vitamin D as part of the pre-transplant evaluation to help guide prevention of further bone density loss and fractures in the peri- and post-transplant period (see Table 11.6). Similarly, society guidelines also recommend regular surveillance bone mineral density (BMD) evaluation with dual-energy X-ray absorptiometry (DXA), with frequency varying based on type of transplant, immunosuppressant pharmacologic regimen, and baseline BMD (see Table 11.6 for details).

Prevention

As with other patients at risk for osteoporosis, solid organ transplant recipients should be counseled on lifestyle measures to decrease the rate of BMD decline and fall risk including avoiding tobacco, limiting alcohol, and engaging in regular

Table 11.6 Major transplant society guidelines for osteoporosis screening and prophylaxis

Society	Pre-transplant screening	Post-transplant screening	Calcium and Vitamin D supplementation, daily	Prophylactic anti-resorptive therapy	Comments
ISHLT	Baseline DXA Consider spine X-rays to evaluate for prevalent vertebral fractures	DXA 1 year post-transplant Repeat DXA every 3 years if normal; or every 2 years if osteopenia present	Calcium 1000–1500 mg Vitamin D 400–1000 IU as needed to main serum 25-OH-D level >30 ng/mL	Recommended for all heart transplant patients through the first post-transplant year	Bisphosphonates are first line; followed by calcitriol or estrogen/progesterone in hypogonadal women. Consider stopping anti-resorptive therapy if corticosteroids have stopped and T score >−1.5
AASLD	N/A	DXA every 2–3 years if BMD normal; or yearly if osteopenia present, for the first 5 years post-transplant. Individualize screening beyond 5 years post-transplant	Calcium 1000–1200 mg Vitamin D 400–1000 IU as needed to main serum 25-OH-D level >30 ng/mL	Consider if T score <−2.5 or history of pathologic fracture OR T score −1.5 to −2.5 and other osteoporosis risk factors present	
KDIGO	N/A	DXA in patients with eGFR >30 mL/min /1.73 m² within 3 months of transplant if receiving corticosteroids or have osteoporosis risk factors. Routine screening not recommended if eGFR <30 mL/min/1.73 m² post-transplant	Vitamin D 400–1000 IU as needed to main serum 25-OH-D level >30 ng/mL	Consider within first year post-transplant if eGFR >30 mL/min/1.73 m² and low bone mineral density	Consider a bone biopsy to guide treatment of osteoporosis, particularly prior to bisphosphonate use. Frequently monitor serum calcium, phosphorus, PTH, alkaline phosphatase, and 25-OH-vitamin D

ISHLT International Society for Heart and Lung Transplantation [43], *AASLD* American Association for the Study of Liver Diseases [44], *KDIGO* Kidney Disease Improving Global Outcomes [45], *DXA* dual-energy X-ray absorptiometry, *BMD* bone mineral density weight-bearing activity. Additionally, professional transplant society guidelines recommend that all solid organ transplant recipients take adequate calcium (1000–1200 mg daily through diet and supplements) and vitamin D (400–1000 IU daily or higher if needed to achieve serum 25-OH vitamin D levels >30 ng/mL) [43–45]. However, the various societies differ in their recommendations for who should receive prophylactic anti-resorptive therapy (see Table 11.6). The International Society for Heart and Lung Transplantation (ISHLT) takes the most aggressive approach, recommending that all heart transplant recipients take anti-resorptive medication during the first post-transplant year [43]. This recommendation is based on data showing the rate of bone loss and fracture risk are highest in the first year following transplant [40]. For kidney transplant recipients, prophylactic and treatment considerations are more nuanced as BMD does not reliably predict fracture risk or type of bone disease in this population [45]. Kidney transplant practice guidelines recommend frequent monitoring of serum calcium, phosphorus, PTH, and 25-OH vitamin D as well as consideration of bone biopsy prior to bisphosphonate use to inform mechanism of low bone mineral density and optimal treatment [45].

Treatment

Osteoporosis-specific medical therapy is recommended for solid organ transplant recipients with either pre- or post-transplantation osteoporosis, defined as either a T score <−2.5 or a history of an osteoporotic (fragility) fracture [39]. All solid organ transplant recipients being treated for osteoporosis should also take adequate calcium (1000–1200 mg daily in divided doses, either through diet or supplement) and vitamin D (400–1000 IU daily; or sufficient to maintain serum 25-hydroxy vitamin D levels above 30 ng/mL) [39]. Modifiable risk factors such as alcohol use and smoking should be addressed.

Similar to the general population, bisphosphonates are the most commonly used first-line osteoporosis treatment agents for solid organ transplant recipients who do not have contraindications such as advanced kidney disease (eGFR <30 mL/min/1.73m^2), high-risk dental disease, or, for oral bisphosphonates, dysphagia. This practice is based primarily on multiple prevention-focused trials that demonstrated decreased rates of bone loss, increasing bone mineral density, and/or decreased fractures in SOT recipients treated with bisphosphonates for the first year after transplant [46]. 25-hydroxy vitamin D levels should be checked and repleted if found to be low prior to starting bisphosphonate therapy.

As per above, the evaluation and treatment of osteoporosis in kidney transplant recipients is more nuanced given the high prevalence of adynamic bone disease related to longstanding kidney disease. In this population, KDIGO recommends consideration of bone biopsy prior to initiating bisphosphonates [45]. Caution should also be taken in premenopausal female solid organ transplant recipients with preserved fertility as bisphosphonates are contraindicated in pregnancy.

Second-line evidence-based options to treat osteoporosis in solid organ transplant recipients who are not candidates for bisphosphonates include calcitriol, estrogen/progesterone in hypogonadal premenopausal women, or testosterone therapy in hypogonadal men. Calcitriol has been shown to reduce rate of bone loss and prevent fractures in solid organ transplant recipients [46]. If calcitriol is used, it is important to monitor for hypercalcemia regularly; either stop calcium supplements or reduce or stop the calcitriol if the hypercalcemia persists.

Other agents that are FDA approved for the treatment of osteoporosis and are considered second line ahead of calcitriol and sex hormonal therapy in the general population, including teriparatide, abaloparatide, and denosumab, unfortunately have not yet been well studied for use in solid organ transplant recipients, and are therefore not recommended for routine use in primary care.

In general, in patients who do not tolerate or have contraindications to bisphosphonate therapy, the primary care provider should consider consultation with an endocrinologist or metabolic bone disease specialist familiar with the care of transplant recipients to optimize therapy.

There are not consensus guidelines on duration of treatment with osteoporosis-specific medications in solid organ transplant recipients. Experts recommend individualized management, with regular (every 1–2 year) surveillance DXA and consideration of changes in the immunosuppressive regimen, other osteoporosis risk factors, incident fractures, and response to therapy to guide management.

Conclusion

As the solid organ transplant recipient population both increases and ages, it is key for primary care providers to become familiar with common metabolic complications that occur in these patients. A general understanding of the pathophysiology of these complications, some of which are unique to transplant recipients and some of which overlap with the general population, as well as specific nuances in their treatment, will aid primary care providers in continuing to promote longevity and quality of life of their patients long after transplantation.

References

1. Sen A, Callisen H, Libricz S, Patel B. Complications of solid organ transplantation: cardiovascular, neurologic, renal, and gastrointestinal. Crit Care Clin. 2019;35(1):169–86.
2. Ghanta M, Kozicky M, Jim B. Pathophysiologic and treatment strategies for cardiovascular disease in end-stage renal disease and kidney transplantations. Cardiol Rev. 2015;23(3):109–18.
3. Konerman MA, Fritze D, Weinberg RL, Sonnenday CJ, Sharma P. Incidence of and risk assessment for adverse cardiovascular outcomes after liver transplantation: a systematic review. Transplantation. 2017;101(7):1645–57. https://doi.org/10.1097/TP.0000000000001710.

4. Gallegos-Orozco JF, Charlton MR. Predictors of cardiovascular events after liver transplantation. Clin Liver Dis. 2017;21(2):367–79.
5. Lund LH, Edwards LB, Kucheryavaya AY, Dipchand AI, Benden C, Christie JD, Dobbels F, Kirk R, Rahmel AO, Yusen RD, Stehlik J, International Society for Heart and Lung Transplantation. The Registry of the International Society for Heart and Lung Transplantation: thirtieth official adult heart transplant report--2013; focus theme: age. J Heart Lung Transplant. 2013;32(10):951–64. https://doi.org/10.1016/j.healun.2013.08.006.
6. Silverborn M, Jeppsson A, Mårtensson G, Nilsson F. New-onset cardiovascular risk factors in lung transplant recipients. J Heart Lung Transplant. 2005;24:1536–43.
7. Christie JD, Edwards LB, Aurora P, et al. Registry of the International Society for Heart and Lung Transplantation: 25th official adult lung and heart/lung transplant report – 2008. J Heart Lung Transplant. 2008;27(9):957–69.
8. Alhaj E, Alhaj N, Rahman I, et al. Uremic cardiomyopathy: an underdiagnosed disease. Congest Heart Fail. 2013;19:E40–5.
9. McCartney SL, Patel C, Del Rio JM. Long-term outcomes and management of the heart transplant recipient. Best Pract Res Clin Anaesthesiol. 2017;31(2):237–48.
10. Munagala MR, Phancao A. Managing cardiovascular risk in the post solid organ transplant recipient. Med Clin North Am. 2016;100(3):519–33.
11. Wei L, MacDonald TM, Walker BR. Taking glucocorticoids by prescription is associated with subsequent cardiovascular disease. Ann Intern Med. 2004;141(10):764–70.
12. Knoll GA, Kokolo MB, Mallick R, Beck A, Buenaventura CD, Ducharme R, et al. Effect of sirolimus on malignancy and survival after kidney transplantation: systematic review and meta-analysis of individual patient data. BMJ. 2014;349:g6679.
13. Kidney Disease: Improving Global Outcomes Transplant Work Group. KDIGO clinical practice guideline for the care of kidney transplant recipients. Am J Transplant. 2009;9(Suppl 3):S1–155.
14. Cross NB, Webster AC, Masson P, O'Connell PJ, Craig JC. Antihypertensive treatment for kidney transplant recipients. Cochrane Database Syst Rev. 2009;3:CD003598.
15. Paoletti E, Bellino D, Marsano L, Cassottana P, Rolla D, Ratto E. Effects of ACE inhibitors on long-term outcome of renal transplant recipients: a randomized controlled trial. Transplantation. 2013;95(6):889–95.
16. Kato T, Tokoro T, Namii Y, Kobayashi T, Hayashi S, Yokoyama I, et al. Early introduction of HMG-CoA reductase inhibitors could prevent the incidence of transplant coronary artery disease. Transplant Proc. 2000;32(2):331–3.
17. Arnett DK, Blumenthal RS, Albert MA, Buroker AB, Goldberger ZD, Hahn EJ, Himmelfarb CD, Khera A, Lloyd-Jones D, McEvoy JW, Michos ED, Miedema MD, Muñoz D, Smith SCJ, Virani SS, Williams KA Sr, Yeboah J, Ziaeian B. 2019 ACC/AHA guideline on the primary prevention of cardiovascular disease: a report of the American College of Cardiology/American Heart Association Task Force on Clinical Practice Guidelines. Circulation. 2019;140(11):e596–646. https://doi.org/10.1161/CIR.0000000000000678.
18. Dad T, Tighiouart H, Joseph A, Bostom A, Carpenter M, Hunsicker L, et al. Aspirin use and incident cardiovascular disease, kidney failure, and death in stable kidney transplant recipients: a post hoc analysis of the folic acid for vascular outcome reduction in transplantation (FAVORIT) trial. Am J Kidney Dis. 2016;68(2):277–86.
19. Gaston RS, Kasiske BL, Fieberg AM, Leduc R, Cosio FC, Gourishankar S, Halloran P, Hunsicker L, Rush D, Matas AJ. Use of cardioprotective medications in kidney transplant recipients. Am J Transplant. 2009;9:1811–5.
20. Haddad EM, McAlister VC, Renouf E, Malthaner R, Kjaer MS, Gluud LL. Cyclosporin versus tacrolimus for liver transplanted patients. Cochrane Database Syst Rev. 2006;4:CD005161.
21. Wilkinson A, Davidson J, Dotta F, Home PD, Keown P, Kiberd B, et al. Guidelines for the treatment and management of new-onset diabetes after transplantation. Clin Transpl. 2005;19(3):291–8.
22. Pham PT, Pham PM, Pham SV, Pham PA, Pham PC. New onset diabetes after transplantation (NODAT): an overview. Diabetes Metab Syndr Obes. 2011;4:175–86.

23. Shah T, Kasravi A, Huang E, Hayashi R, Young B, Cho YW, et al. Risk factors for development of new-onset diabetes mellitus after kidney transplantation. Transplantation. 2006;82(12):1673–6.
24. Luan FL, Steffick DE, Ojo AO. New-onset diabetes mellitus in kidney transplant recipients discharged on steroid-free immunosuppression. Transplantation. 2011;91(3):334–41.
25. Chakkera HA, Kudva Y, Kaplan B. Calcineurin inhibitors: pharmacologic mechanisms impacting both insulin resistance and insulin secretion leading to glucose dysregulation and diabetes mellitus. Clin Pharmacol Ther. 2017;101(1):114–20.
26. Ojo AO, Held PJ, Port FK, Wolfe RA, Leichtman AB, Young EW, et al. Chronic renal failure after transplantation of a nonrenal organ. N Engl J Med. 2003;349(10):931–40.
27. O'Riordan A, Wong V, McCormick PA, Hegarty JE, Watson AJ. Chronic kidney disease post-liver transplantation. Nephrol Dial Transplant. 2006;21(9):2630–6.
28. Voora S, Adey DB. Management of kidney transplant recipients by general nephrologists: core curriculum 2019. Am J Kidney Dis. 2019;73(6):866–79.
29. Sawinski D, Trofe-Clark J. BK virus nephropathy. Clin J Am Soc Nephrol. 2018;13(12): 1893–6.
30. Hirsch HH, Randhawa P, AST Infectious Diseases Community of Practice. BK polyomavirus in solid organ transplantation. Am J Transplant. 2013;13(Suppl 4):179–88. https://doi.org/10.1111/ajt.12110.
31. Stamp L, Searle M, O'Donnell J, Chapman P. Gout in solid organ transplantation: a challenging clinical problem. Drugs. 2005;65(18):2593–611.
32. Abdelrahman M, Rafi A, Ghacha R, Youmbissi JT, Qayyum T, Karkar A. Hyperuricemia and gout in renal transplant recipients. Ren Fail. 2002;24(3):361–7.
33. Sullivan PM, William A, Tichy EM. Hyperuricemia and gout in solid-organ transplant: update in pharmacological management. Prog Transplant. 2015;25(3):263–70.
34. Abbott K, Kimmel P, Dharnidharka V, et al. New-onset gout after kidney transplantation: incidence, risk factors and implications. Transplantation. 2005;80(10):1383–91.
35. https://www.fda.gov/drugs/drug-safety-and-availability/fda-adds-boxed-warning-increased-risk-death-gout-medicine-uloric-febuxostat. Accessed 12/4/2019.
36. Choi HK, Soriano LC, Zhang Y, Rodriguez LA. Antihypertensive drugs and risk of incident gout among patients with hypertension: population based case-control study. BMJ. 2012;344: d8190.
37. Yu TM, Lin CL, Chang SN, Sung FC, Huang ST, Kao CH. Osteoporosis and fractures after solid organ transplantation: a nationwide population-based cohort study. Mayo Clin Proc. 2014;89(7):888–95.
38. Cohen A, Shane E. Osteoporosis after solid organ and bone marrow transplantation. Osteoporos Int. 2003;14(8):617–30.
39. Early C, Stuckey L, Tischer S. Osteoporosis in the adult solid organ transplant population: underlying mechanisms and available treatment options. Osteoporos Int. 2016;27(4): 1425–40.
40. Kulak CA, Cochenski Borba VZ, Kulak J, Ribeiro CM. Osteoporosis after solid organ transplantation. Minerva Endocrinol. 2012;37(3):221–31.
41. van Staa TP, Leufkens HG, Cooper C. The epidemiology of corticosteroid-induced osteoporosis: a meta-analysis. Osteoporos Int. 2002;13(10):777–87.
42. Movsowitz C, Epstein S, Fallon M, Ismail F, Thomas S. Cyclosporin-a in vivo produces severe osteopenia in the rat: effect of dose and duration of administration. Endocrinology. 1988;123(5):2571–7.
43. Costanzo MR, Dipchand A, Starling R, Anderson A, Chan M, Desai S, et al. The International Society of Heart and Lung Transplantation Guidelines for the care of heart transplant recipients. J Heart Lung Transplant. 2010;29(8):914–56.
44. Lucey MR, Terrault N, Ojo L, Hay JE, Neuberger J, Blumberg E, et al. Long-term management of the successful adult liver transplant: 2012 practice guideline by the American Association for the Study of Liver Diseases and the American Society of Transplantation. Liver Transpl. 2013;19(1):3–26.

45. Kasiske BL, Zeier MG, Chapman JR, Craig JC, Ekberg H, Garvey CA, et al. KDIGO clinical practice guideline for the care of kidney transplant recipients: a summary. Kidney Int. 2010;77(4):299–311.
46. Stein EM, Ortiz D, Jin Z, McMahon DJ, Shane E. Prevention of fractures after solid organ transplantation: a meta-analysis. J Clin Endocrinol Metab. 2011;96(11):3457–65.

Chapter 12
Preventive Health in the Adult Solid Organ Transplant Recipient

Leah M. Marcotte and Heidi Powell

Cancer Screening in Solid Organ Transplant Recipients

Cancer is one of the leading causes of death in solid organ transplant recipients, in addition to cardiovascular disease and infections. Overall, solid organ transplant recipients have a twofold increased incidence of all types of cancers and a three- to fivefold increased rate of cancer mortality, as compared with respective rates in the general population. The most extensive cohort study involving 175,732 solid organ transplant recipients (58.4% kidney, 21.6% liver, 10% heart, and 4% lung) in the United States showed a cancer standardized incidence ratio of 2.1 [1]. The risk was increased for a total of 32 different malignancies. The cancers with the highest risk relative to the general population included Kaposi sarcoma (KS); non-Hodgkin lymphoma; and lip, nonmelanoma skin, liver, vulvar, and anal cancers. Immunosuppression is associated with an increased incidence in HPV-related cancers (vulva, vagina, cervix, anus) [2]. Skin cancers are the most frequent malignancy seen in the solid organ transplant population, accounting for more than 40% of post-transplant malignancies [3].

The risk of specific malignancies varies according to the organ transplanted. Lung transplant recipients have a twofold increase in non-Hodgkin lymphoma compared to other solid transplant recipients [1]. Lung cancer is more common in lung and heart transplant recipients than in kidney or liver recipients. Liver and kidney cancers are more common in liver and kidney transplant recipients, respectively. Solid organ transplant recipients with primary sclerosing cholangitis are at increased risk for colorectal cancer and those with alcoholic liver disease are at increased risk for esophageal and head/neck cancers compared with patients undergoing lung transplants for other indications [4].

L. M. Marcotte (✉) · H. Powell
Division of General Internal Medicine, Department of Medicine, University of Washington, Seattle, WA, USA
e-mail: leahmar@uw.edu; powell@uw.edu

© Springer Nature Switzerland AG 2020
C. J. Wong (ed.), *Primary Care of the Solid Organ Transplant Recipient*,
https://doi.org/10.1007/978-3-030-50629-2_12

Risk factors for cancer in solid organ transplant recipients include immunosuppression, oncogenic viruses, and disease-specific associations. Traditional risk factors such as tobacco use, sun exposure, and history of cancer also are important. Donor-derived malignancy rarely occurs.

Cancers in solid organ transplant recipients are more advanced at diagnosis, more aggressive and difficult to treat, and have worse outcomes than the general population [5]. Unfortunately, the optimal screening strategy remains uncertain as randomized controlled cancer screening trials have not been performed in the solid organ transplant population. Furthermore, screening trials that might improve outcomes are unlikely to be conducted since solid organ transplant recipients are relatively few in number compared to the general population.

A systematic review of 12 clinical practice guidelines for adult solid organ transplant recipients found that although most of the guidelines made recommendations for cancer screening, they varied considerably by transplanted organ, were largely based on expert opinion, and were derived primarily from cancer screening guidelines for the general population [6]. However, screening for two types of cancer, cervical and skin, in solid organ transplant recipients deserves further discussion.

Cervical Cancer Screening

Recommendations for cervical cancer screening among non-HIV immunosuppressed women remain limited because of lack of quality studies. The 2018 US Preventive Services Task Force guidelines on cervical cancer screening did not include recommendations for solid organ transplant recipients. In the review of clinical practice guideline recommendations for solid organ transplant recipients, eight of twelve guidelines recommended cervical cancer screening but with varying screening intervals: two recommended screening every 3 years, five recommended annual screening, and one recommended screening every 3–5 years [6].

A panel of cervical cancer researchers concluded that there is a consistent increase in the risk of cervical neoplasia and invasive cervical cancer in kidney, heart/lung, liver, and pancreas transplant recipients, and that using the CDC cervical cancer screening guidelines for HIV-infected women was a reasonable approach for screening and surveillance in the solid organ transplant population [7]. Cervical cancer screening recommendations among HIV-infected women have been supported by evidence from retrospective and prospective studies. The purpose of more frequent screening in high risk populations is to identify low-grade lesions before progression to high-grade squamous intraepithelial lesions or carcinoma. The recommendations are as follows: [7]

1. Women under age 30 should undergo annual cytology tests (i.e., Papanicolaou smear test), and if results of three consecutive cytology tests are normal, then subsequent cytology can be done every 3 years.
2. Women of age 30 and older have two screening options:

    (a) Annual cytology, and if three consecutive tests are normal, then repeat test-
        ing can be done every 3 years

    (b) Cytology and HPV co-testing at baseline, and if both are normal, then repeat
        co-testing can be done every 3 years

3. Continue screening throughout lifetime (do not stop at age 65 even if normal prior
    testing)

The American Society of Transplantation recommends more frequent screening using Pap testing every 6 months for the first year, then annually indefinitely if first tests are negative. These guidelines provide the option of high-risk HPV testing to determine if more frequent testing is indicated. They also recommend considering increasing the frequency back to every 6 months if a patient has been treated for rejection, necessitating an increased level of immunosuppression [8].The direct effect of specific immunosuppressants on gynecologic cancers is not well studied and data is conflicting. Risk factors for developing squamous cell HPV-related cancers of the cervix, vulva, and vagina include multiple sexual partners or male partners with multiple sexual partners, current tobacco use, and infection with other sexually transmitted diseases. Cervical cancer screening (test, type, and frequency) should be discussed with the patient after reviewing the potential benefit, risks of harms, and their personal preferences. The decision to stop screening should be made based on co-morbidities, life expectancy, and personal factors.

Skin Cancer Screening

Nonmelanoma skin cancers are among the most common of all malignancies in solid organ transplant recipients. The risk of cutaneous squamous cell carcinoma (SCC) is 65 times that of the general population and the risk is threefold for malignant melanoma (MM) [3]. Risk factors include male gender, fair skin, sun exposure, geographic location, history of previous nonmelanoma skin cancer, age 50 years or older at the time of transplant, a recipient of a thoracic organ, and having a longer time elapsed since transplant [3].

Squamous cell cancers tend to develop at a younger age, are more aggressive, and metastasize more often [9]. Primary care providers should have a low threshold to biopsy any suspicious lesion and aggressively treat actinic keratoses or other precancerous lesions. Patients should be advised to seek evaluation for any new skin lesion as soon as it is noticed, minimize sun exposure, and always use sunscreen and wear hats. Most clinical practice guidelines for solid organ transplant recipients recommend annual skin and lip cancer screening by either a primary care physician or dermatologist [6]. These recommendations are in contrast to those of the US Preventive Services Task Force for the general population, which cite insufficient evidence to recommend for or against skin cancer screening [10].

A diagnosis of cutaneous SCC is associated with a higher risk of subsequently developing a non-cutaneous SCC [9]. These include cancers of the oral cavity/pharynx, lip, tongue, lung, and HPV- related cancers (anal and female genital cancers). Therefore, it is important for primary care providers to be diligent in evaluating any new symptoms that arise in these areas if a solid organ transplant recipient has a history of SCC.

Adherence to Cancer Screening in Solid Organ Transplant Recipients

Adherence to cancer screening has not been well studied in solid organ transplant recipients but a large study in Canada suggests that adherence is very low [11]. A population cohort was studied between 1997 and 2010 to determine the uptake of breast, cervical, and colorectal cancer screening. They found that 4436 were eligible for colorectal screening, 2252 for cervical cancer screening, and 1551 for breast cancer screening. Of those, 77.5%, 69.8%, and 91.4%, respectively, were not up to date in cancer screening tests during the observed period. More surprisingly, greater than 30% had not been screened at all during the study period for colorectal, cervical, and breast cancer. The screening rates were lower than in the general population. The reason for these low screening rates is not clear but it does suggest that there is room for significant improvement and better communication between transplant specialists and primary care providers in the routine care of these patients.

Table 12.1 summarizes cancer screening in solid organ transplant recipients. See also Chap. 10 for further discussion.

Risk of Cardiovascular Disease and Diabetes

Solid organ transplant recipients are at increased risk for cardiovascular disease (CVD), and in many solid organ transplant populations, cardiovascular disease is a leading cause of non-graft related death [12, 13]. In a review of managing CVD risk [14], the authors categorized risk factors into four categories: pre-transplant risk factors (including usual risk factors, e.g., obesity, hyperlipidemia, diabetes, and smoking), transplant-related risk factors (e.g., immunosuppression, graft dysfunction, rejection, and anemia), donor risk factors (smoking, age of donor, quality of organ donated, ischemic time prior to transplantation), and other risk factors (e.g., increased C-reactive protein, prothrombosis, and proteinuria). Although transplant-related and donor risk factors are generally not modifiable, it is important to consider these non-traditional factors in solid organ transplant recipients so as not to misjudge CVD risk. For example, as a result of unique risk factors related to solid organ transplant, traditional risk models such as the Framingham Heart Study risk score, tend to underestimate CVD risk in solid organ transplant recipients [15].

Table 12.1 Cancer screening in solid organ transplant recipients

Cancer risk	Risk factors	Modified screening recommendations[a]

Overall >2× general population
 	
Most common:
Nonmelanoma skin cancer
	Type of transplant: Lung transplant > other transplants
	
	Immunosuppression (esp. calcineurin inhibitors)
		Cervical cancer screening:[b]
		Women < age 30:
		  Annual cytology
		  If 3 consecutive cytology tests are normal, then repeat every 3 years

Others at increased frequency:
 	
Kaposi sarcoma (KS)
 	
Liver cancer (esp. in liver transplant recipients)
 	
Lung cancer (esp. in lung transplant recipients)
 	
Kidney and urothelial cancer (esp. in kidney transplant recipients)
 	
HPV-associated: Cervical, vulvar, penile, anal, oral squamous cell carcinomas
 	
Post-transplant lymphoproliferative disorder (PTLD)/non-Hodgkin lymphoma
 	
Colorectal cancer
 	
Head and neck cancer
 	
Thyroid cancer
	Exposures:
	
	Smoking
	
	Alcohol (both pre- and post-transplant)
	
	EBV serostatus
	
	HPV infection
		Women ≥ age 30:
		  Annual cytology; if 3 consecutive tests are normal, then repeat testing every 3 years;
		Or
		  Cytology and HPV co-testing at baseline; if both normal, then repeat co-testing every 3 years
		Note some guidelines recommend cytology testing every 6 month for the first year post-transplant, then yearly if testing is negative
		Continue after age 65 if indicated
		Skin cancer screening:
		Annual skin exam

[a]Screening for cancers not listed here is similar to the general population
[b]See text for details; guidelines vary. Shown are recommendations similar to cervical cancer screening for patients with HIV

As multiple non-traditional and often non-modifiable factors contribute to solid organ transplant recipients' overall CVD risk, it is important to identify and manage modifiable risk factors such as hypertension, hyperlipidemia, obesity, and diabetes in primary care. Even adjusting for transplant-specific risk factors, solid organ transplant recipients are at increased risk for the usual risk factors above [14].

Transplant medications can lead to multiple side effects, increasing the risk for hypertension, diabetes, and cardiovascular disease. Calcineurin inhibitors are associated with increased risk of hypertension, diabetes, hyperlipidemia, hypomagnesemia, and hyperuricemia [16]. Corticosteroids are associated with increased risk of hypertension, diabetes, and increased weight. (Also see Chap. 3)

Given the frequency of routine lab testing and office visits for solid organ transplant recipients driven by transplant specialists, much of the data needed for screening for these conditions will be ordered by the transplant team and can be reviewed in primary care as well. However, the primary care provider should ensure that blood pressure is monitored at each visit, lipids are measured, and diabetes is screened for annually. Counseling patients on the benefits of regular exercise and maintaining a healthy diet is very important.

Recommendations for assessment of cardiovascular risk and diabetes at outpatient clinic visits are shown in Table 12.2. Management of cardiovascular risk factors, including the use of aspirin and statins for primary prevention, and treatment of hypertension and dyslipidemia are addressed in Chap. 11.

Metabolic Bone Disease

Solid organ transplant recipients are at significantly increased risk for osteoporosis. Osteoporosis risk includes preexisting factors (e.g., smoking, prednisone use, poor nutrition, and vitamin D deficiency) as well as transplant-specific factors, specifically corticosteroids and possibly calcineurin inhibitors [17]. This risk is particularly increased within the first 6–12 months of organ transplantation coinciding with higher doses of corticosteroids.

Table 12.2 Routine outpatient assessment of cardiovascular risk and diabetes in solid organ transplant recipients

History
Review risk factors including:
Smoking
Exercise
Nutrition
Body-mass index
Exam
Blood pressure, height, weight
Cardiopulmonary exam
Laboratory
Often ordered routinely by the transplant team
Diabetes screening every 3 months for the first year, then yearly if normal
Lipid panel annually if normal
Other testing
Heart transplant recipients: review surveillance for cardiac allograft vasculopathy
Risk stratification
Existing risk tools may underestimate risk in solid organ transplant recipients
Chemoprevention (see Chap. 11)
Aspirin used in all heart transplant recipients; variable use in kidney transplant recipients
Statin therapy used in all heart transplant recipients; commonly used in kidney transplant recipients

All Solid Organ Transplant Recipients—History

At outpatient visits, the primary care provider should assess risk factors:

- Smoking status: Active smoking is a contraindication to lung transplantation, and strongly discouraged prior to other solid organ transplants. Patients should be asked about whether they have started or resumed tobacco use after transplantation.
- Alcohol use: Alcohol use has been most studied in liver transplant recipients who had alcoholic cirrhosis and subsequently return to using alcohol after transplantation. In addition to other health risks, alcohol is associated with osteoporosis [18].
- Weight-bearing exercise: Solid organ transplant recipients should be counseled to maintain weight-bearing exercise, unless contraindicated by their medical conditions.
- Medications: Corticosteroid use is typically lowered over time, and in lower risk transplants (e.g., liver), it often can be discontinued completely. However, patients may be treated with higher doses of corticosteroids for longer periods of time, or indefinitely, if they have had episodes of rejection or other indications for use. Increased exposure to corticosteroids may merit more frequent bone mineral density testing. Other medications not related to transplantation should be reviewed for risk of lowering bone density (e.g., depot medroxyprogesterone for contraception, certain anti-epileptic medications, high-dose acid-suppressive medications, and thiazolidinediones for diabetes).
- Malabsorption: Some solid organ transplant recipients have continued risk factors for malabsorption. For example, a lung transplant recipient for cystic fibrosis may continue to have significant gastrointestinal disease, or a liver transplant recipient for primary sclerosing cholangitis may have ongoing inflammatory bowel disease symptoms after transplantation. Mycophenolate therapy commonly causes mild to moderate diarrhea, but rarely it can cause an enterocolitis with malabsorption.
- Nutrition and body weight: Many solid organ transplant recipients have difficulty maintaining body weight prior to transplantation due to cachexia from their organ failure. After transplantation, they should be monitored closely for maintenance of normal body weight.
- Family history: Although nonmodifiable, the patient's family history of fracture should be reviewed.
- Personal history: Patients should be asked about a prior history of fracture. When the solid organ transplant recipient presents for an initial primary care visit, it is advisable to review the pre-transplant workup, as most transplant recipients will have received bone mineral density testing prior to transplantation (see Chap. 2).

Screening Tests and Preventive Therapy

While guidelines for average risk adults recommend screening dual-energy X-ray absorptiometry (DXA) to assess bone density for women starting at age 65 years, and continuing interval screening depending on baseline risk [19], in general, all solid organ transplant recipients should be screened with DXA scans within the first-year post-transplant. Following initial screening, guidelines vary with regard to suggested interval screening depending on risk factors and which organ is transplanted (Table 12.3).

- Liver transplant recipients: The 2012 American Association for the Study of Liver Diseases (AASLD) and American Society of Transplantation (AST) guidelines [13] recommend continuing screening every 2–3 years for liver transplant recipients without osteopenia and annually if osteopenia is present for the first 5 years following transplant. The AASLD and AST guidelines also recommend all post-liver transplant patients with or at risk for osteopenia take 1000–1200 mg daily calcium supplementation, maintain vitamin D levels above 30 ng/mL, and engage in regular, weight-bearing exercise.
- Heart transplant recipients: Heart transplant practice guidelines [20] recommend screening with a DXA scan as part of the pre-transplant workup with evaluation and treatment of osteoporosis as appropriate prior to transplant. All adult heart transplant recipients are recommended bisphosphonate therapy in the first year after transplant in addition to calcium and vitamin D supplementation and regular, weight-bearing exercise. Following the first year post-transplant, if corticosteroids are discontinued, continuation of bisphosphonate therapy is to be determined based on clinical risk; for example, if BMD > −1.5, guidelines suggest that it is reasonable to stop treatment. These recommendations were mainly based on expert opinion with authors citing insufficient evidence for bisphosphonate therapy in heart transplant patients. A subsequent meta-analysis, however, including 425 heart transplant patients did find efficacy of bisphosphonate therapy in reducing vertebral bone loss without additional medication-associated adverse events; given limitations of data, fracture prevention was not formally evaluated [21].
- Kidney transplant recipients: The risk of osteoporosis in kidney transplant recipients is higher, and screening and treatment are more complicated than in other organ transplant populations due to preexisting metabolic bone disease associated with end-stage renal disease. The fracture risk after renal transplant is estimated to be almost four times higher than that of the general population [22]. Age, female gender, and duration of pre-transplant dialysis increased the risk of hip fracture [22]. Similar to other solid organ transplant recipients, kidney transplant recipients have the most rapid decrease of bone density within the first 6–12 months after transplant. However, unlike other solid organ transplant recipients whose risk of osteoporosis decreases thereafter, the risk in kidney transplant recipients persistently increases at a slower rate following the first year after transplant [23].

Table 12.3 Screening for osteoporosis in solid organ transplant recipients

	Osteoporosis incidence	Screening recommendations	Prevention recommendations
Lung	Common pre-transplant: [26] Osteopenia 36% Osteoporosis 31% At 1-year post-transplant: [26] Osteopenia: 33% Osteoporosis: 40% Osteoporotic fracture rate post-transplant: 19–225 per 1000 person-years [27, 28] (note: Limited data, few studies)	No consensus guideline recommendations Some authors recommend: [29] Baseline DXA (time not specified, most would assess within first year) Osteopenia: Repeat DXA every 2–3 years Osteoporosis: Treat and measure annually	No consensus guideline recommendations Some authors recommend: [29] Calcium 1000–1500 mg/d Vitamin D 400–800 IU/d
Heart*	Osteoporosis 13% pre-transplant [30] Vertebral fractures: 21% at 1-year post-transplant [30] Total osteoporotic fractures: 36% at 1-year-post-transplant [31]	DXA 1-year post-transplant. Normal BMD: Repeat DXA every 3 years Osteopenia: Repeat DXA every 2 years (IIa/C)	Bisphosphonate therapy in first year post-transplant (IB), afterward depending on risk Calcium 1000–1500 mg/d (IC) Cholecalciferol 400–1000 IU/d to maintain 25(OH) vitamin D > 30 ng/mL (IC) Regular weight-bearing exercise (IB)
Liver**	Common pre- and post-transplant At 1-year post-transplant: [32] Osteopenia 39% Osteoporosis: 44%	For the first 5 years after transplant: Osteopenia: Repeat DXA yearly Normal BMD: Repeat DXA every 2–3 years DXA (2B) [13]	If osteopenia or at risk of osteopenia: Calcium 1000–1200 mg/d Maintain 25(OH) vitamin D > 30 ng/mL Regular weight-bearing exercise (1A) [13]
Kidney***	Hip fracture rate: 3.3 per 1000 person-years [22] All fractures: 22.5% within 5-year post-transplant [33]	DXA within 3 months of transplant if treated with corticosteroids or have other risk factors (2D) [24] Insufficient evidence later post-transplant [25]	Take into account if chronic kidney disease mineral and bone disorder is present; consider assessing calcium, phosphate, PTH, alkaline phosphatases, and 25(OH) vitamin D levels (2C) [25]

DXA dual-energy X-ray absorptiometry
BMD bone mineral density
*ISHLT guidelines use the American College of Cardiology/American Heart Association system for Class of Recommendation (I, IIa, IIb, III) and Level of Evidence (A, B, C) prior to its revision in 2015
**AASLD guidelines use a modified version of the GRADE system for strength of recommendation (Strong =1, Weak = 2) and Level of Evidence (High = A, Moderate = B, Low = C)
***KDIGO guidelines use the GRADE system unmodified for strength of recommendation (Strong =1, Weak = 2) and Level of Evidence (High = A, Moderate = B, Low = C, Very low = D)

The 2009 KDIGO guidelines [24] recommend measurement of BMD before and within 3 months of transplant. Updated guidelines in 2017 for metabolic bone disease [25] specifically recommend considering treatment for low BMD with vitamin D, calcitriol, and/or antiresorptive agents within the first year after transplant. However, they cite equivocal evidence for antiresorptive agents in kidney transplant recipients and highlight that there is not sufficient current data to demonstrate decreased fracture risk with antiresorptive treatment in kidney transplant population. They also recommend considering bone biopsy (an ungraded recommendation) in order to characterize bone osteodystrophy to guide treatment in renal transplant patients with osteoporosis and/or elevated fracture risk. The 2017 guidelines state that there is insufficient evidence to make recommendations past the first year after kidney transplant. Because of the complexity of management considerations in kidney transplant recipients, the primary care provider should address modifiable risk factors and if osteopenia or osteoporosis is identified, work with the transplant nephrologist to optimize therapy.

- Lung transplant recipients: There is relatively less data regarding the incidence of osteoporosis in lung transplant recipients (few studies with small number of patients); however, in a retrospective analysis of 72 lung transplant recipients, 36% had osteopenia prior to transplant and 31% had osteoporosis without significant changes in bone mineral density (BMD) a year following transplant; authors therefore recommended DXA scan as part of pre-transplant workup [26]. There are no current guidelines for osteoporosis screening in the lung transplant population.

Contraception and Pregnancy in Solid Organ Transplant Recipients

Contraception

More and more women of child-bearing age are receiving solid-organ transplants. In 2018, there were 13,904 solid organ transplants in women and 35% (4881) of them were of child-bearing age [34]. It is important that primary care providers appropriately counsel their solid organ transplant recipients on their fertility before and after transplantation and their contraception options. Prior to transplantation, many women have decreased fertility, especially those with end-stage renal disease and end-stage liver disease. Dysfunction of the hypothalamic-pituitary-ovarian axis in women with chronic renal failure or severe hepatic disease results in anovulation and reduced fertility. It has been found that conception rates are approximately 0.5% per year in women undergoing peritoneal dialysis or hemodialysis [35]. Fertility is often restored within months of a successful organ transplantation and ovulatory cycles may begin as soon as 1 month after transplantation [36]. Unfortunately, many solid organ transplant recipients are not informed of this change in fertility. In one survey of 309 female solid organ transplant recipients, it was found that 44% were unaware that they could become pregnant after transplant [37]. Another study of 217 female solid organ transplant recipients aged 18–45 found that 33% were unaware of the necessity to use contraception within the first year after transplantation [38]. Approximately one-third of pregnancies are unintended in solid organ transplant recipients, which likely represents an underestimate given that some women may not report pregnancies that were terminated [39].

Contraception is best started before or shortly after receiving the transplanted organ. Pregnancy should be delayed at least 1 year after transplant to stabilize transplant function and reduce immunosuppressant medications to maintenance levels. The risks of an unintended pregnancy after a transplant are much greater than the risks of any contraceptive method. Two forms of contraception should be used until pregnancy is desired with condoms as one of the methods to protect against sexually transmitted infections.

Contraceptive choice will depend on the woman's preference, co-morbidities, side effects, costs, and reversibility. The Centers for Disease Control (CDC) updated the US version of the Medical Eligibility Criteria (US MEC) guide for contraceptive use to evaluate the risks and benefits of contraception among women with certain medical conditions including solid organ transplantation [40].

The category risks are as follows:

Category 1. A condition for which there is no restriction for the use of the contraceptive method.

Category 2. A condition for which the advantages of using the method generally outweigh the theoretical or proven risks.

Category 3. A condition for which the theoretical or proven risks usually outweigh the advantages of using the method.

Category 4. A condition that represents an unacceptable health risk if the contraceptive method is used.

The CDC categorizes a patient's medical condition after transplant as either complicated or uncomplicated. Complicated conditions include acute and chronic graft failure, graft rejection, and cardiac allograft vasculopathy [40]. Table 12.4

Table 12.4 Contraception management in solid organ transplant recipients

Method	Advantages	Disadvantages	CDC category (uncomplicated)	CDC category (complicated)
Copper-T IUD	Most effective, long acting, reversible	Heavy menses	2	Initiation: 3 continuation: 2
Progestin IUD	Most effective, long acting, reversible, decreased anemia	Irregular bleeding	2	Initiation:3 continuation: 2
Depot medroxyprogesterone acetate	Highly effective, decreased anemia	Decrease in BMD, irregular bleeding, possible cholestatic effect	2	2
Progestin implant	Most effective, long acting, no BMD decrease	Irregular bleeding	2	2
COC	Menstrual regulation, decreased anemia	Contraindicated in those with uncontrolled hypertension, active liver disease, and personal history of myocardial infarction, stroke, or DVT; first-pass liver metabolism; gastrointestinal disturbance may decrease absorption	2	4
Contraceptive patch	First-pass liver metabolism avoided	Higher circulating levels of estrogen; contraindicated in those with uncontrolled hypertension, active liver disease, and personal history of myocardial infarction, stroke, or DVT	2	4
Vaginal ring	First-pass liver metabolism avoided, lower circulating estrogen	Contraindicated in those with uncontrolled hypertension, active liver disease, and personal history of myocardial infarction, stroke, or DVT	2	4

Table 12.4 (continued)

Method	Advantages	Disadvantages	CDC category (uncomplicated)	CDC category (complicated)
Progestin-only pill		Less effective than COC; first-pass liver metabolism	2	2
Condoms	No drug interactions, protects from sexually transmitted diseases	Less effective	1	1
Cervical cap/ diaphragm	No drug interactions	Less effective	1	1

Data from Centers for Disease Control and Prevention. Adapted from https://www.cdc.gov/repro-ductivehealth/contraception/mmwr/mec/appendixk.html#transplantation [41]

BMD bone mineral density, *CDC* Centers for Disease Control and Prevention, *COC* combined oral contraceptive, *DVT* deep vein thrombosis, *IUD* intrauterine device

summarizes the different contraceptive options and their advantages/disadvantages and CDC categories for solid organ transplant recipients [41].

For women with *uncomplicated* solid organ transplants, all forms of contraceptive (except barrier methods) are classified as Category 2, meaning that the advantages for using the method generally outweigh the theoretical or proven risks. In women with a *complicated* solid organ transplant, estrogen-containing methods of contraception are considered Category 4 and intrauterine devices (IUDs) are considered Category 3. However, if a woman already has an IUD in place, then it is considered a Category 2 and she should continue with it.

The methods with the lowest failure rate (<1%) include permanent methods (female and male sterilization) and long-acting reversible methods (IUD and the subdermal progestin implant). Male sterilization is safer, less expensive, and less invasive than female sterilization (for women in a monogamous relationship with a male partner). Immunosuppressive medications do not alter the efficacy of the IUD or increase the risk of pelvic inflammatory disease [39]. IUDs are an excellent option for this patient population and should be highly recommended [42]. The subdermal progestin implant is very effective and there is no hepatic first pass effect which results in fewer drug interactions.

Depot medroxyprogesterone is highly effective with correct use (<1%), but with typical use it has a 6% failure rate. A disadvantage is that it reduces bone density which is important in solid organ transplant recipients who may be at high risk for bone loss due to chronic corticosteroid use and renal osteodystrophy (see Section "Metabolic Bone Disease" above). Combined hormonal contraceptives (pills, patches, rings) have a high failure rate with typical use (9%) and therefore are not considered first-line options. If chosen, these combined hormone contraceptives should be initiated at least 6 months after a liver transplant when organ stability is clear. If combined hormone therapy is chosen, then the ring or patch may be better options as they bypass the liver resulting in less drug interactions.

Table 12.5 Classifications for emergency contraception, including the copper-containing intrauterine device, ulipristal acetate, levonorgestrel, and combined oral contraceptives in solid organ transplant recipients [40]

	Cu-IUD	UPA	LNG	COC
Complicated: Graft failure (acute or chronic), rejection, or cardiac allograft vasculopathy	3	1	1	1
Uncomplicated	2	1	1	1

Abbreviations: *COC* combined oral contraceptive, *Cu-IUD* copper-containing intrauterine device, *LNG* levonorgestrel, *UPA* ulipristal acetate

Additionally, it is advisable to inform the transplant team when starting systemic hormonal treatment.

Unfortunately, the most highly effective contraceptive methods may not be used the most by transplant recipients. A cross-sectional survey study of 32 female solid organ transplant recipients found that the most common contraceptive method used in the year before and after transplant was condoms (18% failure rate with typical use) [43]. This finding along with the high unintended pregnancy rate among solid organ transplant recipients highlights the need for primary care physicians to address contraception with their solid organ transplant patients of child-bearing age.

Emergency Contraception

Solid organ transplant recipients can use all the emergency contraception methods (see Table 12.5) currently available which include copper IUD (Cu-IUD), levonorgestrel, ulipristal acetate, and combined oral contraceptive pills [40]. The only exception is that the copper IUD should not be used in women with complicated transplants: graft failure (acute or chronic), rejection, or cardiac allograft vasculopathy.

Pregnancy

Pregnancy in solid organ transplant recipients should be carefully planned and delayed until at least 1 year after transplant [42]. Pregnancy during the first 12 months after a transplant is associated with graft dysfunction, rejection or loss, and pre-term delivery [44]. Solid organ transplant recipients benefit from pregnancy planning by a collaborative multidisciplinary approach with the transplant team, maternal-fetal medicine specialists, and pharmacists. Solid organ transplant recipients have an increased risk of miscarriage, gestational hypertension, preeclampsia, gestational diabetes, fetal prematurity, and low birth weight. It is also important that chronic medical problems such as diabetes or hypertension are well controlled. Immunosuppressive drugs with risks to the fetus need to be discontinued prior to pregnancy. Exposure to mycophenolate is associated with higher rates of miscarriages and birth defects compared to pregnancies without that exposure [45]. Mammalian target of rapamycin inhibitors (everolimus, sirolimus) are associated with increased risks of preterm delivery, decreased fetal weight, and skeletal ossification. The incidence of birth defects in infants exposed to prednisone, azathioprine, cyclosporine, or tacrolimus in utero is about 3–5% which is similar to the general population [46].

The American Society of Transplantation recommends that the following clinical criteria be met prior to pregnancy: [47]

- No rejection within the previous year
- Stable graft function
- No acute infection that might affect the fetus
- Immunosuppressant drugs at stable doses

With appropriate preconception planning and subsequent careful management by the transplant team and high-risk obstetrician, solid organ transplant recipients can have successful pregnancies and healthy infants. Because of demographics and other factors, successful pregnancies are more commonly reported in kidney and liver transplant recipients compared to other solid organ transplant recipients [48]. The primary care provider should ask about family planning in solid organ transplant recipients of child-bearing age and make early referrals to specialty care. Additionally, the primary care provider can assist in the control of other medical conditions, standard preconception care including ensuring adequate folate intake, avoidance of tobacco and alcohol, and reviewing other medications for safety in pregnancy.

Immunizations in Solid Organ Transplant Recipients

Solid organ transplant recipients should receive the same vaccinations as the general population except for live vaccines which are contraindicated. Recommendations are based on the routine schedule for immunocompetent individuals according to age, vaccination status, and exposure history and are summarized in Table 12.6 [49]. Primary care providers and specialists share the responsibility for ensuring that appropriate vaccinations are administered to solid organ transplant recipients and for recommending appropriate vaccinations for household members and close contacts [50].

Since solid organ transplant recipients receive life-long immune suppression, they may have lower rates of serological conversion, lower mean antibody titers, and waning of protective immunity over a shorter period as compared to the general population [51]. Therefore, it is important that vaccines, especially live vaccines, be given to the patient prior to transplant if possible. Live vaccines should be given at least 4 weeks before transplant, whereas inactivated vaccines can be given up to 2 weeks before. Most transplant centers review and update vaccines as part of the pre-transplant evaluation. However, if transplants are done more urgently,

Table 12.6 Vaccine recommendations for adult solid organ transplant recipients

Vaccine	Schedule	Comments
Influenza	One dose annually	Inactivated or recombinant vaccines, trivalent or quadrivalent, high-dose trivalent may be preferred [54]
Tdap	Single dose ≤2 yrs after last Tetanus-diptheria (Td)	Td booster every 10 years
Prevnar® (PCV13)	Once regardless of age	If given after PPSV23, then wait >1 y
Pneumovax® (PPSV23)	≥ 8 weeks after Prevnar	One booster after 5 years and then again ≥ age 65 at least 5 years after most recent booster
Shingrix®	Not yet determined	The CDC has not provided guidance on its use in solid organ transplant recipients
HPV	3 doses through age 26	9-valent
Meningococcal (MenACWY)	1–2 doses depending on the indication	Those treated with eculizumab or another indication Booster every 5 years if ongoing risk
MenB	2 or 3 doses depending on vaccine	Those treated with *eculizumab*
Hepatitis B	2 or 3 doses depending on vaccine	Wants protection or is at risk (consider 40 mcg dose)
Hepatitis A	2–3 doses depending on vaccine	Wants protection or is at risk

vaccinations are not always given. At the initial primary care visit, the patient's pre-transplant vaccination history should be reviewed.

After transplantation, it is extremely important that patients are kept up to date in their immunizations as they are more susceptible to infections and their complications. For example, a systematic review of the incidence of invasive pneumococcal disease (IPD) in immunocompromised patients found that the IPD incidence was 465/100,000 in solid organ transplant recipients vs only 10/100,000 in healthy controls [52]. There is no evidence that vaccines lead to allograft rejection in solid organ transplant recipients, so there should be no hesitation in administering them except for the Shingrix® vaccine (discussed below) [53]. For patients that are non-immune, vaccines can be administered starting 2–6 months after transplant. Vaccinations should be withheld from solid organ transplant recipients during intensified immunosuppression, including the first 2 months after transplant, or in the setting of treatment for rejection, because of the likelihood of inadequate immune response [51]. It is not routine to measure serologic responses to immunizations given after transplant as there is no data showing that booster doses are helpful. Vaccine guidelines change frequently and primary care providers will need to check updated recommendations from either the CDC or the WHO, as well as their local public health organizations. The following information is relevant for solid organ transplant recipients regarding specific vaccines:

- *Pneumococcal vaccine.* The current recommendations for solid organ transplant recipients are one dose of PCV13 followed by one dose of PPSV23 at least 8 weeks later. Another dose of PPSV23 should be given at least 5 years after the previous PPSV23. At age 65 years or older, one dose of PPSV23 should be given if it has been at least 5 years since the last PSV23. No further doses are indicated. If pneumococcal vaccines are given prior to transplantation, they do not need to be repeated after transplantation.
- *Influenza vaccine.* There are two types of inactivated vaccines: trivalent and quadrivalent. The high-dose trivalent is safe and immunogenic in solid organ transplant recipients. It is recommended that it be given 1–3 months after transplant as immunogenicity may be reduced if given earlier. However, it can be administered within 1 month after transplant during an influenza outbreak and revaccination at 3–6 months after transplant if outbreak is ongoing [50]. In one study, the high-dose trivalent vaccine demonstrated significantly better immunogenicity than the standard dose in adult transplant recipients and may be the preferred influenza vaccine for this population [54].
- *Meningococcal vaccine.* Meningococcal disease does not occur at higher rates after transplant, so it is not routinely prescribed for solid organ transplant recipients except for those with risk factors. Risk factors include those receiving eculizumab which is used for treatment of antibody-mediated rejection post-transplant [55], history of splenectomy, military recruits, or travel to high-risk areas. The quadrivalent conjugated vaccine (MenACWY) is preferred as it provides a T-cell-dependent immune response, immune memory, and long-term protection. It requires two doses at 0 and 2 months. Those treated with eculizumab should also receive MenB.
- *Zoster vaccine.* Although Shingrix® is a recombinant vaccine, it has not yet been approved for solid organ transplant recipients due to a concern that its immunogenicity may affect allografts by causing rejection.

In addition to keeping up to date in vaccinations, solid organ transplant recipients need to take many precautions due to their high risk for infections. Food and water safety are very important. They must take care to minimize direct contact with pathogens, so frequent handwashing and avoidance of others with respiratory or gastrointestinal illnesses are recommended. Household members and other close contacts should be up to date in their vaccinations. They can receive both live and inactivated vaccines except for the live polio vaccine which is easily transmitted via the oral-fecal route and therefore is unsafe for the solid organ transplant recipients [49]. With the COVID-19/SARS-CoV-2 worldwide pandemic, solid organ transplant recipients are considered in the highest risk category, and they should follow local public health guidelines to avoid exposure. At the time of this publication, data are continuing to be analyzed to better characterize the risk to solid organ transplant recipients. Recommendations are summarized in Table 12.7.

Table 12.7 Strategies for disease prevention in solid organ transplant recipients [56]

Foodborne illness:
Avoid unpasteurized dairy products, undercooked meats, unwashed fruits/vegetables, raw seafood (*Vibrio vulnificus*). A handout on food safety can be found at: http://wwwfda.gov/Food/FoodborneIllnessContaminants/PeopleAtRisk/ucm312570.htm
Water sources
Avoid drinking water from private wells and ingesting water exposed to human or animal waste
Hand hygiene
Wash hands after eating or preparing food, touching plants or dirt, using the restroom, changing diapers, touching animals, etc.
Avoid exposures
Avoid visiting prisons, homeless shelters, or other TB high-risk areas, tattooing, self-piercing, sharing needles, and close contact with individuals with respiratory/gastrointestinal illnesses or herpes zoster outbreak*

*SOT recipients should follow guidelines for high risk populations during the COVID-19/SARS-CoV-2 pandemic. These guidelines are expected to continue to evolve

Travel Immunizations and Recommendations

Solid organ transplant recipients are living longer and traveling internationally—it is important that they receive the appropriate travel advice, as they are at increased risk of developing opportunistic and non-opportunistic infections. Surveys of transplant centers found significant rates of illness in transplant recipients during foreign travel with insufficient rates of pre-travel counseling and interventions [57]. Travel clinics provide the best comprehensive care for solid organ transplant recipients, but these are not always available, so primary care providers need to be able to appropriately counsel and provide medical care for them. Travel recommendations change frequently as international conditions change; therefore, primary care providers should check for updated guidelines prior to making recommendations.

- *Immunizations:* All individuals should be up to date in routine immunizations (tetanus, influenza, pneumococcal). The specific vaccines needed for travel will depend on the travel agenda, including the specific areas in the countries that will be visited and exposure risks, and the patient's vaccination status. In general, solid organ transplant recipients should avoid traveling to countries with yellow fever or other endemic outbreaks such as typhoid, dengue, measles, polio, and chikungunya. Ideally, vaccines should be given several months before travel to allow for an optimal immune response. Comprehensive information regarding travel vaccines for solid organ transplant recipients can be found at the Centers for Disease Control and Prevention Traveler's Health website [58], but a few recommendations are highlighted below:
- Hepatitis A. For those who have not been vaccinated or are on higher levels of immunosuppression and plan to travel within 2 weeks, IM pooled immunoglobulins should be given as they provide 85–90% protection against hepatitis A. A

dose of 0.02 ml/kg provides up to 3 months of protection. The first dose of the hepatitis A vaccine should also be given.

- Typhoid. This must be given in the inactivated IM form and is protective for 2 years. It should be given at least 2 weeks before departure.
- Hepatitis B. High-dose hepatitis B (40 mcg) should be used. Also, accelerated schedules 0, 7, 21, and 28 days or 0, 1, and 2 months (both with a booster at 6 months) are acceptable.
- Measles. If solid organ transplant recipients must travel to an endemic area, their immunity should be checked (those born before 1957, evidence of two vaccinations, positive IgG titer, or clear h/o clinical disease). If non-immune, then immunoglobulin may be administered for short-term protection.

Travel Precautions

Ideally, solid organ transplant recipients should not travel for 1 year after transplant or during treatment for rejection. Once they are on maintenance doses of immunosuppressants and the allograft has stabilized, then it is safer for them to travel. It is important for them to carefully follow food and water precautions to prevent infections. They should drink only boiled or bottled water, and avoid ice in drinks, raw food, and food rinsed with tap water. Solid organ transplant recipients need to minimize their sun exposure as they are at high risk for developing skin cancers, especially squamous cell cancer. Diarrhea, the most common illness of travelers, can be life threatening for solid organ transplant recipients. Dehydration can lead to decreased renal function, especially those taking tacrolimus. Complications include bacteremia and altered absorption and metabolism of immunosuppressive drugs. Patients should be prescribed ciprofloxacin or azithromycin to take at the onset of symptoms; however, these medications can potentially interact with transplant medications and should be discussed with the transplant team first. The threshold for treatment is more than three unformed stools in 24 hours. Anti-motility agents should be used with caution. Bismuth-containing antidiarrheal medications should be avoided as they put solid organ transplant recipients at risk for salicylate toxicity if the patients have decreased renal function. Patient should not take an antibiotic prophylactically as this can lead to antibiotic resistance, *C. difficile* infection, and drug interactions. Additionally, the COVID-19/SARS-CoV-2 pandemic has restricted travel for high risk populations. Solid organ transplant recipients who desire to travel during this pandemic should follow public health guidelines and should be strongly cautioned against travel that would increase exposure to areas with high rates of infection, or travel via indoor settings in which they cannot sufficiently reduce their risk of exposure. Table 12.8 summarizes the recommendations for solid organ transplant recipients who plan to travel internationally.

Table 12.8 Travel advice for solid organ transplant recipients [59]

Review precautions: *Food and water, mosquito, traveler's diarrhea and when to take antibiotics, sun exposure, sex/blood-borne

Healthcare: Make a list of facilities where medical care can be obtained if needed, consider obtaining evacuation insurance, carry a list of medications/medical problems

Supplies: Insect repellent, sunscreen, basic first aid kit, and antibacterial hand wipes or an alcohol-based hand cleaner

Medications: Malaria prophylaxis if indicated, all regular medications to cover the entire trip, antibiotics for diarrhea, OTC PRN medications

*Please see text above re: risk of travel during the COVID-19/SARS-CoV-2 pandemic

Behavioral Health and Substance Use in Transplant Recipients

Behavioral Health

Behavioral health diagnoses are prevalent in solid organ transplant recipients, although further research is needed to better characterize the incidence and impact of these conditions following solid organ transplant. The most evidence is for depression. Solid organ transplant recipients are at higher risk for developing depression post-transplant compared to the general population. In a survey of liver transplant recipients, approximately 50% of those surveyed met criteria consistent with at least mild depression based on Patient Health Questionnaire-9 (PHQ-9) responses [60]. A diagnosis of depression post-transplant is correlated with worse outcomes. A 2015 systematic review and meta-analysis found that post-transplant depression was associated with a 65% greater risk of mortality. The same analysis examined the impact of anxiety on post-transplant mortality and found a non-significant increased risk; however, the authors noted that these data were likely unreliable due to far fewer studies and less precision of results as compared to those for depression [61].

There is emerging data regarding post-traumatic stress disorder (PTSD) following solid organ transplant. A systematic review found 10–17% cumulative incidence of post-transplant PTSD. Poor social support and pre-existing psychiatric diagnoses were correlated with post-transplant PTSD. Post-transplant PTSD was associated with worse mental health-related quality of life [62].

There is no consensus recommendation for screening for psychiatric diagnoses post-transplant, although many recommend at least regular interval screening for depression [63].

Substance Use

Substance use is screened and monitored heavily as part of pre-transplant evaluations. After solid organ transplant, substance use (e.g., alcohol and tobacco) is associated with higher rates of graft failure [64, 65]. Although precise estimates are unknown, a meta-analysis of studies in solid organ transplant recipients found a 1–4% rate of post-transplant substance use (defined as tobacco, alcohol, or illicit drug use) [66]. Still, comprehensive screening guidelines are lacking for the solid organ transplant population.

Substance use after transplant is best studied in patients who received liver transplant for alcoholic liver disease. In a study surveying 67 liver transplant recipients, approximately 20% reported alcohol use; however, only 4.5% reported at-risk behavior (as defined by the Alcohol Use Disorders Identification Test (AUDIT)), 30% reported tobacco use, and a minority (3%) reported non-marijuana drug use [60].

Alcohol use after liver transplant is associated with worse outcomes regardless of reason for transplant [67]. The AASLD and AST guidelines [13] recommend that patients who receive a liver transplant for alcoholic liver disease should be encouraged to abstain from alcohol. However, there are not specific guidelines for screening patients who do not have a prior diagnosis of alcoholic liver disease. Guidelines for care of kidney transplant recipients include avoidance of alcohol and other behaviors associated with worse outcomes in the evaluation of adherence; however, no specific screening recommendations are given [24].

Tobacco use in solid organ transplant recipients is associated with poorer graft function and significantly worse survival [68]. Currently, only lung transplant guidelines cite tobacco use as an absolute contraindication to transplant [69]. While there are not clear guidelines regarding screening for tobacco use in solid organ transplant recipients, it is recommended, given the clear correlation with worse outcomes and the demonstrated substantial rates of recurrent use in recipients who smoked prior to transplant [64].

Increasingly, states are legalizing medical and recreational marijuana, yet there is little guidance as to how to screen and counsel solid organ transplant recipients regarding use. Studies that have looked at the effect of marijuana use in solid organ transplant recipients have not found significant differences in graft function and/or survival as compared to non-marijuana users [70, 71, 72]. However, there remain concerns regarding marijuana's potential inhibition of metabolic pathways that could lead to medication toxicity, infectious risks in the context of immunosuppression, end organ risks that may be amplified in immunosuppression, as well as addiction behaviors and impacts on cognition that might worsen adherence to medical therapy [73].

Conclusion

Solid organ transplant recipients are at increased risk for a broad spectrum of common conditions, several of which are discussed in this chapter. We emphasize the importance of contraception and pregnancy planning in women and vaccinations for all recipients. Travel planning and precautions are also addressed.

For many of the conditions reviewed, there are still unclear or absent guidelines with respect to screening. For example, we were unable to find any guidelines for screening for osteoporosis in lung transplant recipients, although there is an increased risk. This can cause uncertainty, especially among primary care physicians, as to what to recommend to patients. More frequently updated guidelines and further research is needed to establish effective screening modalities and intervals for different medical problems in the solid organ transplant population.

Primary care providers play an important role in providing optimal healthcare for solid organ transplant recipients. The checklist below (Table 12.9) summarizes most

Table 12.9 Preventive health checklist for solid organ transplant recipients (see text for details)

Screening/prevention category	Recommendations
Cancer[a]	☐ Cervical cancer screening: Cytology +/− HPV at 1–3 year intervals; continue after age 65 if indicated *(see Table 12.1 for additional detail and age-specific recommendations)*
	☐ Skin cancer screening: Annual skin and lip cancer screening
Cardiovascular disease and diabetes	☐ Monitor blood pressure each visit ☐ Annual lipids ☐ Exercise and diet counseling ☐ Diabetes screening every 3 months for first year, then annually
Osteoporosis	☐ DXA at least within the first year of transplant ☐ Consider calcium/vitamin D supplementation *(see Table 12.3 for additional detail and transplanted-organ specific recommendations)*
Pregnancy	If pregnancy desired: ☐ Contraception at least through first-year post-transplant; delay pregnancy until graft and immunosuppressive medications are stable (LARC preferred) ☐ After the first year, early involvement with maternal-fetal medicine specialist in pregnancy planning If pregnancy not desired: ☐ Address contraception (see Table 12.4)
Immunizations	☐ Influenza: annually ☐ PCV13: once ☐ PPSV23: ≥ 8 weeks after Prevnar; one booster after 5 years (additional booster ≥65 years and 5 years since prior booster) ☐ TdaP: Single dose ≤2 yrs after last Td and then Td booster every 10 years Shingrix®: not yet approved for solid organ transplant recipients – avoid until further guidance *(see Table 12.6 for additional vaccine recommendations)*
Behavioral health	☐ Depression screening (PHQ-2 and/or PHQ-9) at least annually[b]
Substance use	☐ Alcohol screening at least annually[b] ☐ Tobacco screening at least annually[b]

[a]Only cancer screening recommendations that are different than for the general population are shown
[b]No consensus guidelines

topics covered in this chapter and can serve as a tool for primary care physicians to ensure solid organ transplant recipients receive regular screening and appropriate preventive care.

References

1. Engels EA, et al. Spectrum of cancer risk among US solid organ transplant recipients. JAMA. 2011;306(17):1891–901.
2. Liao JB, Fisher CE, Madeleine MM. Gynecologic cancers and solid organ transplantation. Am J Transplant. 2019;19(5):1266–77.
3. Garrett GL, et al. Incidence of and risk factors for skin cancer in organ transplant recipients in the United States. JAMA Dermatol. 2017;153(3):296–303.
4. Mukthinuthalapati PK, Gotur R, Ghabril M. Incidence, risk factors and outcomes of de novo malignancies post liver transplantation. World J Hepatol. 2016;8(12):533–44.
5. Miao Y, et al. De novo cancers arising in organ transplant recipients are associated with adverse outcomes compared with the general population. Transplantation. 2009;87(9):1347–59.
6. Acuna SA, et al. Cancer screening recommendations for solid organ transplant recipients: a systematic review of clinical practice guidelines. Am J Transplant. 2017;17(1):103–14.
7. Moscicki AB, et al. Guidelines for cervical cancer screening in immunosuppressed women without HIV infection. J Low Genit Tract Dis. 2019;23(2):87–101.
8. Chin-Hong PV, Reid GE, AST Infectious Disease Community of Practice. Human papillomavirus infections in solid organ transplant recipients: Guidelines from the American Society of Transplantation Infectious Diseases Community of Practice. Clin Transplant. 2019;00:e13590.
9. Zamoiski RD, et al. Risk of second malignancies in solid organ transplant recipients who develop keratinocyte cancers. Cancer Res. 2017;77(15):4196–203.
10. Bibbins-Domingo K, Grossman DC, Curry SJ, Davidson KW, Ebell M, Epling JW Jr, García FA, Gillman MW, Kemper AR, Krist AH, Kurth AE, Landefeld CS, Mangione CM, Phillips WR, Phipps MG, Pignone MP, Siu AL, US Preventive Services Task Force. Screening for skin cancer: US preventive services task force recommendation statement. JAMA. 2016;316(4):429–35. https://doi.org/10.1001/jama.2016.8465.
11. Acuna SA, et al. Uptake of cancer screening tests among recipients of solid organ transplantation. Am J Transplant. 2017;17(9):2434–43.
12. Briggs JD. Causes of death after renal transplantation. Nephrol Dial Transplant. 2001;16(8):1545–9. https://doi.org/10.1093/ndt/16.8.1545.
13. Lucey MR, Terrault N, Ojo L, Hay JE, Neuberger J, Blumberg E, et al. Long-term management of the successful adult liver transplant: 2012 practice guideline by the American Association for the Study of Liver Diseases and the American Society of Transplantation. Liver Transpl. 2013;19:3–26. https://doi.org/10.1002/lt.23566.
14. Munagala MR, Phancao A. Managing cardiovascular risk in the post solid organ transplant recipient. Med Clin North Am. 2016;100(3):519–33. https://doi.org/10.1016/j.mcna.2016.01.004.
15. Ducloux D, Kazory A, Chalopin JM. Predicting coronary heart disease in renal transplant recipients: a prospective study. Kidney Int. 2004;66(1):441–7. https://doi.org/10.1111/j.1523-1755.2004.00751.x.
16. Wong CJ, Pagalilauan G. Primary care of the solid organ transplant recipient. Med Clin North Am. 2015;99(5):1075–103. https://doi.org/10.1016/j.mcna.2015.05.002.
17. Sakhaee K. Osteoporosis following organ transplantation: pathogenesis, diagnosis and management. Expert Rev Endocrinol Metab. 2011;6(2):157–76. https://doi.org/10.1586/eem.10.86.

18. Cheraghi Z, Doosti-Irani A, Almasi-Hashiani A, Baigi V, Mansournia N, Etminan M, et al. The effect of alcohol on osteoporosis: a systematic review and meta-analysis. Drug Alcohol Depend. 2019;197:197–202. https://doi.org/10.1016/j.drugalcdep.2019.01.025.
19. Final Recommendation Statement: Osteoporosis to Prevent Fractures: Screening. U.S. Preventive Services Task Force. 2019. https://www.uspreventiveservicestaskforce. org/Page/Document/RecommendationStatementFinal/osteoporosis-screening1. Accessed 1 Dec 2019.
20. Costanzo MR, Dipchand A, Starling R, et al. The International Society of Heart and Lung Transplantation Guidelines for the care of heart transplant recipients. J Heart Lung Transplant. 2010;29(8):914–56. https://doi.org/10.1016/j.healun.2010.05.034.
21. Zhao J, Wang C, Hu Z. Efficacy and safety of bisphosphonates for osteoporosis or osteopenia in cardiac transplant patients: a meta-analysis. Transplant Proc. 2015;47(10):2957–64. https:// doi.org/10.1016/j.transproceed.2015.10.049.
22. Ball AM, Gillen DL, Sherrard D, Weiss NS, Emerson SS, Seliger SL, et al. Risk of hip fracture among dialysis and renal transplant recipients. JAMA. 2002;288(23):3014–8. https://doi. org/10.1001/jama.288.23.3014.
23. Julian BA, Laskow DA, Dubovsky J, et al. Rapid loss of vertebral mineral density after renal transplantation. N Engl J Med. 1991;325:544–50. https://doi.org/10.1056/ NEJM199108223250804.
24. Kasiske BL, Zeier MG, Craig JC, Ekberg H, Garvey CA, Green MD, et al. KDIGO clinical practice guideline for the care of kidney transplant recipients. Am J Transplant. 2009;9:S1– S155. https://doi.org/10.1111/j.1600-6143.2009.02834.x.
25. Isakova T, Nickolas TL, Denburg M, et al. KDOQI US Commentary on the 2017 KDIGO Clinical Practice Guideline Update for the Diagnosis, Evaluation, Prevention, and Treatment of Chronic Kidney Disease–Mineral and Bone Disorder (CKD-MBD). Am J Kidney Dis. 2017;70(6):737–51. https://doi.org/10.1053/j.ajkd.2017.07.019.
26. Wang TKM, O'Sullivan S, Gamble GD, Ruygrok PN. Bone density in heart or lung transplant recipients-a longitudinal study. Transplant Proc. 2013;45(6):2357–65. https://doi. org/10.1016/j.transproceed.2012.09.117.
27. Aris RM, Neuringer IP, Weiner MA, Egan TM, Ontjes D. Severe osteoporosis before and after lung transplantation. Chest. 1996;109(5):1176–83. https://doi.org/10.1378/chest.109.5.1176.
28. Yu TM, Lin CL, Chang SN, Sung FC, Huang ST, Kao CH. Osteoporosis and fractures after solid organ transplantation: a nationwide population-based cohort study. Mayo Clin Proc. 2014;89(7):888–95. https://doi.org/10.1016/j.mayocp.2014.02.017.
29. Adegunsoye A, Strek ME, Garrity E, Guzy R, Bag R. Comprehensive care of the lung transplant patient. Chest. 2017;152(1):150–64. https://doi.org/10.1016/j.chest.2016.10.001.
30. Leidig-Bruckner G, Hosch S, Dodidou P, Ritschel D, Conradt C, Klose C, et al. Frequency and predictors of osteoporotic fractures after cardiac or liver transplantation: a follow-up study. Lancet. 2001;357(9253):342–7. https://doi.org/10.1016/S0140-6736(00)03641-2.
31. Shane E, Rivas M, Staron RB, Silverberg SJ, Seibel MJ, Kuiper J, et al. Fracture after cardiac transplantation: a prospective longitudinal study. J Clin Endocrinol Metab. 1996;81(5):1740–6. https://doi.org/10.1210/jcem.81.5.8626827.
32. Guichelaar MM, Kendall R, Malinchoc M, Hay JE. Bone mineral density before and after OLT: long-term follow-up and predictive factors. Liver Transpl. 2006;12(9):1390–402. https:// doi.org/10.1002/lt.20874.
33. Nikkel LE, Hollenbeak CS, Fox EJ, Uemura T, Ghahramani N. Risk of fractures after renal transplantation in the United States. Transplantation. 2009;87(12):1846–51. https://doi. org/10.1097/TP.0b013e3181a6bbda.
34. US Department of Health and Human Services. Organ procurement and transplantation network. 21 Apr 2019.; Available from: https://optn.transplant.hrsa.gov/data/view-data-reports/ national-data.
35. Hou S. Pregnancy in chronic renal insufficiency and end-stage renal disease. Am J Kidney Dis. 1999;33(2):235–52.
36. Gill JS, et al. The pregnancy rate and live birth rate in kidney transplant recipients. Am J Transplant. 2009;9(7):1541–9.

37. French VA, et al. Contraception and fertility awareness among women with solid organ transplants. Obstet Gynecol. 2013;122(4):809–14.
38. Szpotanska-Sikorska M, Pietrzak B, Wielgos M. Contraceptive awareness and birth control selection in female kidney and liver transplant recipients. Contraception. 2014;90(4): 435–9.
39. Al-Badri M, Kling JM, Vegunta S. Reproductive planning for women after solid-organ transplant. Cleve Clin J Med. 2017;84(9):719–28.
40. Curtis KM, et al. U.S. medical eligibility criteria for contraceptive use, 2016. MMWR Recomm Rep. 2016;65(3):1–103.
41. CDC. Summary of classifications for hormonal contraceptive methods and intrauterine devices. 25 Apr 2019. Available from: https://www.cdc.gov/reproductivehealth/contraception/mmwr/mec/appendixk.html#transplantation.
42. Krajewski CM, Geetha D, Gomez-Lobo V. Contraceptive options for women with a history of solid-organ transplantation. Transplantation. 2013;95(10):1183–6.
43. Rafie S, et al. Contraceptive use in female recipients of a solid-organ transplant. Prog Transplant. 2014;24(4):344–8.
44. Deshpande NA, et al. Pregnancy after solid organ transplantation: a guide for obstetric management. Rev Obstet Gynecol. 2013;6(3-4):116–25.
45. Kim M, Rostas S, Gabardi S. Mycophenolate fetal toxicity and risk evaluation and mitigation strategies. Am J Transplant. 2013;13(6):1383–9.
46. Coscia LA, et al. Immunosuppressive drugs and fetal outcome. Best Pract Res Clin Obstet Gynaecol. 2014;28(8):1174–87.
47. McKay DB, et al. Reproduction and transplantation: report on the AST Consensus Conference on Reproductive Issues and Transplantation. Am J Transplant. 2005;5(7):1592–9.
48. Mastrobattista JM, Gomez-Lobo V, Society for Maternal-Fetal Medicine. Pregnancy after solid organ transplantation. Obstet Gynecol. 2008;112(4):919–32. https://doi.org/10.1097/AOG.0b013e318187d00c.
49. Stucchi RSB, Lopes MH, Kumar D, Manuel O. Vaccine Recommendations for Solid-Organ Transplant Recipients and donors. Transplantation. 2018;102:S72–80. https://doi.org/10.1097/TP.0000000000002012.
50. Rubin LG, Levin MJ, Ljungman P, Davies EG, Avery R, Tomblyn M, Bousvaros A, Dhanireddy S, Sung L, Keyserling H, Kang I. Infectious diseases society of America. 2013 IDSA clinical practice guideline for vaccination of the immunocompromised host. Clin Infect Dis. 2014;58(3):309–18. https://doi.org/10.1093/cid/cit816.
51. Arora S, Kipp G, Bhanot N. KK. Vaccinations in kidney transplant recipients: Clearing the muddy waters. World J Transplant. 2019;9(1):1–13. https://doi.org/10.5500/wjt.v9.i1.1.
52. van Aalst M, Lotsch F, Spijker R, et al. Incidence of invasive pneumococcal disease in immunocompromised patients: A systematic review and meta-analysis. Travel Med Infect Dis. 2018;24:89–100. https://doi.org/10.1016/j.tmaid.2018.05.016.
53. Chong PP, Avery RK. A comprehensive review of immunization practices in sold organ transplant and hematopoietic stem cell transplant recipients. Clin Ther. 2017;39(8):1581–98. https://doi.org/10.1016/j.clinthera.2017.07.005.
54. Natori Y, Shiotsuka M, Slomovic J, Hoschler K, Ferreira V, Ashton P, Rotstein C, Lilly L, Schiff J, Singer L, Humar A, Kumar D. A double-blind, randomized trial of high-dose vs standard-dose influenza vaccine in adult solid-organ transplant recipients. Clin Infect Dis. 2018;66(11):1698–704. https://doi.org/10.1093/cid/cix1082.
55. Struijk GH, Bouts AH, Rijkers GT, Kuin EA, ten Berge IJ, Bemelman FJ. Meningococcal sepsis complicating eculizumab treatment despite prior vaccination. Am J Transplant. 2013;13(3):819–20. https://doi.org/10.1111/ajt.12032.
56. Blair BM. Safe living following solid organ transplantation. Surg Clin North Am. 2019;99(1):153–61.
57. Buchan CA, Kotton CN, AST Infectious Diseases Community Practice. Travel medicine, transplant tourism, and the solid organ transplant recipient—Guidelines from the American

Society of Transplantation Infectious Diseases Community of Practice. Clin Transplantation. 2019;e13529:1–16. https://doi.org/10.1111/ctr.13529.

58. Center for Disease Control. Traveler's health. https://wwwnc.cdc.gov/travel/destinations/list/.
59. Kotton CN, Hibberd PL. Travel medicine and transplant tourism in solid organ transplantation. Am J Transplant. 2013;13(Suppl 4):337–47.
60. Sacco P, Sultan S, Tuten M, Powell JM, Connelly M, Barth RN, et al. Substance Use and Psychosocial Functioning in a Sample of Liver Transplant Recipients with Alcohol-Related Liver Disease. Transplant Proc. 2018;50(10):3689–93. https://doi.org/10.1016/j.transproceed.2018.07.003.
61. Dew MA, Rosenberger EM, Myaskovsky L, DiMartini AF, DeVito Dabbs AJ, Posluszny DM, et al. Depression and anxiety as risk factors for morbidity and mortality after organ transplantation: a systematic review and meta-analysis. Transplantation. 2015;100(5):988–1003. https://doi.org/10.1097/TP.0000000000000901.
62. Davydow DS, Lease ED, Reyes JD. Posttraumatic stress disorder in organ transplant recipients: a systematic review. Gen Hosp Psychiatry. 2015;37(5):387–98. https://doi.org/10.1016/j.genhosppsych.2015.05.005.
63. Corbett C, Armstrong MJ, Parker R, Webb K, Neuberger JM. Mental health disorders and solid-organ transplant recipients. Transplantation. 2013;96(7):593–600.
64. Anis KH, Weinrauch LA, D'Elia JA. Effects of smoking on solid organ transplantation outcomes. Am J Med. 2019;132(4):413–9. https://doi.org/10.1097/TP.0b013e31829584e0.
65. Ursic-Bedoya J, Donnadieu-Rigole H, Faure S, Pageaux GP. Alcohol use and smoking after liver transplantation; complications and prevention. Best Pract Res Clin Gastroenterol. 2017;31(2):181–5. https://doi.org/10.1016/j.bpg.2017.03.005.
66. Dew MA, DiMartini AF, De Vito Dabbs A, et al. Rates and risk factors for nonadherence to the medical regimen after adult solid organ transplantation. Transplantation. 2007;83(7):858–73. https://doi.org/10.1097/01.tp.0000258599.65257.a6.
67. Faure S, Herrero A, Jung B, et al. Excessive alcohol consumption after liver transplantation impacts on long-term survival, whatever the primary indication. J Hepatol. 2012;52(2):306–12. https://doi.org/10.1016/j.jhep.2012.03.014.
68. Corbett C, Armstrong MJ, Neuberger J. Tobacco smoking and solid organ transplantation. Transplantation. 2012;94(10):979–87. https://doi.org/10.1097/TP.0b013e318263ad5b.
69. Weill D, Benden C, Corris PA, et al. A consensus document for the selection of lung transplant candidates: 2014—An update from the Pulmonary Transplantation Council of the International Society for Heart and Lung Transplantation. J Heart Lung Transplant. 2015;34(1):1–15. https://doi.org/10.1016/j.healun.2014.06.014.
70. Greenan G, Ahmad SB, Anders MG, Leeser A, Bromberg JS, Niederhaus SV. Recreational marijuana use is not associated with worse outcomes after renal transplantation. Clin Transpl. 2016;30(10):1340–6. https://doi.org/10.1111/ctr.12828.
71. Mohite PN, Zeriouh M, Sáez DG, Popov A-F, Sabashnikov A, Zych B, et al. Influence of history of cannabis smoking in selected donors on the outcomes of lung transplantation. Eur J Cardiothorac Surg. 2017;51(1):142–7. https://doi.org/10.1093/ejcts/ezw255.
72. Ranney D, Acker W, Al-Holou S, Ehrlichman L, Lee D, Lewin S, et al. Marijuana use in potential liver transplant candidates. Am J Transplant. 2009;9(2):280–5. https://doi.org/10.1111/j.1600-6143.2008.02468.x.
73. Rai HS, Winder GS. Marijuana use and organ transplantation: a review and implications for clinical practice. Curr Psychiatry Rep. 2017;19:91. https://doi.org/10.1007/s11920-017-0843-1.

Chapter 13
Palliative Care in the Adult Solid Organ Transplant Recipient

Katherine G. Hicks, Eleanor Curtis, and Melissa A. Bender

Introduction: Overview of Palliative Care

Palliative care is specialized medical care for people living with serious illness that focuses on quality of life for both the patient and family [1]. Palliative care interventions can be provided regardless of prognosis and have been associated with improvements in quality of life, symptom burden, and patient and caregiver satisfaction [1, 2]. A common misconception is that palliative care cannot be delivered if a patient is being actively treated for a disease; rather, palliative care is completely compatible with disease-directed therapies. Additionally, palliative care interventions increase rates of advance care planning and decrease overall healthcare utilization [1, 3, 4].

The Institute of Medicine's 2014 report *Dying in America* calls for training all clinicians in the core principles of palliative care: pain and symptom management, communication skills to determine patient/family goals, and coordination of care to achieve those goals [5, 6]. The term "primary palliative care" refers to basic palliative care skills that all clinicians should learn regardless of specialty, such as aligning medical treatment with patient goals and basic symptom management [3]. When

K. G. Hicks
Department of Medicine, Division of General Internal Medicine, University of Washington School of Medicine, Seattle, WA, USA
e-mail: katgh@uw.edu

E. Curtis
Department of Trauma, Burns and General Surgery, University of California, Davis, Sacramento, CA, USA
e-mail: ecurtis@ucdavis.edu

M. A. Bender (✉)
Department of Family Medicine, University of Washington School of Medicine, Seattle, WA, USA
e-mail: benderma@uw.edu

© Springer Nature Switzerland AG 2020
C. J. Wong (ed.), *Primary Care of the Solid Organ Transplant Recipient*,
https://doi.org/10.1007/978-3-030-50629-2_13

Table 13.1 Primary versus specialty palliative care

Primary palliative care	Specialty palliative care
Basic palliative care skills	Advanced palliative care skills
Pain and symptom management	Treating refractory symptoms
Communication skills, especially	Facilitating complex medical decision-making
eliciting patient and family goals,	around approaching end of life, worsening health
coordinating care	status or organ dysfunction, or cognitive decline
May be delivered by primary care	Navigating challenging family dynamics
providers, specialists, or any member of	Performed by practitioners who have completed
a patient's care team	additional training, e.g., fellowship, board
Both inpatient and outpatient	certification
	Both inpatient and outpatient

patients with serious illness present to their primary care clinicians, this may be an opportunity to incorporate palliative care interventions into their medical care. Referral to specialty palliative care may be needed in cases of refractory symptoms, worsening health status or cognitive decline, approaching end of life, consideration of a high-risk procedure or other advanced therapy, complex existential distress, or conducting a challenging family meeting (Table 13.1) [3, 4].

Palliative Care in the Solid Organ Transplant Recipient

Palliative care has been proposed for patients with advanced organ failure beginning at diagnosis and continuing through transplant and beyond, given the associated high morbidity and mortality awaiting transplantation and post-transplantation [4, 7–12]. Palliative care interventions in patients awaiting solid organ transplantation have been associated with improvement in patient symptoms and increased documentation of advance care planning discussions [4]. There is some evidence to suggest that palliative care after transplantation may also improve symptoms [13].

Primary care providers have a unique opportunity to incorporate palliative care interventions, such as revisiting advance care planning and basic symptom management, into the care of solid organ transplant recipients. As noted in previous chapters, the increasing number of solid organ transplant recipients creates a larger role for primary care providers. Furthermore, palliative care specialists are few in number and do not have the capacity to provide consultation on all transplant recipients before and after transplantation. Therefore, primary care providers with palliative care skills ideally would fill this need whenever possible [3]. Depending on a patient's transplantation course, the transplant specialist's time may be completely occupied by managing immunosuppression, treating infectious complications, warding off rejection, and checking for graft dysfunction. Primary care providers often have the advantage of having a long-term therapeutic relationship, in some cases both before and after transplantation. The primary care provider typically continues to manage chronic and acute medical problems, provide preventative care, and may have a history of knowing the patient's decision-making preferences and values, as well as familiarity with a patient's social situation. Studies have consistently shown that patients want the physicians caring for them, rather than outside specialists, to discuss advance care planning [14, 15]. While solid organ transplant recipients may have a close relationship with their transplant specialists, they may be hesitant to bring up palliative concerns with their transplant specialist because of concern for disappointing them—some patients may feel more comfortable broaching this topic with the primary care provider.

Advance Care Planning

Advance care planning (ACP) is the ongoing process by which patients share personal values, goals, and preferences regarding current and future medical care [16]. These preferences should then be documented in the medical record and in an advance directive (AD). Conversations between patients and their physicians regarding preferences for care in the setting of serious illness have been associated with increased goal-concordant care, decreased use of unwanted life-sustaining treatments, higher incidence of preferred place of death, and increased hospice use at end of life [17–20].

Advance Directives

An advance directive (AD) is a legal document that indicates a person's preferences for medical care if he or she were to become seriously ill or incapacitated [21, 22]. Having written documentation of a person's wishes can promote more goal-concordant care, unburden caregivers with having to guess the wishes of their loved one in a health crisis, and help avoid unwanted medical care [17, 18, 23, 24]. An advance directive typically includes preferences for life-sustaining treatments in the setting of serious illness (Living Will) and addresses who would be the person's surrogate decision maker if he or she were to become incapacitated (Durable Power of Attorney for Healthcare, DPOA-HC).

Whereas an advance directive can be completed by an adult at any age or stage of health, a "Provider Orders for Life Sustaining Treatment" form is an optional document in the United States (terminology varies, also called POLST, MOLST, POST, MOST, COLST, or TPOPP) that focuses on adults with serious illness or frailty. The POLST serves as a physician's order to guide care outside of the hospital. Unlike an AD which is completed by a patient and signed by a witness or notary, a POLST form must be completed and signed by the patient and a physician or advanced practice provider. These forms serve distinct purposes and are complementary, not duplicative [21].

There are many types of advance directive documents available, some specific to a given state or institution [21, 22].

Table 13.2 Types of advance directives in the United States[a]

Type of AD	Comments
Living Will [21, 22]	Typically includes wishes related to life support, CPR, ventilator use, artificial nutrition, and hydration in different circumstances, such as a persistent vegetative state or terminal illness Requirements for these documents are based on state-specific regulations; most require signatures from two witnesses with many restrictions on who can serve as witness (e.g., excluding patient's family members, health care power of attorney, and medical providers and staff) and some require a notarized signature
Five Wishes	Only available in some states https://fivewishes.org/
Veterans Affairs Documentation	For patients who receive care through the United States Veterans Affairs healthcare system https://www.va.gov/geriatrics/Guide/LongTermCare/Advance_Care_Planning.asp#
End of Life Washington	Example of state-specific advance directive (United States) https://endoflifewa.org/advance-directive/
Provider Orders for Life Sustaining Treatment (POLST)	https://polst.org/

[a]May vary by state; other countries often have similar types of documents, although local laws may vary. For example, the following websites are available in the United Kingdom: https://mydecisions.org.uk/ and https://compassionindying.org.uk/library/advance-decision-pack/

Table 13.2 summarizes advance directive documents used commonly in the United States.

Internationally, while the fundamental concept of advance directives is similar (a patient's right to self-determination of health), laws and practices differ with regard to duration of effect, surrogate decision-makers, and government oversight [25]. Additionally, advance care planning tools and research are largely based on Western concepts of autonomy and decision-making [26]. Advance care planning discussions should be approached with cultural and narrative humility, including consideration of cultural and religious beliefs and acknowledgment of the provider's roles and responsibilities in a patient's story and that "patients' stories are not objects we can comprehend or master" [27].

Advance Care Planning in Solid Organ Transplant Recipients

Solid organ transplant recipients have unique aspects to their advance care planning. First, they have all, by definition, dealt with (and survived) life-threatening organ failure. Their pre-transplant illness may vary considerably, however. Many patients who have successively received a solid organ transplantation have indeed had a difficult pre-transplantation course, including progressive decline in health, multiple hospitalizations for organ failure, complications, difficult symptom control, and healthcare-associated trauma. However, a relatively smaller subset of patients may have had a comparatively smoother course. For example, some patients with end-stage renal disease are able to successfully live through dialysis and kidney transplantation and still maintain a good quality of life prior to transplantation. A patient with fulminant hepatic failure from an ingestion may have had a severe but brief illness, with good health prior to liver transplantation. If the primary care provider did not know the patient prior to transplantation, it is important to review the patient's pre-transplant history for duration of illness, quality of life, and complications (see Chap. 2).

Second, because advance care planning discussions should recur as health or life circumstances change [6, 16], a major life event such as solid organ transplantation should prompt revisiting of advance care planning. In addition to reviewing the pre-transplant history, the primary care provider should review the post-transplant course the patient has experienced before returning to primary care. As with the pre-transplant course, the perioperative and early postoperative experience can vary widely by individual; some patients may enjoy a relatively smooth journey free of complications, while others may have early difficulties with graft function, rejection, infections and other hospital complications. Although patients may have had pre-transplant conversations with their clinicians and/or families about their preferences, their goals and wishes may change during the transplant process. Goals of care may evolve following transplant, and it is recommended that any prior documentation is reviewed with patients once they have recovered and returned to primary care. It is important not to assume that prior discussions or advance care planning documents still represent the patient's current wishes; therefore, even in those with prior discussions and directives, it is important to revisit them as the patient's preferences may have changed. If patients have not had advance care planning discussions or completed an advance directive, it should be encouraged.

Third, while the life expectancy and quality of life of solid organ transplant recipients have significantly improved over time, these patients are still at increased risk for complications such as infections, graft dysfunction, organ failure, and malignancy [28, 29]. One feature of effective ACP programs is repeated discussions over time, and this is certainly merited post-transplantation given these risks [16]. Approximately one in three adults in the United States has completed any advance care planning documentation with rates highest among patients over age 65; notably, although age is no longer a strict contraindication to transplantation in most centers, only 12% of transplant recipients are over 65 years old [30, 31].

Despite these clear rationales to address advance care planning in the care of solid organ transplant recipients, there is sparse literature with specific guidance on ACP post-transplantation. Nevertheless, given the experience of end-organ failure, transplantation, and ongoing risks of complications, it is reasonable to have advance care planning be a part of a routine post-transplantation care for all solid organ transplant recipients. There is some data to support using a disease-specific approach for ACP discussions. Studies of patients with heart failure or with end-stage renal disease on dialysis suggest that disease-specific approaches result in better surrogate understanding of patients' goals and more goal-concordant care decisions at

Table 13.3 Primary care assessment after organ transplantation: advance care planning and cues to further discuss palliative care

Topic	Example questions

Post-transplant primary care—Routine assessment at initial visit(s)
    Review pre- and post-transplant course
    Duration of illness, complications, end-of-life or near-death experiences, hospitalizations, healthcare trauma
	How has the transplant experience been for you?
	 What surprised you about the experience?
	 Was anything more difficult than you expected?
	 Was anything easier than you expected?

Symptom assessment at all visits	*Do you have any symptoms that are troubling you?/Tell me about any symptoms that may be bothering you.*

Previous advance care planning
    Documents, including advance directive, power of attorney for healthcare
    Prior discussions
	Are you familiar with advance care planning?
	 Have you discussed advance care planning before transplantation? Would you be willing to talk about it today?
	 Have you reviewed your advance care planning documents since your transplant?
	 Who are the important people with you in your health and wellness? Who are your sources of support?

Situations in which revisiting palliative care discussions is indicated:
    Organ dysfunction
    Irreversible graft failure
    Discussion of re-transplantation or needing a different organ transplantation
    Ongoing problems with symptom control
    Recurrent hospitalizations	

the end of life [32, 33]. Table 13.3 summarizes suggested assessment of advance care planning and palliative care needs for solid organ transplant recipients in the primary care setting.

Challenges with Advance Care Planning in the Primary Care Setting

Challenges to ongoing advance care planning and completion of advance directives in the primary care setting include inadequate time during patient visits, lack of education and resources related to advance care planning, billing concerns, and problems with documentation and access in electronic health records (EHRs) [34, 35]. In the United States, as of January 2016, Medicare reimburses physicians and advanced practice providers for advance care planning counseling under a separate billing code; however, estimates suggest that use of this reimbursement remains low [36, 37].

Documentation of advance care planning conversations is essential for the information to be used by patients over time and should be accessible to clinicians in various settings and across the care continuum. Ongoing efforts are being made by EHR vendors to enable clinicians to store and find advance care planning information so that it is easily accessed. Despite this, there are ongoing challenges, such as lack of training and no centralized and consistent location for advance care planning information in the EHR [34].

Resources for Improving Advance Care Planning Skills

There are decision aids for patients and resources to help clinicians build their skills in having conversations about patient's preferences regarding future medical care and personal values (Tables 13.4 and 13.5).

Symptom Management in Solid Organ Transplant Recipients

Advanced chronic disease, including in solid organ transplant recipients, can lead to symptoms of fatigue, depression, anxiety, pain, shortness of breath, peripheral edema, ascites, nausea, pruritus, decreased appetite, sleep disturbances, and encephalopathy [4, 9–12]. Patients may have symptoms post-transplantation due to surgical recovery, toxicity from immunosuppressive medications, or graft dysfunction

Table 13.4 Resources for advance care planning conversations

Resource	Description	Links
Advance Care Planning Decisions	Non-profit subscription service for providers with free videos on advance care planning for patients	For clinicians: https://acpdecisions.org/ For patients: https://acpdecisions.org/patients/
IHI Conversation Project	Guide in multiple languages for families to use in having the initial conversation	https://theconversationproject.org/
VitalTalk	Communication frameworks for goals of care conversations and delivering difficult news	https://www.vitaltalk.org VitalTips App (Apple or Android)
CAPC Communication Skills	Online course on communication skills Membership required and CME available	https://www.capc.org/training/communication-skills/
Conversation Resources Dying in America: Improving Quality and Honoring Individual Preferences Near the End of Life	Variety of Resources from the National Academies of Sciences, Engineering, Medicine	http://nationalacademies.org/HMD/Reports/2014/Dying-In-America-Improving-Quality-and-Honoring-Individual-Preferences-Near-the-End-of-Life/The-Conversation.aspx%20

Table 13.5 Helpful questions and statements for discussing advance care planning

Exploring
"How do you feel things are going with your health?"
"Can you talk more about what you mean when you say…?"
"Will you tell me more about…?"

Responding to emotion
"This must be frustrating, I know you've been waiting a long time for…"
"Will you tell me more about what you're worried about?"
"I know this can be hard to talk about…"

Support
"I would like regular appointments with you to continue to support you in this."
"I appreciate your willingness to talk about this."

[4, 12]. Lung transplantation is associated with high symptom burden [12]. In the early post-transplant period, the transplant team and/or pain specialists manage symptoms. When patients return to primary care, the primary care provider may begin to manage pain and other symptoms.

A symptom screening tool, such as the Edmonton Symptom Assessment System (ESAS), may be helpful for screening and longitudinal monitoring of symptoms in solid organ transplant recipients [38]. If the etiology of a symptom is unknown, diagnostic evaluation may be warranted to determine the underlying cause.

Symptom management goals often differ pre-transplantation, in the immediate post-operative recovery period, and long-term post-transplantation. Whenever possible, it is recommended to treat the underlying cause of pain and other symptoms. This is dependent on whether an effective treatment is available and on the patient's prognosis and goals of care. For patients who have undergone successful solid organ transplantation and have a resulting improvement in symptoms, the focus may be on discontinuing opioids and other symptom medications. In one study, patients receiving palliative care while awaiting lung transplantation had opioids discontinued in a timely manner postoperatively [4]. Non-pharmacologic and less-invasive measures should be utilized to treat pain and other symptoms whenever possible.

Patients with persistent symptoms from post-transplantation complications or other causes may require opioids or other medications. Opioids are effective in treating pain and dyspnea, common symptoms in advanced chronic disease, but caution is warranted due to the risks of addiction and opioid overdose that may result in death, and other adverse effects such as worsening encephalopathy and constipation [38]. Patients with liver and kidney dysfunction have a higher risk of adverse medication side effects, including with opioids, due to impaired clearance of drugs and their metabolites. Initiation or escalation of opioid therapy, for any symptom indication, may be a good time to revisit goals of care discussions with patients.

Pain

Pain management in the solid organ transplant recipient can be a significant challenge. Transplant recipients may have pain related to transplantation or chronic or acute pain due to other causes. After evaluation and treatment, if appropriate, of the underlying cause of pain, non-pharmacologic interventions should be considered. Non-pharmacologic interventions associated with improvement in chronic and/or postoperative pain include manipulative therapy, acupuncture, massage therapy, mindfulness-based stress reduction (MBSR), cognitive behavioral therapy (CBT), physical therapy, biofeedback, and movement therapies such as yoga [39].

When medications are utilized, it is recommended to start with non-opioid analgesics. Over-the-counter pain medications such as acetaminophen may benefit some patients, even those with liver failure. Short-term use of acetaminophen at 4 g/day may be appropriate; one study showed no adverse effects when acetaminophen was given to patients with stable liver disease [40]. Recommendations for longer term use include decreasing the dose to 2–3 g/day and should always be discussed with transplant team before using doses that exceed 3 g/day in the liver transplant recipient [11]. Nonsteroidal anti-inflammatory drugs (NSAIDs) are not recommended in patients with liver or kidney failure because of increased risk of kidney injury, hepatorenal syndrome, and bleeding, and they interfere with the effect of diuretics [11]. Furthermore, chronic kidney disease is common in solid organ transplant recipients, and NSAIDs are often routinely avoided in this population because of the high risk of kidney disease (see Chap. 11). Heart transplant recipients receive routine aspirin therapy and the use of NSAIDs increase the risk of bleeding and cardiovascular disease (see Chap. 6). Gabapentin and pregabalin should be dose-reduced or discontinued in renal failure patients, in particular in end-stage renal disease (ESRD) patients when dialysis is stopped [41].

For patients with moderate to severe acute or persistent pain, opioids may be appropriate to manage pain. Initiation or escalation of opioid therapy for persistent or worsening pain or other symptoms may warrant a discussion of goals of care. If oxycodone, morphine, or hydromorphone is prescribed in the setting of end-stage liver disease, dose reduction and increased dosing intervals are recommended due to impaired elimination [11]. In kidney and liver failure, toxic morphine and hydromorphone metabolites accumulate and may cause adverse effects [11, 41]. Morphine should be avoided in patients with both liver and renal dysfunction due to the resulting risk of neurotoxicity [11].

Fentanyl and methadone are good options for patients with severe liver or kidney disease as they do not have known altered kinetics. The recommendation is to start with low doses and titrate slowly, and methadone should be prescribed by those with adequate clinical experience with its use [11, 41]. If these medications need to be used, consider consultation with a pain specialist or palliative care specialist.

Dyspnea, Cough

Solid organ transplant recipients may experience dyspnea and cough from advanced chronic disease or complications of transplantation. The underlying cause should be determined and treated whenever possible. Dyspnea can be difficult to manage and can be a sign of advanced disease or graft failure. In cases of refractory or difficult-to-manage dyspnea, especially when initiating or escalating opioids or benzodiazepines, patients' goals of care should be revisited.

Management of dyspnea should often include nonpharmacologic measures in conjunction with medications. Nonpharmacologic measures that can improve symptoms include upright positioning and/or use of a fan (or open window) to increase air movement [42]. For patients with hypoxia, oxygen therapy may help ease their discomfort. Opioids often provide relief from dyspnea refractory to the treatment of the underlying cause [42]. In opioid-naive patient, start with low doses of an oral opioid such as morphine. Patients who are opioid tolerant often need higher doses. Benzodiazepines can also be considered for breathlessness, though they may have more sedating effects than opioids and are considered second- or third-line treatment [43].

Diarrhea, Nausea, and Constipation

Diarrhea is common in solid organ transplant recipients and can lead to serious complications and impact the quality of life. It is important to determine the cause of diarrhea in solid organ transplant recipients since they have a higher incidence of opportunistic infections, chronic diarrhea, and diarrhea as a medication side effect (see Chaps. 3, 8, and 9). Targeted treatment against pathogen(s) identified and fluid replacement should be prioritized [44]. Reduction of transplant medication dose or changing to other immunosuppressive regimens can be attempted by the transplant team when pathogens are ruled out [44]. For patients that have a negative test for *C. difficile* and no evidence of megacolon or inflammatory diarrhea, empiric anti-motility agents should be considered [44].

Nausea and constipation are common symptoms in advanced chronic disease. As with other symptoms, the underlying cause must be evaluated and treated whenever possible. Nausea and constipation may be the result of a medication side effect and discontinuation is recommended if possible. Acupuncture, ginger, pyridoxine (vitamin B6), or a low-fat or liquid diet may provide relief from nausea [45]. The cause of nausea may be helpful in choosing an antiemetic, though the etiology may be multifactorial or uncertain. Types of antiemetics include anticholinergics, antihistamines, benzodiazepines, atypical and typical antipsychotics (for example, haloperidol and olanzapine), cannabinoids, corticosteroids, phenothiazines, serotonin 5HT3 antagonists, and pro-motility drugs such as metoclopramide. Due to side effects and drug-drug interactions, caution is recommended with choosing an antiemetic. Phenothiazines and metoclopramide can cause extrapyramidal side effects.

Serotonin antagonists, such as ondansetron, have constipation as a side effect [45]. If uncertain, the primary care provider should consult with the transplant team or a transplant pharmacist to minimize the risk of adverse drug effects or interactions.

Non-pharmacologic measures for constipation may provide some relief, though evidence is limited, and include scheduled toileting, exercise, and increased water and fiber intake [46]. Pharmacologic options for constipation include osmotic laxatives, such as polyethylene glycol and lactulose, and stimulant laxatives, such as senna and bisacodyl. For opioid-induced constipation refractory to other laxatives, a mu-opioid antagonist may provide relief [45]. Stool softeners such as docusate have not been shown to be effective in treating constipation [47].

Edema

Heart, liver, or kidney failure can all lead to fluid accumulation, which can build up in many areas including the abdomen, lungs, and extremities. Diuretics and sodium restriction are the mainstays of treatment for edema in patients with heart failure and liver disease, with close monitoring needed for volume status, electrolyte abnormalities, and renal function. The symptom burden of edema, and the need or desire for medical optimization of volume status, should be balanced against the potential inconveniences of pill burden, frequent urination, and laboratory monitoring. Refractory ascites may require procedural interventions for management, depending on feasibility and a patient's goals of care.

Depression and Anxiety

Depression is the most prevalent psychiatric disorder in the post-transplantation population [48]. Current recommendations for screening for depression and anxiety in the outpatient setting include use of patient-reported measures, such as Patient Health Questionnaire-9 (PHQ-9) and General Anxiety Disorder -7 (GAD-7) [49]. Solid organ transplant recipients may experience feelings of guilt for the donor or other patients who are still on the waiting list or did not survive [50]. It is important to differentiate guilty feelings from depression (which can include guilt) based on history, presence of other depressive symptoms, and examination findings. Adjustment-related symptoms can also occur. Medication therapy includes a selective serotonin reuptake inhibitor (SSRI), with preference for escitalopram and sertraline because of fewer drug interactions with anti-rejection medications [48]. Citalopram may be used, but it may cause QT prolongation; the maximum dose of citalopram recommended for patients over the age of 60 or with liver impairment is 20 mg/day and caution is advised for patients with congestive heart failure, bradyarrhythmia, and if receiving other medications that prolong the QT interval [51]. Venlafaxine, duloxetine, and mirtazapine are also reasonable options since they appear to have few effects on cytochrome P450 and therefore not likely to significantly interact with immunosuppressants [50, 52]. Mirtazapine can be considered a second-line treatment in post-cardiac transplant patients with cachexia, since they may benefit from its side effect of appetite stimulation [50]. For patients with renal and/or liver dysfunction, caution is advised, and for some antidepressants dose reduction is recommended [50, 52, 53] (see Chap. 3). Mindfulness-based stress reduction techniques can help decrease depressive symptoms and increase quality of life in solid organ transplant recipients [54]. Psychotherapy with an SSRI has been shown to be effective in treating patients with depression after cardiac transplantation [50].

Palliative Care Resources for Clinicians

There are resources available for palliative care clinical questions that include symptom management topics (Table 13.6).

Transplant Failure

Even with perfect preparation, technical skill, postoperative care, and medical management, some transplants will fail. Any solid organ transplant failure should trigger additional conversations around goals of care as they may shift over time. Consider palliative care consultation in any patient with organ failure with any of the following signs: significant change in health status, significant change in functional status or cognitive decline, high or increasing symptom burden, worsening disease based on disease-specific classification or markers, consideration of advanced therapies, frequent visits to the ER or ICU admissions, patient or family request, or approaching the end of life [4]. Most importantly, primary care providers should have a low threshold to consult with a palliative care provider if there are ongoing symptoms or potential changes in goals of care, both of which are likely to occur with end-stage disease. Palliative care consults are often called late

Table 13.6 Palliative care resources for symptom management

Resource	Description
Palliative Care Network of Wisconsin: Fast Facts and Concepts	Search palliative care topics via website or mobile app https://www.mypcnow.org/fast-facts/
Primer of Palliative Care, 7th edition (American Academy of Hospice and Palliative Medicine)	Pocket-sized handbook with a variety of palliative care topics, which includes opioid conversation table
CAPC Symptom Management Courses	https://www.capc.org/training/ symptom-management/

in the course of organ transplant failure or not at all, but are likely most beneficial when patients have a therapeutic relationship with palliative care providers prior to graft failure [4].

Each solid organ transplant presents different considerations with respect to readdressing advanced care planning if graft failure occurs.

Kidney transplant recipients more frequently are able to receive another transplant compared to other solid organ transplant recipients—in the United States in 2017, retransplants represented 11% of adult kidney transplant recipients [55]. This comparatively high rate may be due to patient factors, donor availability, and the option of dialysis. However, decisions surrounding the initiation (or re-initiation) of dialysis and pursuing retransplantation are appropriate opportunities for reassessing a patient's goals of care. Even if a patient is familiar with dialysis from prior to transplantation, the post-transplantation dialysis goals of care may have changed: the patient will now be older, may have had more health complications, and is now immunosuppressed—these experiences may factor into the decision-making pertaining to dialysis and retransplantation. If dialysis and retransplantation are not options or not chosen, then management should include relieving the symptoms of end-stage renal disease, including treatment of volume overload and uremia.

Liver transplant recipients sometimes receive re-transplantation, more commonly early after initial transplantation—for example due to vascular complications—and less commonly performed in the late period after transplantation [56]. Unlike kidney transplant recipients, they do not have dialysis or other bridging therapies as options. In patients with end-stage liver disease who are not candidates for or who do not pursue retransplantation, symptom management will likely include care of volume overload, encephalopathy, and bleeding.

Heart retransplantation is less common than kidney or liver retransplantation, representing only 2–3% of heart transplants based on registry data [57]. The use of mechanical circulatory support such as left ventricular assist devices is generally not an option in the post-heart transplant setting because of anatomy, thrombosis, and risk of infection. Given the relative infrequency of retransplantation, early involvement with palliative care should be considered for heart transplant recipients with graft failure. Dyspnea and volume management will be necessary to improve quality of life.

Similar to heart transplant recipients, retransplantation is uncommon in lung transplant recipients, representing 2–3% of lung transplants [58], and is associated with poorer outcome compared with initial transplantation [59, 60]. Because of these outcomes, early palliative care involvement is recommended, as the patient will most likely need management of dyspnea as respiratory failure progresses.

Discussions of comfort-focused care and/or hospice in patients with end-stage disease after solid organ transplantation failure are appropriate if retransplantation is not an option or not desired.

Conclusion

Palliative care is specialized medical care for people living with serious illness that focuses on quality of life for both the patient and family [1]. Palliative care has been proposed for patients with advanced organ failure beginning at diagnosis and continuing through transplant and beyond, given the associated high morbidity and mortality awaiting transplantation and post-transplantation [4, 7–12]. When solid organ transplant recipients present to the outpatient clinic, it may be an opportunity for the primary care provider to incorporate primary palliative care interventions into their medical care. Primary palliative care interventions include advance care planning and basic pain and symptom management. There are clinical resources available for advance care planning, communication skills, and symptom management. Advance care planning discussions should recur as health circumstances change, including post-transplantation, with worsening health status, or cognitive decline. Initiation or escalation of opioid therapy for managing refractory symptoms is an appropriate time to readdress patients' goals of care. Referral to a palliative care specialist may be needed in cases of refractory symptoms, worsening health status including graft failure, cognitive decline, approaching end of life, or challenging decision-making when considering high-risk procedures.

References

1. About palliative care. https://www.capc.org/about/palliative-care/. Accessed 7 Feb 2019.
2. Kavalieratos D, Corbelli J, Zhang D, Dionne-Odom JN, Ernecoff NC, Hanmer J, et al. Association between palliative care and patient and caregiver outcomes: a systematic review and meta-analysis. JAMA. 2016;316(20):2104–14. https://doi.org/10.1001/jama.2016.16840.
3. Quill TE, Abernethy AP. Generalist plus specialist palliative care—creating a more sustainable model. N Engl J Med. 2013;368:1173–5.
4. Wentlandt K, Weiss A, O'Connor E, Kaya E. Palliative and end of life care in solid organ transplantation. Am J Transplant. 2017;17(12):3008–19.
5. Institute of Medicine. https://www.capc.org/topics/iom/. Accessed 7 Feb 2019.
6. Institute of Medicine: Committee on Approaching Death. Dying in America: improving quality and honoring individual preferences near the end of life. Washington, DC: The National Academies Press; 2014.
7. A strategy for the simultaneous provision of pre-operative palliative care for patients awaiting liver transplantation – Rossaro – 2004 – Transplant International – Wiley Online Library [Internet]. [cited 8 Apr 2019]. Available from: https://onlinelibrary.wiley.com/doi/abs/10.1111/j.1432-2277.2004.tb00473.x.
8. Freeman N, Le LW, Singer LG, Colman R, Zimmermann C, Wentlandt K. Impact of a transplant palliative care clinic on symptoms for patients awaiting lung transplantation. J Heart Lung Transplant. 2016;35(8):1037–9.
9. Larson AM, Curtis JR. Integrating palliative care for liver transplant candidates: "too well for transplant, too sick for life". JAMA. 2006;295(18):2168–76.
10. Baumann AJ, Wheeler DS, James M, Turner R, Siegel A, Navarro VJ. Benefit of early palliative care intervention in end-stage liver disease patients awaiting liver transplantation. J Pain Symptom Manag. 2015;50(6):882–6.

11. Potosek J, Curry M, Buss M, Chittenden E. Integration of palliative care in end-stage liver disease and liver transplantation. J Palliat Med. 2014;17(11):1271–7.
12. Colman R, Singer LG, Barua R, Downar J. Characteristics, interventions, and outcomes of lung transplant recipients co-managed with palliative care. J Palliat Med. 2015;18(3):266–9.
13. Wentlandt K, Dall'Osto A, Freeman N, Le LW, Kaya E, Ross H, Singer LG, Abbey S, Clarke H, Zimmermann C. The transplant palliative care clinic: an early palliative care model for patients in a transplant program. Clin Transpl. 2016;30(12):1591–6. https://doi.org/10.1111/ctr.12838.
14. Wenrich MD, Curtis JR, Ambrozy DA, Carline JD, Shannon SE, Ramsey PG. Dying patients' need for emotional support and personalized care from physicians: perspectives of patients with terminal illness, families, and health care providers. J Pain Symptom Manag. 2003;25(3):236–46.
15. Dow LA, Matsuyama RK, Ramakrishnan V, et al. Paradoxes in advance care planning: the complex relationship of oncology patients, their physicians, and advance medical directives. Clin Oncol. 2010;28(2):299–304. https://doi.org/10.1200/JCO.2009.24.6397.
16. Sudore RL, Lum HD, You JJ, Hanson LC, Meier DE, Pantilat SZ, Matlock DD, Rietjens JAC, Korfage IJ, Ritchie CS, Kutner JS, Teno JM, Thomas J, McMahan RD, Heyland DK. Defining advance care planning for adults: a consensus definition from a multidisciplinary Delphi panel. J Pain Symptom Manag. 2017;53:821–32.
17. Jimenez G, Tan WS, Virk AK, Low CK, Car J, Ho AHY. Overview of systematic reviews of advance care planning: summary of evidence and global lessons. J Pain Symptom Manage. 2018;56(3):436–459.e25.
18. Teno JM, Gruneir A, Schwartz Z, Nanda A, Wetle T. Association between advance directives and quality of end-of-life care: a national study. J Am Geriatr Soc. 2007 Feb;55(2):189–94.
19. Detering KM, Hancock AD, Reade MC, Silvester W. The impact of advance care planning on end of life care in elderly patients: randomised controlled trial. BMJ. 2010;340:c1345.
20. Wright AA, Zhang B, Ray A, Mack JW, Trice E, Balboni T, et al. Associations between end-of-life discussions, patient mental health, medical care near death, and caregiver bereavement adjustment. JAMA. 2008;300(14):1665–73.
21. Sabatino CP. The evolution of health care advance planning law and policy. Milbank Q. 2010;88(2):211–39.
22. American Bar Association. Living wills, health care proxies, & advance health care directives [Internet]. ABA. 2019 [cited 15 May 2019]. Available from: https://www.americanbar.org/groups/real_property_trust_estate/resources/estate_planning/living_wills_health_care_proxies_advance_health_care_directives/.
23. Molloy DW, Guyatt GH, Russo R, Goeree R, O'Brien BJ, Bedard M, et al. Systematic implementation of an advance directive program in nursing homes: a randomized controlled trial. JAMA. 2000;283(11):1437–44.
24. Silveira MJ, Kim SYH, Langa KM. Advance directives and outcomes of surrogate decision making before death. N Engl J Med. 2010;362(13):1211–8.
25. Veshi D, Neitzke G. Advance directives in some Western European countries: a legal and ethical comparison between Spain, France, England, and Germany. Eur J Health Law. 2015;22(4):321–45.
26. Russell S. Paying attention to cultural context matters in advance care planning and palliative care. Evid Based Nurs. 2019. https://doi.org/10.1136/ebnurs-2019-103206.
27. Tsevat RK, Sinha AA, Gutierrez KJ, DasGupta S. Bringing home the health humanities: narrative humility, structural competency, and engaged pedagogy. Acad Med. 2015;90(11):1462–5.
28. Rana A, Gruessner A, Agopian VG, Khalpey Z, Riaz IB, Kaplan B, et al. Survival benefit of solid-organ transplant in the United States survival benefit of solid-organ transplant survival benefit of solid-organ transplant. JAMA Surg. 2015;150(3):252–9.
29. Kugler C, Gottlieb J, Warnecke G, Schwarz A, Weissenborn K, Barg-Hock H, et al. Health-related quality of life after solid organ transplantation: a prospective, multiorgan cohort study. Transplantation. 2013;96(3):316–23.

30. Yadav KN, Gabler NB, Cooney E, Kent S, Kim J, Herbst N, et al. Approximately one in three US adults completes any type of advance directive for end-of-life care. Health Aff (Millwood). 2017;36(7):1244–51.
31. United Network for Organ Sharing. Transplants by age of recipient [Internet]. UNOS. [cited 25 June 2019]. Available from: https://unos.org/data/transplant-trends/transplants-by-age-of-recipient/.
32. Schellinger S, Sidebottom A, Briggs L. Disease specific advance care planning for heart failure patients: implementation in a large health system. J Palliat Med. 2011;14(11):1224–30.
33. Kirchhoff KT, Hammes BJ, Kehl KA, Briggs LA, Brown RL. Effect of a disease-specific planning intervention on surrogate understanding of patient goals for future medical treatment. J Am Geriatr Soc. 2010;58(7):1233–40.
34. Fulmer T, Escobedo M, Berman A, Koren MJ, Hernández S, Hult A. Physicians' views on advance care planning and end-of-life care conversations. J Am Geriatr Soc. 2018;66(6):1201–5.
35. Lamas D, Panariello N, Henrich N, Hammes B, Hanson LC, Meier DE, et al. Advance care planning documentation in electronic health records: current challenges and recommendations for change. J Palliat Med. 2018;21(4):522–8.
36. Tsai G, Taylor DH. Advance care planning in Medicare: an early look at the impact of new reimbursement on billing and clinical practice. BMJ Support Palliat Care. 2018;8(1):49.
37. Pelland K, Morphis B, Harris D, Gardner R. Assessment of first-year use of Medicare's advance care planning billing codes assessment of first-year use of Medicare's advance care planning billing codes letters. JAMA Intern Med. 2019;179(6):827–9.
38. Hui D, Bruera E. The Edmonton symptom assessment system 25 years later: past, present, and future developments. J Pain Symptom Manag. 2017;53(3):630–43.
39. Tick H, Nielsen A, Pelletier KR, Bonakdar R, Simmons S, Glick R, Ratner E, Lemmon RL, Wayne P, Zador V, Pain Task Force of the Academic Consortium for Integrative Medicine and Health. Evidence-based nonpharmacologic strategies for comprehensive pain care: the consortium pain task force white paper. Explore (NY). 2018;14(3):177–211.
40. Hayward KL, Powell EE, Irvine KM, Martin JH. Can paracetamol (acetaminophen) be administered to patients with liver impairment? Br J Clin Pharmacol. 2016;81(2):210–22. https://doi.org/10.1111/bcp.12802.
41. Davison SN, Rosielle DA. Fast Fact #208. Clinical care following withdrawal of dialysis [Internet]. Palliative Care Network of Wisconsin Fast Facts. [cited 24 Apr 2019]. Available from: https://www.mypcnow.org/blank-ikz6.
42. Weissman DE. Fast Fact #37. Dyspnea at end-of-life. Palliative Care Network of Wisconsin Fast Facts. [cited 24 Apr 2019]. Available from: https://www.mypcnow.org/blank-mbri1.
43. Benzodiazepines for the relief of breathlessness in advanced malignant and non-malignant diseases in adults – Simon, ST – 2016. Cochrane Library [Internet]. [cited 18 June 2019]. Available from: https://www.cochranelibrary.com/cdsr/doi/10.1002/14651858.CD007354.pub3/full.
44. Ginsburg PM, Thuluvath PJ. Diarrhea in liver transplant recipients: etiology and management. Liver Transpl. 2005;11:881–90. https://doi.org/10.1002/lt.20500.
45. Angarone M, Snydman DR, AST ID Community of Practice. Diagnosis and management of diarrhea in solid-organ transplant recipients: Guidelines from the American Society of Transplantation Infectious Diseases Community of Practice. Clin Transplant. 2019:e13550. https://doi.org/10.1111/ctr.13550.
46. Scorza K, Williams A, Phillips JD, Shaw J. Evaluation of nausea and vomiting. Am Fam Physician. 2007;76(1):76–84.
47. Mounsey A, Raleigh M, Wilson A. Management of constipation in older adults. Am Fam Physician. 2015;92(6):500–4.
48. Kim J, Phongsamran P, Park S. Use of antidepressant drugs in transplant recipients. Prog Transplant. 2004;14(2):98–104.
49. Maurer DM, Raymond TJ, David BN. Depression: screening and diagnosis. Am Fam Physician. 2018;98(8):508–15.

50. Fast Fact #273. Treating depression after heart transplantation [Internet]. Palliative Care Network of Wisconsin Fast Facts. [cited 24 Apr 2019]. Available from: https://www.mypcnow. org/blank-ileos.
51. FDA Drug Safety Communication: abnormal heart rhythms associated with high doses of Celexa (citalopram hydrobromide). https://www-fda-gov.offcampus.lib.washington.edu/ drugs/drug-safety-and-availability/fda-drug-safety-communication-abnormal-heart-rhythms-associated-high-doses-celexa-citalopram. Accessed 15 July 2019.
52. Mullish BH, Kabir MS, Thursz MR, Dhar A. Review article: depression and the use of anti-depressants in patients with chronic liver disease or liver transplantation. Aliment Pharmacol Ther. 2014;40(8):880–92.
53. Shirazian S, Grant CD, Aina O, Mattana J, Khorassani F, Ricardo AC. Depression in chronic kidney disease and end-stage renal disease: similarities and differences in diagnosis, epidemiology, and management. Kidney Int Rep. 2016;2(1):94–107. https://doi.org/10.1016/j. ekir.2016.09.005.
54. Mindfulness-based stress reduction for solid organ transplant recipients: a randomized controlled trial [Internet]. Available from: https://www.ncbi.nlm.nih.gov/pmc/articles/ PMC3076132/. Accessed 24 Apr 2019.
55. Hart A, Smith JM, Skeans MA, Gustafson SK, Wilk AR, Castro S, Robinson A, Wainwright JL, Snyder JJ, Kasiske BL, Israni AK. OPTN/SRTR 2017 annual data report: kidney. Am J Transplant. 2019;19(Suppl 2):19–123. https://doi.org/10.1111/ajt.15274.
56. Marudanayagam R, Shanmugam V, Sandhu B, et al. Liver retransplantation in adults: a single-centre, 25-year experience. HPB (Oxford). 2010;12(3):217–24. https://doi. org/10.1111/j.1477-2574.2010.00162.x.
57. Lund LH, Khush KK, Cherikh WS, Goldfarb S, Kucheryavaya AY, Levvey BJ, Meiser B, Rossano JW, Chambers DC, Yusen RD, Stehlik J, International Society for Heart and Lung Transplantation. The Registry of the International Society for Heart and Lung Transplantation: thirty-fourth adult heart transplantation report-2017; Focus Theme: Allograft ischemic time. J Heart Lung Transplant. 2017;36(10):1037–46. https://doi.org/10.1016/j.healun.2017.07.019. (eSlide 7 available at: https://ishltregistries.org/registries/slides.asp).
58. Kawut SM. Lung retransplantation. Clin Chest Med. 2011;32(2):367–77. https://doi. org/10.1016/j.ccm.2011.02.013.
59. Ren D, Kaleekal TS, Graviss EA, et al. Retransplantation outcomes at a large lung transplantation program. Transplant Direct. 2018;4(11):e404. https://doi.org/10.1097/ TXD.0000000000000844.
60. Hall DJ, Belli EV, Gregg JA, Salgado JC, Baz MA, Staples ED, Beaver TM, Machuca TN. Two decades of lung retransplantation: a single-center experience. Ann Thorac Surg. 2017;103(4):1076–83. https://doi.org/10.1016/j.athoracsur.2016.09.107.

Index

Printed in the United States
by Baker & Taylor Publisher Services